ABOUT THE AUTHOR

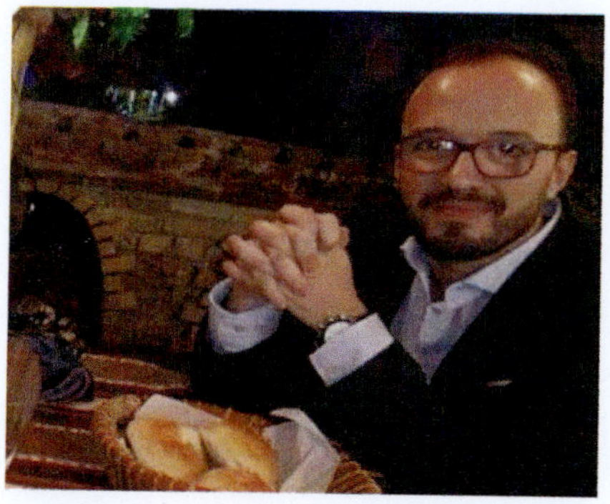

Amine Kerdoun is a dedicated healthcare professional with a comprehensive background in toxicology, academia, and research. Currently serving as a Hospital-university Lecturer in Toxicology at the Faculty of Medicine, Kasdi Merbah University, Ouargla, Algeria, he imparts knowledge to future medical professionals while conducting groundbreaking research in the field. With meticulous attention to detail, Amine analyzes toxic substances, contributes to pathology reports, and delves into epidemiological studies. Amine's academic journey includes earning a Doctorate in Medical Sciences with a focus on Toxicology, as well as diplomas in Pharmacy and Special Medical Studies from esteemed Algerian universities. Committed to lifelong learning, Amine actively engages in research activities and scientific communications, shaping him into a compassionate and skilled healthcare leader.

CLINICAL TOXICOLOGY

Mohamed Amine Kerdoun

ALLIED HEALTH PRESS

Clinical Toxicology

Author: **Mohamed Amine Kerdoun**

Allied Health Press
4164 Lakeshore Road
Burlington ON L7L 1A4
Canada
www.alliedhealthpress.com
Email: orders@arclereducation.com

ISBN: 978-1-77956-248-7

Word Roots, Prefixes, and Suffixes by Chapter

Chapter 1 Clinical Toxicology: An Overview

bi-: Bifurcation

brady-:Bradycardia

cardio-: Cardioversion

-centesis: Thoracocentesis

cephal-: Cephalic

contra-: Contraindicated

-cyst: Cystoscopy

-cyt(e,o)-: Cytoplasm

Chapter 2 Factors Affecting Toxicology

dys-: Dysuria

-ectomy: Hysterectomy

endo-: Endometrium

erythr(o)-: Erythrocyte

extra-: Extracellular

gastr(o)-: Gastro

gen(esis)-:Pathogen

Chapter 3 Principles of Poison Management

Apo-: apoptosis

-aemia: bacteraemia

Brachy-: brachycephalic

Brady: bradycardia

Brev-: Brevundimonas diminuta

-bacillus, bacilli: Bacillus

-blast: osteoblasts

Chapter 4 Toxicokinetics and Toxicodynamics

-asone: corticosteroid

-afil: phosphodiesterase (PDE) inhibitor

-asone: corticosteroid

-bicin: antineoplastic; cytotoxic agent

-bital: barbiturate (sedative)

-caine: local anesthetic

cef-, ceph-: cephalosporin antibiotic

-cillin: penicillin antibiotic

cort: corticosteroid

-cycline: tetracycline antibiotic

-dazole: anthelmintic; antibiotic; antibacterial

Chapter 5 Classes of Toxicants

A-, An-:AnemiaAndr/o-:Androgen Anti-:Anticholinergic drugsAuto-:AutocrineBio- Biology Chem/o-:ChemotherapyContra-:Contraception ac:Cardiac

-blast, -blasto, -blastic: Myeloblast

-cyte, -cytic: Thrombocyte

-dynia:Thoracodynia

Chapter 6 Toxicology of Food and Foodborne Diseases

Bacill-:Bacillus cereus

Cocci-:Staphylococcus aureus

Entero-:Enterotoxin

-toxin:Neurotoxin, Enterotoxin

-itis:Gastroenteritis

-osis;Listeriosis

-phage:Bacteriophage

-gen:Pathogen

Chapter 7 Geriatric Toxicology

Geri-: Geriatrics

Tox-: Toxicology

Pharm-: Pharmacology

-it is: Dermatitis

-osis: Fibrosis

-emia: Toxemia

-opathy: Neuropathy

-lysis: Hemolysis

Chapter 8 Pediatric Toxicology

Toxo-:Toxoplasmosis

Cyto-: Cytotoxic

Neuro-: Neurotoxin

Hepato-:Hepatotoxic

Nephro-:Nephrotoxic

-emia: Bacteremia

-itis: Hepatitis

-pathy: Neuropathy

-toxin: Endotoxin, Exotoxin

-gen: Pathogen

Chapter 9 Role of Analytical Toxicology

-emia: Toxemia

-itis: Hepatitis

-scope: Microscope

-graphy: Chromatography

-meter: Spectrometer

Bio-: Bioanalytical

Chromo-: Chromatography

Spectro-:Spectroscopy

Chapter 10 Toxicology of Drug and Metabolism

-asone: betamethasone; dexamethasone

-afil: avanafil; sildenafil; tadalafil; vardenafil

-asone: betamethasone; dexamethasone;

-bicin: doxorubicin; epirubicin; idarubicin; valrubicin

-bital: butabarbital; butalbital; phenobarbital; secobarbital

-caine:bupivacaine; lidocaine; mepivacaine; prilocaine; proparacaine

cef-, ceph-: cefaclor; cefdinir; cefixime; cefprozil; cephalexin

-cillin: amoxicillin; ampicillin; dicloxacillin; nafcillin; oxacillin

cort: clocortolone; fludrocortisone; hydrocortisone

-cycline: demeclocycline;

-dazole: albendazole; tinidazole

-dipine: amlodipine; nisoldipine

Table of Contents

5 Classes of Toxicants 137

6 Toxicology of Food and Foodborne Diseases 175

7 Geriatric Toxicology 225

LIST OF FIGURES

LIST OF TABLES

PREFACE

Clinical toxicology encompasses the research, prevention, and treatment of diseases caused by exposure to chemicals, drugs, and toxins. It focuses on understanding the levels of chemical exposure and the resultant effects on individuals. This field is particularly crucial in cases of poisoning or overdose and is, therefore, invaluable for medical practitioners and emergency responders. Clinical toxicology can be classified into two main branches: clinical chemistry and toxicology.

Chemical compounds are ubiquitous in our environment, ranging from medications to pollutants, and can have diverse effects depending on the compound and the dosage. Clinical chemistry involves analyzing the composition of bodily fluids, employing molecular diagnostics, and interpreting test results. It plays a vital role in medical testing and utilizes chemical processes to assess patient health, especially in situations involving poisoning or overdose.

Toxicology is a scientific discipline that investigates the adverse effects of chemicals on living organisms, typically focusing on the human body. Risk assessment, a component of toxicology, involves evaluating the potential harmful risks associated with exposure to various substances and aids in establishing regulations to safeguard public health.

Clinical toxicologists often pioneer new methods to ascertain the harmful effects and dosage thresholds of chemicals and drugs. They also conduct research on specific substances to determine safe usage guidelines. However, a comprehensive understanding of clinical toxicology is not limited to clinical toxicologists; physicians, nurses, physician assistants, first responders, and poison control center professionals often study this field to enhance their ability to manage cases involving poisoned or overdosed individuals. Given the rising incidence of drug overdose, which has become the leading cause of injury-related death, clinical toxicology holds immense significance today.

The objective of the textbook "Clinical Toxicology" is to provide a comprehensive and accessible overview of the principles and practices in the field of toxicology. It aims to equip medical professionals, including physicians, nurses, and physician assistants, as well as first responders and poison control center professionals, with the knowledge and skills necessary to effectively manage cases of poisoning and overdose.

The book covers a wide range of topics, including the mechanisms of toxicity, the identification and assessment of toxic agents, and the principles of toxicology testing and management. It also addresses the ethical and legal issues related to toxicology, and the role of toxicology in public health and policy.

Through its detailed explanations and practical guidance, "Clinical Toxicology" seeks to enhance the understanding and practice of clinical toxicology among healthcare professionals. It aims to improve patient outcomes by promoting timely and accurate diagnosis and treatment of toxicological emergencies.

Chapter 1

CLINICAL TOXICOLOGY: AN OVERVIEW

Contents

Introduction

A subspecialty of toxicology called clinical toxicology deals with the bedside management of poisoned patients. This includes making a conclusive toxicological diagnosis, determining the severity and long-term prognosis of the condition, and choosing the best course of treatment, including antidotes. A clinical toxicologist can take part in the planning and avoidance of chemical intoxications by having knowledge of possible drug and chemical hazards. Clinical disease is primarily caused by toxicants. As a result, clinical toxicology is a branch of internal medicine that greatly benefits from other specialties. Pharmacology is a prerequisite for clinical toxicology. On the other hand, a clinical toxicologist might work with tens of thousands of substances, whereas pharmacology deals with thousands. Toxicodynetics is the newest of the subdisciplines that have emerged from clinical toxicology as a result. Enhancing the identification, avoidance, and management of intoxications requires close collaboration between toxicological scientists and clinical toxicologists. For a conclusive diagnosis, it is necessary to clarify the mechanism of toxicity in cases of suspected intoxications. All that exists as an antidote is the benefit of understanding the exact pathophysiology of a poisoning incident.

Orientation and Directional Terms:

Term	Definition	Illustration
New psychoactive substances	New psychoactive substances (NPS) are a complex and diverse group of substances often known as either designer or synthetic drugs, or by the more popular but misleading colloquial term of 'legal highs'.	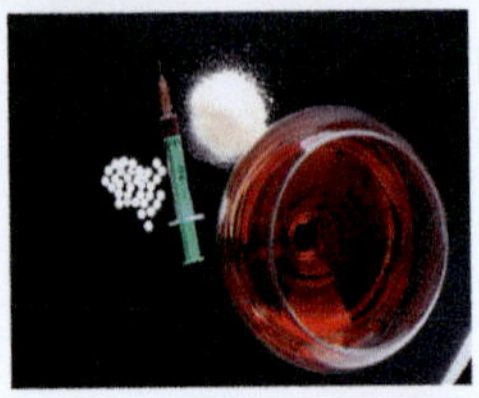
Synthetic drug	Synthetic drugs refer to substances that are artificially modified from naturally-occurring drugs and are capable of exhibiting both therapeutic and psychoactive effects.	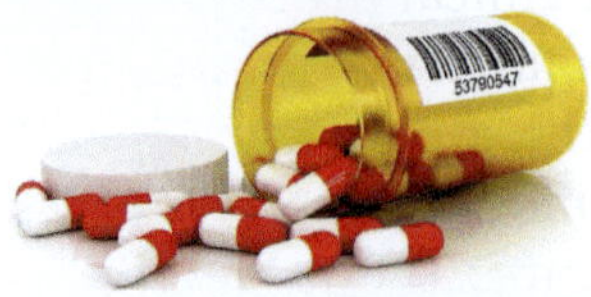
Phencyclidine	An infamous hallucinogenic sought for its ability to induce the illusion of euphoria, omnipotence, superhuman strength, and social and sexual prowess.	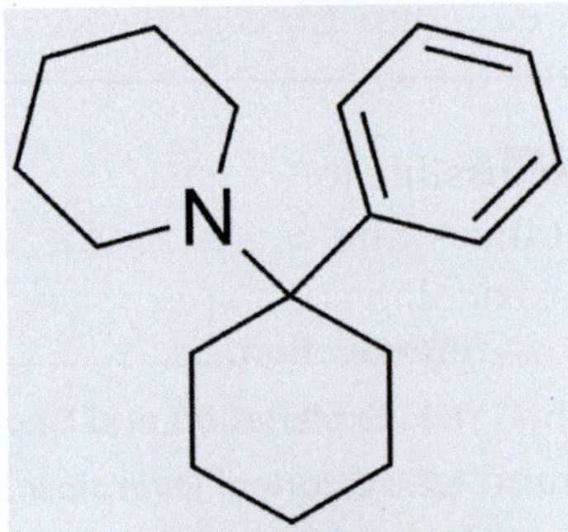
Micrograms	A microgram or microgramme is a unit of mass equal to one millionth (1×10^{-6}) of a gram.	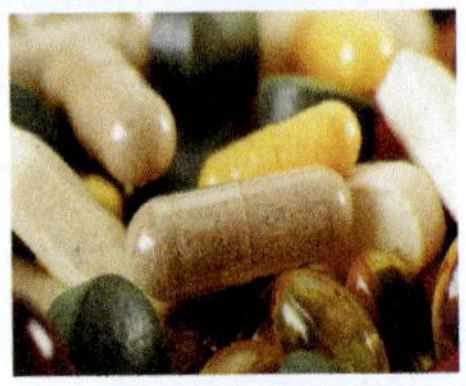
Tetrahydrogestrinone	A synthetic and orally active anabolic–androgenic steroid which was never marketed for medical use. It was developed by Patrick Arnold and was used by a number of high-profile athletes such as Marion Jones, Barry Bonds, and Dwain Chambers.	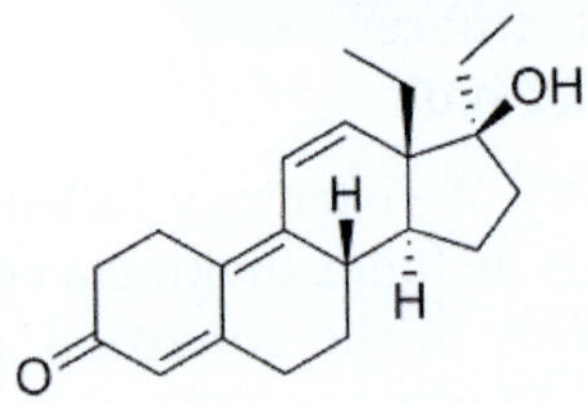

1.1. Explanation and Scope of Clinical Toxicology

Clinical toxicology is the study, prevention, and management of illnesses brought on by poisons, drugs, and chemicals. Levels of chemical exposure and the potential effects on humans are given particular consideration. Clinical toxicology is helpful for first responders and medical professionals because it is particularly helpful when handling poisoned or overdosed individuals. Clinical chemistry and toxicology are the two components that make up clinical toxicology. Chemicals are present in everything we touch, including medications and pollutants, and their effects vary based on the type of chemical and its dosage. Analyzing bodily fluid composition, examining molecular diagnostics, and interpreting test results are all part of clinical chemistry. It entails assessing patient health through chemical processes and medical testing. In both inpatient and outpatient medical settings, clinical chemistry plays a crucial role in managing patients who have overdosed or been poisoned. The scientific field of toxicology investigates the detrimental effects of chemicals on living things, most commonly the human body. Risk assessment, a component of toxicology (Goldfrank et al., 2019), identifies potentially dangerous risks associated with substance exposure. Toxicologists can evaluate substances or circumstances that put people's health at risk and help create laws to safeguard the general public's health.

It is possible for clinical toxicologists to create new techniques for identifying the negative effects of substances and medications, along with the dosage at which these effects occur. Additionally, clinical toxicologists research particular chemicals and their safe uses. Nonetheless, the relevance of clinical toxicology studies does not require one to become a clinical toxicologist. Clinical toxicology is a subject that doctors, nurses, and physician assistants frequently study in order to better understand patients who have overdosed or been poisoned. To better prepare for their careers, professionals working in poison control centers and first responders may choose to pursue studies in clinical toxicology.

1.1.1. Scope of Clinical Toxicology

Wide range of actions pertaining to the detection, evaluation, treatment, and avoidance of toxic exposures and poisonings in people. Essentially, clinical toxicology is the study of the harmful effects that different substances—such as chemicals, drugs, natural toxins, pollutants from the environment, biological agents, and pollutants—have on human health. Pharmacology, toxicology, medicine, pathology, epidemiology, and public health are just a few of the disciplines whose knowledge is integrated in this field to understand toxicity mechanisms, evaluate the risks of toxic exposure, and create prevention and treatment plans. Evaluating and treating acute poisonings and toxic emergencies is a crucial part of clinical toxicology's range of practice. With a methodical approach to evaluating the type and extent of poisoning, identifying the toxic agent(s) involved, and launching the necessary interventions to minimize damage and encourage recovery, clinical toxicologists are trained to detect and react to toxic exposures quickly. Depending on the precise toxins and clinical symptoms present, this may entail performing in-depth patient assessments, acquiring comprehensive exposure histories, doing physical exams, arranging diagnostic testing, and putting treatment plans into place.

Clinical toxicology deals with chronic toxicities and long-term health effects linked to different substances in addition to acute poisonings. This covers the treatment of drug overdoses, drug addiction disorders, environmental contaminants, occupational exposures, and other long-term toxic conditions that need for continual monitoring, treatment, and rehabilitation. Clinical toxicologists collaborate with other medical professionals, toxicology experts, poison control facilities, and public health organizations to create all-encompassing treatment regimens, offer patient counseling and education, and organize multidisciplinary care for people impacted by toxic exposures. A key aspect of clinical toxicology's purview is prevention, which includes initiatives to detect and reduce toxic hazards, increase public knowledge of possible risks, encourage safe behaviors, and create laws and regulations to safeguard the public's health. Clinical toxicologists participate in surveillance programs to track trends in toxic exposures, spot new dangers, and assess how well preventative measures are working. Reducing the frequency and effects of poisonings, may entail research studies, creating public health campaigns, putting regulatory standards into place, and supporting laws that encourage safer goods, settings, and practices.

Within the field of clinical toxicology, research plays a significant role in expanding scientific understanding, refining diagnostic and treatment methodologies, and tackling new problems in the practice of toxicology. Studies on toxic mechanisms, pharmacokinetics, toxicogenomics, exposure and effect biomarkers, the creation of counteragents and treatment modalities, and assessments of the effectiveness and safety of interventions are all included in this. In order to put research into practice and create evidence-based toxicology practice guidelines, clinical toxicologists collaborate with academic institutions, business partners, and governmental organizations in addition to publishing scientific articles and attending conferences.

1.1.2. Duration and Frequency of Exposure

Experimental animals may be exposed to chemicals in four different ways: acute, sub-acute, chronic, and lifetime. Acute exposure is defined as chemical exposure lasting longer than 24 h. Some examples of exposure pathways include topical application, oral intubation, intraperitoneal (IP), intravenous (IV), and subcutaneous injections. Although the word "exposure" usually refers to a single dosage, some drugs that are almost benign or marginally hazardous can require several exposures over the course of a 24-h period. A continuous exposure of less than twenty-four hours, usually 4 h, is referred to as an acute exposure by inhalation.

Sub-acute, sub-chronic, and chronic exposure are the three categories into which repeated exposure falls:

- Sub-acute exposure is defined as repeated chemical exposure lasting one month or less.
- Sub-chronic exposure is the recurrent ingestion of a chemical throughout one to three months.
- Repeated chemical exposure lasting more than three months is referred to as chronic exposure (usually, this refers to studies with at least one year of repeated dosing).

All three of these types of repeated exposure are possible, but the most common is the oral route, which involves adding the chemical directly to food. Compared to carefully controlled animal experiments, the frequency and duration of exposure are usually not as well defined in human exposure scenarios. But there are essentially the same terms used to characterize common exposure conditions. Exposures that occur at work or in the environment can, therefore, be categorized as acute, which stems from a single event or episode, sub-chronic, which occurs repeatedly over weeks or months, or chronic, which occurs repeatedly over an extended period, like years.

1.1.3. Classifications of Toxicants

It is possible to classify toxic substances in a variety of ways, contingent upon the goals and preferences of the classifier. The ideal classification system may include a combination of methods based on multiple criteria, as no single classification can encompass the entire spectrum of hazardous chemicals. The classification of poisons may take into account the chemical and biological properties of the agent, but exposure characteristics are also significant in the field of toxicology. The physical states of toxic substances (gaseous, dust, liquid, and solid), their target organs and systems (nephrotoxicants, pulmotoxicants, neurotoxicants, hepatotoxicants, hematotoxicants, and dermatotoxicants), their chemical structure and nature (nonmetals, metals, acids, and alkalies), their organic toxicants (carbon compounds other than oxides of carbon, metallic carbides, cyanides, and the carbonates), their analytical behavior (volatile toxicants, metalloid extractive toxicants, and metals), and their type of toxicity (acute, subacute, chronic, etc.), use (insecticides, herbicides, rodenticides, fungicides, food additives, etc.), and toxic effects (carcinogens, teratogens, mutagens, and clastogens), mode of action, and factors related to public health and the environment (Goldfrank, 2019).

A "toxicity rating" system has been developed for common poisons to assist medical professionals and provide them with some understanding regarding hazardous nature of certain poisons when administered to humans. The more dangerous a chemical is rated on a scale of one to sixteen for its toxicity, the more powerful it is.

1.1.4. Factors Affecting Toxicology

It is well known that not every species is equally vulnerable to the negative effects of xenobiotics. For example, unlike most mammals, rabbits can ingest large amounts of the extremely deadly medication belladonna (*Atropa belladonna*). It is also well known that different people may react differently to a given level of toxin exposure within a population because there are several factors that can alter the overall toxic reaction. Age plays a big role in determining the chemical toxicity of most substances. Younger people tend to be more toxic for a variety of reasons, including, among others, a decreased ability to biotransform and remove xenobiotics. The way the body responds to foreign substances can be influenced by a variety of factors, such as environmental, personal, or even the xenobiotic itself.

The following categories can be used to group some of the factors that can influence chemical toxicity:

- Host factors (factors related to the subject)
- Factors related to toxicant or associated with xenobiotics
- Environmental conditions

Hence, individual and non-individual factors may impact how any drug or chemical reacts with the body.

1.1.4.1. Host Factors

- **The weight and size of a person:** It is essential to figure out how much chemical agent is required to cause a particular reaction. If the same chemical is given to people of different sizes, the concentration of the chemical in their tissues will differ, changing the effect that is produced. A larger dose can be tolerated by larger individuals than by smaller ones. Consequently, the acceptable daily intake (ADI) or chemical amount to be given is expressed as a unit of body weight for each chemical amount or dosage. Because body surface area is directly correlated with metabolism and activity, this function has been used to calculate ADI and establish tolerance thresholds for a variety of chemical agents.

- **Age:** Infants and young animals are especially susceptible to relatively safe toxins in the future. Different early life responses result from a variety of factors, such as the immaturity of the blood-brain barrier (BBS), relative inefficiency of certain excretory and metabolic pathways, increased tissue sensitivity, and others. Many enzyme systems are known to be incompletely formed at birth. Though much less than in an adult, the systems for chemical agent excretion or biotransformation are present. This impairment is, therefore, mainly quantitative. Newborns exhibit significantly lower activity levels in the oxidative pathways involved in the metabolism of various chemical substances when compared to adult counterparts. For example, substances that depend on the activity of glucuronyl transferase for detoxification become more toxic when there is a build-up of unbound bilirubin, which can result in jaundice. Immaturity of the kidneys, brain, or other organs may also increase a child's susceptibility to drugs or environmental contaminants. Chemical agents of the central nervous system (CNS) may be able to enter the brain more easily in immature BBS than in adult brains.
- **Strains and species:** Differences in species can have a major impact on a substance's toxicity. The relative toxicity of certain compounds, such as endosulfan, varied significantly when tested on multiple species. Diverse tissues can undergo different types of biotransformation, which frequently results in varying toxicities. A substance may be rapidly transformed by one species into a harmless or, on rare occasions, a more poisonous one; however, if the same substance is given to another, it may be digested very slowly or even by a different process, producing a different metabolite.
- **Acute toxicity:** Experiments conducted on diverse inbred mouse strains have demonstrated that variances in animal strains also lead to variations in chemical agent reactions. The human species is extraordinarily diverse. Therefore, the rate at which a given substance is metabolized by each individual can differ significantly.
- **Sex:** The toxicity of a chemical agent is frequently influenced by the gender of the animal. The endocrine system directly influences notable variations. In male mice, the nephrotoxic effects of chloroform can be reduced by castration and estrogen therapy; in female mice, these effects are amplified by androgen therapy. Sex hormones

may influence a chemical's enzymatic biotransformation in specific circumstances, which could explain why there are differences in sex. Women usually require a lower dosage than men because of their smaller stature. It is imperative to exercise caution when using medications or chemical agents during pregnancy, as there is a documented risk of teratogenic effects on females due to variations in toxicity caused by sex. Particularly, some substances secreted during lactation may have an impact on the offspring. Therefore, it is preferable to determine acute toxicity in both male and female animals of any species.

- **Feed and feeding:** The makeup of the feed or food may affect the results of toxicity testing. While diets high in fat can make animals more vulnerable to the hepatotoxic effects of chloroform, diets high in carbohydrates and protein can shield against those effects. It is noteworthy that mice fed a low-protein diet exhibited decreased activity of their liver's drug-metabolizing enzyme systems, and that vitamin C deficiency has been demonstrated to affect drug metabolism in guinea pigs. Acute poisoning in animals given synthetic meals has been observed to cause altered reactions. Certain foods may even have a deleterious effect when taken with medication. For example, cheese with a high tyramine content and monoamine oxidase inhibitors cause sympathomimetic effects. These findings imply that standard meals sufficiently nutrient-dense must be provided in toxicity studies. However, some toxicity studies involve animals that have certain nutritional deficiencies (e.g., protein). For example, oral toxicity testing typically detects a reduction in the amount of chemicals absorbed from the animal feed prior to intubation. To ensure equal absorption, it is customary to withhold the feed for 1618 h prior to intubation. However, the consequences of poisoning may also be impacted by the catabolic effects of hunger. It is common practice to go without food overnight for practical reasons. Free water is available both before and after the dose.
- **Changes in the internal environment:** Toxicity tests are performed on healthy animals because it is well known that a number of physiological factors, such as physical activity, stress, an animal's hormonal state, and internal organ degradation, can affect a compound's toxicity. Modifications in body composition or metabolism can impact toxicological responses during major surgery, lactation, and pregnancy.
- **Chemical toxicity alteration:** Importantly, it is triggered by a substance that is administered prior to the one under study. For example, certain drugs may increase the synthesis of liver microsomal enzymes and alter how another drug is metabolized. Chemical agents can also interfere with the ability of a

chemical to bind to proteins, inhibit a chemical's renal clearance, or stop a chemical from being metabolized by drugs or other chemicals (Hoffman et al., 2021).

- **Pathologic conditions:** Because animals or people react to the same chemical in various ways when they are healthy compared to when they are unwell, chemical agents are frequently modified to a very substantial level. Any one of these conditions will significantly increase medication or chemical toxicity.
- **Habitually used drugs:** It has been demonstrated that people who regularly use some psychoactive substances are more or less susceptible to negative drug reactions. Many drinks, including tea, coffee, and sodas with alcohol and nicotine, contain caffeine. Another common misuse of caffeine is for social purposes. Habitual, especially excessive, use of these compounds may affect a person's sensitivity to toxic doses of pharmaceuticals and other chemicals.
- **Idiosyncratic reaction/toxicity:** Occasionally, unique toxicity that affects only a specific individual or a small number of people, rather than the general population, has been observed. Idiosyncratic toxicity is rare, occurring in as few as 1 in 100,000 to 1 in 10 people. These reactions often occur after a person has been sensitized to a drug and exposed to it multiple times. Some medications, such as amoxicillin clavulanic acid, can cause symptoms to appear weeks after finishing a short course of treatment, but the symptoms may appear more quickly with subsequent doses. Drugs like halothane, diclofenac, phenytoin, and sulfonamides have been linked to immune-mediated idiosyncratic reactions in some individuals. Skin reactions, such as hives, asthma, swelling, and severe allergic reactions, have also been reported in response to certain chemicals or medications taken internally.

Hemolysis may occur when certain medications or meals are consumed by individuals who do not have the enzyme glucose-6-phosphate dehydrogenase. Despite having a lengthy (up to 12 months) latency period, some unique drug reactions do occasionally happen, and their reactions to a subsequent challenge are unpredictable. They fall under the category of peculiar non-immune-mediated reactions. Medication combinations such as troglitazone, ketoconazole, valproate, disulfiram, amiodarone, and isoniazid have all been connected to this unusual reaction. However, there is a chance that some allergic processes are at play.

1.1.4.2. Factors Related to Toxicant

The toxicant's physical condition and chemical characteristics, such as:

- Water solubility
- Vegetable oils solubility
- The suspending medium
- The size of the particle
- Rates of breakdown of chemical compositions
- The chemical agent's chemical stability
- The crystal form

- The gritty nature of inert chemicals used in large doses.

For instance, finer particles absorb more readily than coarser ones (this is especially true for irritant-containing poisons like zinc phosphide and naphthylthiourea). Because smaller particles can reach a larger portion of the stomach mucosa, they may cause protective vomiting. Some substances are readily converted to dichlorvos in alkaline solutions, which has an eight-fold lower oral LD50 in rats than the original drug. Dichlorvos is a wettable powder that can be used to treat external parasites. Solvents and other components used in commercial preparations may also influence the active principle's overall toxicity (s). Nonpolar solvents have the potential to dramatically speed up the absorption of lipophilic toxins, particularly when topical exposure is considered. Routes and administration speed: A drug's level of toxicity increases with the speed at which it enters the bloodstream. When most xenobiotics are administered parenterally as opposed to orally, the bioavailability occurs more quickly and completely, often leading to a lower LD50. The hazardous IV dosage is significantly influenced by the injection rate. Different ways for an ingredient to pass through the digestive tract can be absorbed. The differences in the parenteral and oral LD50 values reveal how much of a drug is absorbed. Additionally, poisons taken orally may undergo first-pass metabolism, which in certain cases may lead to nearly complete detoxification. For example, because of significant gut hydrolysis in mammalian species, pyrethrum-based pesticides are virtually safe, but not in fish because of the potential for significant molecular ingestion through the gills.

The toxicity of several xenobiotics can be modulated by a wide range of chemicals, including pesticides, plant toxins, drugs, and environmental pollutants. These compounds can act as either enzyme inducers or inhibitors, boosting or decreasing the expression or activity of hepatic and extrahepatic phase I and phase II enzyme systems involved in biotransformation reactions. This can occur prior to or coincidentally with other compounds (drug-drug interactions). This is achieved by either raising or lowering these enzyme systems' expression or activity, respectively. Therefore, simultaneous administration of two or more compounds with different structures at the same time may cause a summation, negative summation, potentiation, or additive effect. When two agents act on the same tissue or organ, an additive effect is produced, and the impact is the algebraic sum of the agents' individual actions. When something induces the induction of an enzyme, it usually happens slowly and necessitates constant exposure to the inducing molecule or molecules. Changing the biotransformation capacity prescribed for a particular toxin may yield different clinically significant outcomes based on the toxin's nature and the metabolite(s) that are produced. If the parent molecule is the source of any negative effects, then the overall toxicity level is expected to decrease; on the other hand, if one or more (re)active metabolites generated during biotransformation reactions are the source of toxic injury, then the opposite is true.

On the other hand, enzyme inhibition can have beneficial effects in cases of toxicant poisonings that require metabolic activity. In certain situations, inhibitors may be used as a therapeutic approach. For example, cimetidine is recommended for treating acetaminophen toxicity in dogs and cats because it inhibits the production of the reactive metabolite NAPQI, which can cause severe liver damage in poisoned animals. Enzyme inhibition may also enhance the effectiveness of compounds that act directly (without requiring metabolic activation), leading to potential drug interactions. These interactions can occur in the bloodstream, especially with anticoagulant rodenticides like bromadiolone, warfarin, and brodifacoum, which have prolonged plasma half-lives due to their high plasma protein binding. Additionally, the co-administration of certain medications can alter the toxicity of toxins by acting at the receptor level. For example, drugs that block neuromuscular transmission through nicotinic receptors, such as d-tubocurarine or succinylcholine, can increase the toxicity of carbamates or organophosphates. In contrast, the use of parasympatholytic agents like atropine, which is commonly used as an antagonist in clinical practice, may decrease the toxicity of certain toxins.

- **Tolerance:** An animals harmful response to a medication dose can decrease, stay the same, or increase when that dose is administered again. Hyper-susceptibility denotes an increase in harmful responses, whereas tolerance denotes a decrease in them. When a drug is administered repeatedly, tolerance to it is often developed through high enzyme activity or enzyme induction, which are processes involved in drug detoxification and elimination. Tolerance is known to result from decreased sensitivity of an end-organ to the deleterious effects of the drug. For instance, in healthy albino rats, chlorpromazine lowers the central nervous system and reduces locomotor activity. When chlorpromazine is administered repeatedly, the areas of the brain that the drug had previously depressed become more excitatory in response, and the sensitivity of those regions to the drug's depressive effects gradually decreases. Abruptly stopping a medication causes excitatory feedback to be unbalanced by the depressive effect of the drug, which leads to a significant increase in brain activity, increased motor activity, and insomnia.

1.1.4.3. Environmental Conditions

An environment can impact how animals and humans react to substances. In environment of laboratory animals employed in toxicity testing, there are three essential elements:

- An existence of other animal species, with humans being the most prevalent of these. Depending on the researcher's methods, the animals used in experiments can acquire feelings that range from hostility to apathy to affection. The disposition of the animal can influence adverse reaction it has to drugs.
- An existence of other creatures of same species. A harmful reaction to certain substances can be influenced by the presence of another female or male of same species, most likely owing to hostility or fear.
- **Physical environment:** The physical environment in which a toxicity test is carried out significantly influences the toxic reaction (e.g., temperature, light, relative humidity, and so forth). The LD50 values of rats for various compounds have also been demonstrated to be influenced by temperature, with differences observed between values at 37°C and 26°C. It has been demonstrated that a warm, humid atmosphere enhances skin absorption and

influences toxicity, specifically in inhalation toxicity tests. The number of animals in the cage, the design of the cage, seasonal variations, and the cycles of light and dark throughout the day all affect how toxic the environment is. Since it is rarely feasible to investigate the effects of every variation in the environmental factors, it is critical to document the conditions of an experiment in order to identify potential causes of variance in the event that the experiment is repeated and yields different results.

Chlorophenols and nitrophenols, for example, are more toxic in high ambient temperatures because they decouple mitochondrial oxidative phosphorylation and produce more heat. However, cats can die from hypothermia caused by the rodenticide/avicide chloralose, which acts on hypothalamic thermoreceptors. Because of this, exposure to toxins can have different effects based on a variety of factors. Variations in food, species, breed, and physio-pathological features of previous or ongoing exposure to multiple foreign chemicals can all affect the expression of proteins or enzymes involved in poison kinetics, which is typically the cause of variance in the toxic reaction. Researchers now have a better understanding of the mechanisms underlying many previously unexplained differences in how the body reacts to foreign substances thanks to recent substantial advancements in molecular techniques.

1.2. Historical Overview

One could argue that the study of poisons and counteragents was the original form of clinical toxicology. For more than 2000 years of human history, the application of poisons and the development of counter-measures have been recorded. Power struggles throughout civilization's history have frequently involved poisoning opponents to usurp their position of authority. Over overt physical violence, poisoning—a more subtle and difficult-to-prove method of murder—was favoured. Another popular suicide strategy was poisoning, which frequently involved the use of plant toxins like hemlock. The Greek writer Homer made the first mention of the science of poisons and countermeasures around 600 BCE. In his epic poem "Odyssey," Homer described how Ulysses was counseled to take a preventative potion made from the cholinesterase-inhibiting plant Galanthus nivalis to guard against Circe's poison, which contained the anticholinergic plant Datura stramonium. Greek physician, surgeon, and philosopher Galen (129–210 ACE) wrote multiple treatises on antidote mixtures to guard against more than 70 recognized poisons during his time in the Roman Empire. The first person to describe inducing emesis by stimulating the hypopharynx or using chemical emetics to lessen the absorption of ingested poisons was Nicander, a Greek physician and poet who lived in the second century. Similarly, charcoal was used in ancient Greece and Rome to treat a variety of poisonings. Notably, the use of particular poison antidotes and parenteral charcoal or induction of emesis as a means of preventing toxicant absorption continue to be mainstays in the treatment of human poisoning to this day. It is obvious that the earliest methods of poisoning prevention and treatment are closely related to the roots of contemporary clinical toxicology.

1.2.1. Middle East and North African Clinical Toxicology Association (Menatox)

The U.S.A recognized and incorporated the Middle East and North Africa Clinical Toxicology Association (MENATOX). S. 2014 saw the founding and president at the time, Dr. Ziad Kazzi, take over. MENATOX obtained federal tax exemption status from the U.S. government in

May 2018, within the framework of a 501(c) non-profit. The Middle East and North Africa (MENA) region is geographically defined as Algeria, Bahrain, Djibouti, Egypt, Iran, Iraq, Israel, Jordan, Kuwait, Lebanon, Libya, Malta, Morocco, Oman, Palestinian Authority, Qatar, Saudi Arabia, Sudan, Syria, Tunisia, United Arab Emirates, and Yemen. MENATOX is a professional organization devoted to the care of poisoned patients in this region. MENATOX is dedicated to the investigation of issues pertaining to toxicological exposures in all their forms. MENATOX will work on multidisciplinary research projects, provide education, and treat and prevent human poisonings from chemicals, illicit drugs, pharmaceuticals, and other toxins. In addition, MENATOX will carry out multidisciplinary research, instruction, and the management of ionizing radiation exposures.

In pursuance of these objectives, MENATOX will (taken from the website):

- Foster a better understanding of the principles and practice of clinical toxicology in order to prevent poisoning and to promote better care for the poisoned patient, particularly through poison information and treatment centers;
- Unite individuals whose professional activities are concerned with clinical toxicology whether in a poison center, academic institution, health care facility or in government or industry;
- Encourage basic and clinical research in all aspects of poisonings and overdoses;
- Facilitate the collection, exchange, and dissemination of relevant information among individual members, poison centers and organizations interested in clinical toxicology;
- Promote training in and set standards for the practice of clinical toxicology and encourage high standards in poison centers and in the management of poisoned patients generally;
- Work together with global organizations such as the Asia-Pacific Association of Medical Toxicology, the American College of Medical Toxicology, the American Academy of Clinical Toxicology, the World Health Organization, and the European Association of Poisons Centers and Clinical Toxicologists, among others.
- Form and uphold productive partnerships with governmental entities, associations of professionals, non-profits, and other pertinent entities or persons engaged in the application, instruction, and study of clinical toxicology.

1.2.2. Middle Ages and Renaissance

Toxicology as a scientific field was founded on the substantial advances made by academics and alchemists during the Middle Ages and Renaissance regarding the knowledge of poisons, toxic plants, and chemical agents. Throughout medieval Europe, the effects and uses of poisons were frequently combined with superstition, folklore, and real-world applications in the fields of medicine, law enforcement, and warfare. Alchemists experimented with a variety of materials, such as metals, minerals, and plant extracts, in an attempt to turn base metals into gold and find the elixir of life. This unintentionally led to the early understanding of toxicology. During this time, there was an increasing interest in the pharmacological and toxicological characteristics of chemical agents, as evidenced by the descriptions of poisonous substances, antidotes, and poison detection techniques found in alchemical texts and manuscripts.

Paracelsus (1493–1541), a Swiss physician, alchemist, and philosopher whose groundbreaking work transformed the field of toxicology, is one prominent person from this era. In contrast to the conventional wisdom of medieval medicine, Paracelsus placed a strong emphasis on empirical data, experimentation, and observation when attempting to understand how drugs affect the human body. He popularized the idea that "the dose makes the poison," arguing that any substance could be harmful if consumed in excess and that the secret to comprehending toxicity was figuring out the right dose-response relationship for each one. In addition, Paracelsus experimented with different substances and minerals, recording the effects on both humans and animals and promoting the application of particular remedies and countermeasures in poisoning situations.

Progress in chemistry, pharmacology, and botany during the Renaissance increased our comprehension of toxicology. Herbalists and botanists compiled herbals and botanical texts that explained the applications, side effects, and toxicities of different botanical substances, cataloguing the medicinal and toxic qualities of plants. The techniques for creating and compounding pharmaceutical formulations for treating poisonings and antidotes were developed by pharmacists and apothecaries. Alchemical treatises and manuscripts persisted in their circulation among academics, imparting knowledge of laboratory procedures, chemical reactions, and experimental results that were pertinent to the field of toxicology. The field of toxicology began systematically studying the characteristics, effects, and nature of substances that are toxic to living things during the Middle Ages and Renaissance, when early toxicology texts and treatises appeared. These seminal works bridged the gap between alchemy, medicine, and natural philosophy and laid the foundation for the modern scientific field of toxicology. Even though many of the theories and methods of medieval toxicology were not grounded in scientific rigor but rather in empirical observation and real-world experience, they did set the groundwork for later developments in toxicological research, analytical methods, and regulatory standards meant to safeguard the environment and public health from the dangers of toxic substances.

1.2.3. Development of Toxicology as a Scientific Discipline

Toxicology changed dramatically in the 19th and early 20th centuries, moving from a largely descriptive and observational field to a distinct scientific discipline based on pharmacology, biochemistry, and pathology. This era saw a number of important discoveries that transformed our knowledge of toxic substances and how they affect living things, laying the groundwork for modern toxicology. The establishment of experimental pharmacology as a scientific field, which offered the framework for researching the functions and impacts of medications and toxins on biological systems, was one significant advancement. Animal experimentation was first used by German pharmacologist Rudolf Buchheim, who is frequently recognized as the father of experimental pharmacology, to study the physiological and pharmacological characteristics of pharmaceuticals. His work established the foundation for methodical investigations into drug metabolism, dose-response relationships, and toxicological testing, forming the basis for contemporary toxicological research techniques. Simultaneously, 19th-century developments in biochemistry and physiology offered fresh perspectives on the molecular and cellular mechanisms underlying drug toxicity and action. Understanding the biochemical processes involved in drug metabolism and detoxification is made possible by the research conducted by German physiologist and chemist Justus von Liebig on metabolism and the chemical makeup of living tissues. The field of biochemical toxicology emerged as a result of Liebig's work and later discoveries in enzyme kinetics and metabolic pathways. This field aimed to clarify the mechanisms underlying drug metabolism, detoxification, and biochemical changes induced by toxicants. The discipline of pathology's establishment to examine the anatomical and functional alterations linked to disease and toxic injury was another crucial development. The concept of cellular pathology, developed by German pathologist Rudolf Virchow, stressed the significance of cellular changes in the pathogenesis of disease, including toxicological conditions. By enabling researchers to see and describe the morphological changes brought about by toxic substances in tissues and organs, Virchow's groundbreaking work in histopathology and microscopy shed light on the mechanisms underlying toxicity and the effects that are specific to particular organs.

The field's evolution underwent a sea change when experimental toxicology emerged as a separate scientific discipline in the late 19th and early 20th centuries. The development of toxicological testing techniques, including carcinogenicity assays, acute and chronic toxicity studies, and reproductive toxicity assessments, set the stage for evaluating the safety and risk of chemicals, pharmaceuticals, and consumer goods. The significance of toxicological research in safeguarding public health and safety was further highlighted by regulatory initiatives such as the establishment of regulatory agencies like the Food and Drug Administration (FDA) and the passing of the Pure Food and Drug Act in the United States in 1906.

1.2.4. Poison Control Centers and Public Health Initiatives

Considerable progress was made in public health and poison control programs in the middle of the 20th century with the goal of lowering the number of poisonings and increasing public safety. The establishment of poison control centers (PCCs) in numerous parts of the world, which functioned as centralized resources for poison prevention, education, and emergency response, was one of the major turning points during this time. Dr. Edward Press, a pediatrician, established the nation's first poison control center in Chicago in 1953 after realizing the need for a specialized facility to handle poison-related emergencies. The Illinois Poison Center was one of the first poison control centers in the nation, and it served as a model for others to open. The American Association of Poison Control Centers (AAPCC) was established in 1958 with the goal of standardizing procedures for poison management and prevention and coordinating the efforts of poison control centers across the country.

Alongside the opening of poison control centers, educational campaigns and poison prevention programs were created to educate the public about common poisons, encouraging safe handling and storage techniques, and disseminating knowledge about emergency response and poison first aid. These programs used media campaigns, community outreach activities, school-based programs, and public service announcements to reach a variety of audiences, including educators, parents, caregivers, healthcare professionals, and the general public. To address the risks associated with poisoning and advance public safety, regulatory measures were also put into place. To prevent accidental poisonings, especially among young children, the Poison Prevention Packaging Act (PPPA) was passed in the United States in 1970 and mandated that certain household products and medications be packaged in a way that is child-resistant. The frequency of pediatric poisonings brought on by the ingestion of medicines, household chemicals, and other dangerous materials has significantly decreased as a result of the PPPA.

Improvements in medical toxicology and toxicological research, in addition to poison control centers and laws, have helped to better diagnose, treat, and manage poisonings. When it came to handling complicated poison-related cases and organizing emergency medical services, cooperation between poison control centers, medical professionals, toxicologists, and emergency responders allowed for quick access to professional advice and consultation.

1.2.5. Advances in Analytical Toxicology

The field of toxicology has advanced significantly due to the use of analytical techniques and instrumentation, which have made it possible to identify, detect, and quantify toxic substances in a variety of matrices, such as biological samples, environmental samples, and forensic specimens. These analytical techniques have transformed toxicological research, forensic investigations, environmental monitoring, and clinical practice, which enable more precise risk assessment, toxic exposure diagnosis, and management. The development of techniques for identifying and measuring toxic substances in biological samples, such as blood, urine, hair, and tissues, is one of the analytical techniques' most significant contributions to the field of toxicology. Techniques for analysis like chromatography (e.g., mass spectrometry (MS), gas and liquid chromatography (LC), and other analytical techniques have been crucial in isolating and characterizing distinct constituents in intricate blends, thereby enabling accurate quantification of carcinogens and their byproducts at minute concentrations. These techniques are commonly employed in forensic toxicology labs to examine biological specimens gathered during autopsies or criminal investigations, as well as in clinical toxicology labs to screen for drugs, toxins, and other chemical agents in patients presenting with suspected poisonings or drug overdoses.

Analytical methods have been used in environmental toxicology to track and evaluate the presence of hazardous materials in soil, water, air, and food samples. Environmental samples have been analyzed using methods like high-performance liquid chromatography (HPLC), gas chromatography-mass spectrometry (GC-MS), and inductively coupled plasma-mass spectrometry (ICP-MS) to check for a variety of pollutants, such as pesticides, heavy metals, industrial chemicals, and persistent organic pollutants (POPs). To inform regulatory decisions and pollution control strategies, these analytical methods offer important information on environmental contamination levels, exposure pathways, and potential health risks to human populations and ecosystems. In forensic toxicology, postmortem samples taken from deceased people are analyzed using analytical techniques to see if any drugs, alcohol, poisons, or other toxic substances were present that could have caused the death. In order to identify and measure particular substances in biological fluids and tissues, forensic laboratories frequently use immunoassays, chromatographic procedures, and spectroscopic methods for screening and confirmation tests during toxicological analyses. These analyses are essential for establishing the cause and manner of death, assisting with criminal investigations, and supplying proof in court cases.

1.3. Basic Principles of Toxicology

Toxicology is defined as "the study of poisons." "Toxic" first appeared in English around 1655. It was borrowed from the Late Latin word "toxicus," which means "poisonous," and was derived from the ancient Greek word "toxikón," which refers to poisons used to dip arrows. The application of different poisons was the historical focus of toxicology, and most people still think of "toxic substances" as a class of chemicals to which even a small amount of exposure inevitably leads to death or some serious long-term adverse effect, like cancer. Over the years, toxicology has developed into a highly developed field of study that examines all potential negative health effects of drugs. The following definitions are provided to help the reader grasp a number of basic ideas. The term "toxicity" describes any negative (harmful) effects that a chemical or physical substance may have on a living thing. The study of the detrimental effects (toxicities) that chemicals or occupational exposure may have on living things under specific exposure circumstances is known as toxicology.

It is a science that looks for every threat (i.e., organ toxicities) associated with a substance while also seeking to measure the exposure conditions that give rise to those risks or toxicities. The scientific study of the occurrence, nature, incidence, mechanism, and risk factors for the harmful effects of hazardous chemicals is known as toxicology chemicals effects on how substances interact with living things. A toxicologist is trained to forecast the occurrence of these effects and to look into their nature, including their cellular, biochemical, and molecular modes of action.

1.3.1. Toxicology's Disciplines

A mechanistic toxicologist investigates the molecular, cellular, and biochemical mechanisms by which toxins injure living things. When designing and producing safer chemicals and developing logical treatments for chemical toxicity and illness, mechanical data may be helpful. Mechanistic evidence in risk assessment can be useful in proving that a negative outcome observed in lab animals has direct application to humans. Mechanistic toxicologists can identify genetically sensitive individuals, shield them from hazardous environmental exposures, and customize drug therapy based on their specific genetic makeup thanks to toxicogenomics. Before starting pharmaceutical therapy, sensitive people can be identified using a range of genetic tests. Involved directly in toxicity testing, which provides information for safety evaluation and regulatory requirements, is a descriptive toxicologist. The goal of toxicity studies on laboratory animals is to gather information that can be utilized to evaluate the risks that particular chemicals pose to humans and the environment.

Drawing from the evidence provided by mechanistic and descriptive toxicologists, a regulatory toxicologist is responsible for determining whether a medicine or other chemical poses a low enough risk to be sold for a particular purpose. Regulatory toxicologists develop standards for the amount of chemicals that are permitted in pharmaceuticals, food products, industrial settings, ambient air, and drinking water. In order to address the medicolegal ramifications of chemical toxicity in humans and animals, forensic toxicology integrates analytical chemistry with fundamental toxicologic principles. The field of clinical toxicology focuses on illnesses that are either directly caused by or closely associated with dangerous chemicals.

Examples of toxicology disciplines related to human toxicology are:

- **Toxicology of animals:** the study of the detrimental effects of chemicals, medicines, and other substances on mammals to anticipate their consequences on humans.
- **Toxicology of Reproduction and Development:** the study of the

detrimental effects of chemicals, medicines, and other substances on mammalian reproduction and development.

- The study of the adverse effects of chemicals, medicines, and other compounds on genetic material, such as DNA and RNA.
- **Immunotoxicology** studies the immunotoxic effects of chemicals, medicines, and other substances.
- **Neurotoxicology** studies the adverse effects of chemicals, medicines, and other substances on the central and peripheral neurological systems (PNS).

1.3.2. Principles

The study, diagnosis, treatment, and prevention of human poisonings and toxic exposures are governed by a set of basic ideas and principles known as clinical toxicology principles (Van Der Linden et al., 2018). These principles offer a framework for comprehending the effects of toxic substances on the body and handling toxicological emergencies. They are drawn from a variety of disciplines, including pharmacology, toxicology, medicine, emergency care, and public health.

Some key principles of clinical toxicology include:

- **Toxicokinetics:** Understanding the absorption, distribution, metabolism, and excretion (ADME) of toxic substances within the body is essential for predicting their effects and guiding treatment decisions. Toxicokinetic principles help clinicians assess the rate and extent of exposure, estimate tissue distribution, and evaluate the potential for toxicity based on factors such as route of exposure, dose, duration, and individual variability.
- **Toxicodynamics:** Understanding how toxic substances interact with cellular and molecular targets within the body to produce harmful effects is central to the principles of toxicodynamics. This involves determining the crucial molecular targets, clarifying the toxicity mechanisms, and describing dose-response relationships in order to forecast the beginning, intensity, and length of toxic effects.
- **Clinical Assessment:** In order to determine the type and extent of toxic exposures and to provide guidance for appropriate management, a methodical approach to evaluating poisoned patients is imperative. A comprehensive history of exposure, a physical examination to identify symptoms and indicators of toxicity, and diagnostic testing to identify the presence of toxicants and evaluate organ function are all part of the clinical assessment process.
- **Poison Management:** Timely identification, stabilization, and treatment of toxic exposures are necessary for the effective management of poisoned patients. The fundamentals of managing poisoning involve starting the proper supportive care measures, applying decontamination methods (e.g., providing antidotes or targeted treatments for recognized toxins (e.g., gastric lavage, activated charcoal), and keeping an eye on

patients for indications of toxicity resolution or progression.

- **Prevention:** Clinical toxicology's primary focus is prevention, which includes methods to lower the risk of toxic exposures and decrease the frequency of poisonings. This entails advancing poison prevention education and awareness campaigns, supporting safe handling and storage procedures for dangerous materials, implementing legal restrictions to limit access to toxicants, and creating public health initiatives to address occupational and environmental risks.
- **Collaboration and Consultation:** To provide comprehensive care for patients who have been poisoned, clinical toxicologists frequently collaborate with multidisciplinary teams that include emergency physicians, toxicologists, pharmacists, nurses, and poison control specialists. Toxicology specialists and poison control centers can offer invaluable advice on handling complicated cases, interpreting toxicological data, and selecting the best course of treatment.
- **Research and Education:** Continued research, instruction, and training are necessary to advance understanding and proficiency in clinical toxicology. Clinical toxicology research and education are based on the principles of conducting studies to clarify toxic mechanisms, create novel therapeutic and diagnostic approaches, and assess the efficacy of preventive measures. Healthcare providers, toxicologists, and public health professionals can benefit from education and training programs that spread knowledge, improve clinical skills, and advance best practices in toxicology practice.

By adhering to these principles, clinical toxicologists can effectively manage poisonings and toxic exposures, promote public health and safety, and contribute to the advancement of knowledge in the field of toxicology.

1.3.3. Using Toxic Syndrome Recognition for Rapid Diagnosis and Empiric Therapy

- Chemical classes.
  - Toxic chemicals can often be grouped into classes, whereby all the chemicals in each class cause similar human health effects.
  - These constellations of toxic effects or toxic syndromes comprise a set of clinical "fingerprints" for groups of toxins.
  - All of the toxins associated with a given toxic syndrome are treated similarly.
- Emergency treatment.
  - During the early phases of a toxic chemical emergency, when the exact chemical is often unknown, identifying the toxic syndromes present can be a useful decision-making tool.
  - Toxic syndromes are easily identified with only a few observations, such as:
  - Vital signs
  - Mental status

  - Pupil size
  - Mucous membrane irritation
  - Lung exam for wheezes or rales
  - Skin for burns, moisture, and color
- The identification of the constellation of signs and symptoms is all that is needed to diagnose and treat a life-threatening condition (e.g., respiratory arrest).
- Once the life-threatening crisis has been averted and time passes, more specific information from the history or diagnostic test results will guide additional therapeutic decisions and patient disposition.

1.3.4. Route of Exposure is a Determinant of Toxicity

- A chemical's physical state and the route of exposure influence toxicity.
- The chemical's state often determines the route of exposure.
- For many chemicals, the toxic effects occur at the site of absorption.
  - Inhalation exposure: Inhalation risks include gases, vapors, airborne powders, and aerosolized liquids.
  - Irritant gases attack the water in the respiratory mucosa and eye, causing burning pain, irritation, and copious secretions at the site of contact.
  - Inhalation exposure also allows some rapid entry into the systemic circulation, causing toxic effects distant from the entry route.
  - Hydrogen cyanide is a gas that rapidly enters the circulation through the lung and causes loss of consciousness, seizures, cardiac dysrhythmias, hypotension, and possible death in a matter of minutes after the exposure.
- Dermal exposure: Chemicals in contact with the skin can cause local effect but may also enter the systemic circulation and cause effects at distant sites from the entry route.
  - Organophosphate insecticides are fat-soluble chemicals that rapidly penetrate the skin and enter the bloodstream to circulate to distant sites.
  - Skin exposure can delay the onset of systemic effects compared to the rapid entry through the lung.

1.3.5. The Dose Makes the Poison

- Dose - response
  - Evaluating clinical effects based on the amount of exposure is a basic toxicology principle called dose-response.
  - The dose is the total amount of chemical absorbed during an exposure.
  - Dose depends on the concentration of the chemical and duration (contact time) of the exposure. Chemicals cause predictable toxic effects based on the dose.
  - Ethanol is a good example. Incremental increases in blood ethanol levels result in predictable increases in

alteration of consciousness (signs of inebriation), poor coordination, and eventually coma/respiratory depression, and finally death.

- Exposure
  - Duration of exposure is one important factor affecting the dose.
  - High concentrations over a long duration are more likely to produce adverse health effects than the same or lower concentration over a shorter exposure period.
  - Example 1, Dermal exposure: an acid placed on the skin will cause more tissue destruction the longer it stays in contact with the tissues. The injury is limited if the acid is immediately washed off the skin.
  - Example 2, Inhalation exposure: The longer a victim is allowed to breathe toxic chemicals, the greater the dose of exposure.
- Application of dose-response principles
  - Applying the above dose-response principles can guide patient assessment of toxic chemical exposures.
  - Patients who have higher concentrations and longer durations of exposure result in greater doses to the victim and will more likely have harmful effects.
  - Those receiving larger doses need more urgent attention and possibly life-saving interventions than those receiving smaller doses (especially if asymptomatic).

1.4. Laboratory Developed Tests in Clinical Toxicology

A branch of laboratory medicine called clinical toxicology examines bodily fluids to look for chemicals, medications, or poisons. This testing can give medical professionals important information for patient diagnosis and care. It can be quantitative or qualitative, and it can be applied to a variety of clinical situations, such as identifying inappropriate drug use, detecting toxicity, and confirming prescription compliance. Therapeutic drug monitoring (TDM) and medicolegal testing are frequently linked to clinical toxicology; however, they are not covered in this mini-review article and merit separate discussion. The application of laboratory developed tests (LDT) in clinical toxicology is the main topic of this chapter.

1.4.1. In Vitro Diagnostics and Laboratory Developed Tests in Clinical Toxicology

Commercial in vitro diagnostic (IVD) assays are available and governed as medical devices by the US Food and Drug Administration (FDA) for the majority of general laboratory testing. The manufacturer's usage instructions, which specify which sample types are tested and how the assay is used clinically, must be followed by laboratories (e.g., urine, serum, etc.). The performance characteristics of the assay, as specified by the assay manufacturer, are maintained by this rigidity. When an FDA-approved or cleared test is unable to satisfy clinical requirements, a certified laboratory may use an LDT to close the gap in clinical care or enhance clinical workflow. Additionally, for lower testing volumes, an LDT might be less expensive than an IVD. Labs can develop LDTs in several ways thanks to the Clinical Laboratory Improvement Amendments (CLIA), including by altering an IVD test that has been approved or cleared by the FDA (e.g., testing a sample type that isn't covered in the product insert), following a test protocol created as an LDT by another organization, or developing a brand-new test. The performing laboratory must evaluate each LDT's performance characteristics—normally set by the IVD manufacturer—and confirm that it is appropriate for use in patient care. Since LDTs are classified as high complexity, laboratories need to adhere to stricter quality standards, personnel requirements, and proficiency testing guidelines. While it may be more convenient for laboratories to use IVD assays instead of LDTs when they are available and practical, these tests are necessary to meet changing clinical testing requirements.

The laboratory medicine community is concerned about the possibility that legislative reform will increase oversight of LDTs. The proposed regulatory framework may make it prohibitively expensive to implement LDTs and may make it more difficult for laboratories to promptly address emerging patient care needs. The clinical toxicology landscape might alter significantly if this reform is implemented, which would probably have a detrimental effect on laboratories' capacity to offer state-of-the-art clinical toxicology testing. Since they are frequently used as first-line screening tests for the presence of drugs and toxic substances, IVD assays are essential to clinical toxicology. They do, however, have a number of drawbacks that are especially pertinent to the field of clinical toxicology. Immunoassays, which generally have low specificity or insufficient detection sensitivity for the target drug or toxin, make up the great majority of toxicology IVDs. Despite the fact that Europe offers a number of mass spectrometry (MS)-based toxicology IVD assays, their current use in the US is restricted to TDM applications. Additionally, IVD assays might not be commercially available for all but the most common drugs and toxins. Even though IVD assays have been a mainstay of clinical toxicology testing for many years, they are currently unable to satisfy all clinical needs. LDTs solve the flaws in IVD assays and give labs the testing assistance they need to accurately evaluate patients with toxicology.

The most common LDTs in clinical toxicology, according to data from literature and proficiency testing surveys, are chromatographic techniques like GC or LC coupled to MS and high-resolution MS. However, a comprehensive database listing all LDTs in clinical use is not yet available. In terms of analytical performance, they typically outperform IVD immunoassays. While other testing methodologies are also available for LDTs, MS-based LDTs continue to be the gold standard in clinical toxicology and have become increasingly more popular in the last ten years. The 'Drug Monitoring for Pain Management' proficiency testing surveys, conducted in 2022 by the College of American Pathology, involved approximately 500 participants. Of these, about 80% produced quantitative results and 15% produced qualitative results through chromatographic methods (i.e., LCMS as well as HPLC). This illustrates how deeply integrated MS-based LDTs are into clinical toxicology. The next section addresses the gaps currently recognized between clinical requirements and current toxicology IVD assays, along with instances of how LDTs have been utilized to close these gaps.

1.4.2. LDTs Are Bridging the Gaps Between Patient Needs and Available Toxicology In Vitro Diagnostics

1.4.2.1. Controlled Substance Monitoring

By determining the presence of the prescribed controlled substance, the absence of non-prescribed medications, and the absence of illicit drugs, toxicology testing can be used to assess compliance with a controlled substance prescription regimen. This can reduce risk for the patient as well as the healthcare provider. The most popular method for conducting drug testing for this clinical indication is a two-step procedure that starts with an immunoassay-based qualitative drug screen and ends with a confirmatory test for particular drugs or drug classes that screen positive. IVD immunoassays are generally used for initial screening, although LDT immunoassays can be employed when an IVD solution is not available. Although less common, qualitative toxicology screening can also be conducted with MS-based LDT techniques. To lower the possibility of false-positive results, these screening results are typically reported as "presumptive" or "preliminary" positive and are verified by a more sophisticated analytical technique. Because of their superior sensitivity and specificity, quantitative MS-based LDTs have traditionally been used for confirmatory or "definitive" testing. Interestingly, despite MS LDTs being the gold standard for confirmatory testing and a mainstay of clinical drug testing for decades, there are no FDA-cleared confirmatory assays.

IVD immunoassays have a number of benefits, including fast turnaround times for results, affordability, and high levels of automation that make them simple to use. But they also have several drawbacks that make determining prescription compliance difficult. For example, with many IVD amphetamine drug screens, drugs of abuse immunoassays can produce false-positive results due to cross-reaction with compounds that are structurally or chemically like their target. Examples of such compounds include some over-the-counter nasal decongestants and the prescription drug bupropion. Further testing with an MS LDT is required to ascertain whether the initial screening result was a true or false positive. This gives the doctor more assurance when determining whether to continue or stop prescribing. Additionally, a positive test result does not reveal the specific compound(s) that are present in the sample because many qualitative IVD immunoassays are made to detect an entire class of medications. On the other hand, MS LDTs can identify the individual drugs and metabolites that are present as well as their relative concentrations. This information can be useful in determining prescription compliance as well as the possibility of abusing several drugs in one class. Toxicology MS LDTs can currently give clinicians crucial information that IVD techniques cannot.

Compared to MS-based LDTs, immunoassays are more likely to produce false-negative results because IVD manufacturers set higher cutoffs for positivity. Cutoffs for many IVD drugs of abuse in clinical settings are orders of magnitude higher than the MS-based LDT cutoff. For instance, levels ≤ 20 ng/mL can be readily quantified using MS-based LDTs, whereas the standard cutoff for benzodiazepine immunoassays in clinical laboratories is 200 ng/mL. When it comes to situations where there is a high positivity rate, such as medication adherence monitoring, the traditional screening with reflex approach to drug testing minimizes false-positive results. However, in these situations, a testing strategy that lowers false-negative results is necessary. With a longer detection window and the ability to precisely detect lower drug/metabolite concentrations, MS-based LDTs greatly reduce the number of false-negative results.

The various medications and metabolites in a class of drugs have variable cross-reactivities with one another, and immunoassays intended to screen for the entire class of drugs are calibrated using a representative compound. Because of this, some drugs may not be detected at all, while others may require higher concentrations to be detected. As an excellent illustration, consider opiate assays, which are made to have good cross-reactivity with naturally occurring opiates (e.g., morphine, and codeine), but exhibit less cross-reactivity with opioids that are semi-synthetic (e.g., oxycodone) and very few with opioids that are entirely synthetic (e.g., fentanyl, tramadol). Because of this, clinical labs frequently provide distinct, more focused immunoassay drug screens to identify frequently prescribed and misused semi-synthetic and synthetic opioids. Because of the large number of benzodiazepines and their complex metabolism, benzodiazepine assays are also a good example. Immunoassay screens frequently miss commonly prescribed benzodiazepines like clonazepam and alprazolam because they are not sensitive enough to identify the drug's metabolites, which are the relevant forms, given that only a small portion of the drug is eliminated as the parent or unchanged. Because MS-based drug testing methods target individual compounds and can differentiate between parent compounds and metabolites, they are more dependable when it comes to detecting drugs within a class. They are therefore better suited to assess drug adherence. While variations exist in the lower limits of quantitation amongst compounds in MS-based methods, they are not as significant as those found in immunoassays and are unlikely to influence clinical judgments.

Many have argued that MS-based toxicology techniques should be used as the first line of testing methodology for drugs that are frequently prescribed for pain management, such as opioids and benzodiazepines, because they are superior to immunoassays in this regard. Using the advantages of both technologies, some have embraced a hybrid strategy that combines MS-based testing for some drugs with immunoassay screening for others, based on assay performance and predicted positivity rates. Whether a hybrid or traditional approach is taken, the literature shows that toxicology LDTs invariably enhance the quality of results and patient care in this population.

1.4.2.2. Addiction Medicine

Drug testing is a helpful tool in addiction medicine for identifying substance use, organizing treatment, and assessing how well patients with addiction or those at risk for addiction are responding to treatment. Because IVD toxicology immunoassays yield results faster than multiplex methods, they are frequently utilized in this clinical setting for both initial and ongoing patient assessments. Furthermore, MS-based LDTs can be used to verify the cessation of specific substances (e.g., ethanol, opioids) or identify relapse because they are able to identify even minute amounts of substances that might be below an immunoassay's cutoff threshold. In addition, MS LDTs can be used to identify the recreational use of substances not picked up by screening tests, like designer drugs like synthetic cannabinoids or herbal supplements that contain mitragynine (i.e., kratom). For many newly developed drugs of abuse, non-FDA-cleared immunoassay kits are also available. These kits can be used to expedite the laboratory's LDT development and validation process, although their development takes longer than that of MS-based versions because of the difficulties in producing and assessing diagnostic antibodies.

When evaluating adherence to medication-assisted treatment (MAT) regimens, such as methadone or buprenorphine, which are used to treat opioid substance use disorders, MS-based LDTs are frequently employed in clinical settings. Additional information about whether the medication is taken as directed can be obtained through the quantitative assessment of the parent compound to metabolite ratio. When compared to its metabolite, norbuprenorphine, a compliant patient on a buprenorphine regimen will have a comparatively low level of buprenorphine. Conversely, a patient who tries to falsify their urine sample to appear compliant will have a very high level of buprenorphine in comparison to the norbuprenorphine metabolite. In general, a ratio of <0.02 for norbuprenorphine to buprenorphine concentration indicates that the medication was degraded in the urine sample rather than taken. IVD immunoassays cannot provide this extra degree of information for tracking treatment adherence and spotting potential drug diversion because they are unable to discern the parent drugs from their metabolites. By strengthening the drug testing utilized to support the assessment, diagnosis, treatment, and recovery of patients with substance use disorders, toxicology LDTs enhance patient care.

1.4.2.3. Routine Care

Mass spectrometry-based laboratory-developed tests (LDTs) can play a crucial role in preventing harmful drug interactions by identifying and measuring substances that can impact patient care but may go undetected by standard drug screenings. These tests are also beneficial in improving patient safety in routine care, such as assessing substance exposure before medical procedures. For instance, patients may undergo testing to confirm they have abstained from tobacco products before elective surgery, as nicotine has been linked to delayed wound healing in postoperative recovery. These tests can detect and measure the major nicotine metabolites, allowing differentiation between active and passive exposure based on concentration levels. Furthermore, they can also measure tobacco-specific alkaloids to distinguish between nicotine replacement therapy and tobacco use. This added information empowers physicians to make more informed clinical decisions regarding nicotine exposure and enables a more accurate assessment of patient risk.

Toxicology LDTs can assess if substance use or withdrawal may be a factor in psychiatric symptoms, which can help with unexplained symptoms, unexpected responses to treatment, and potential mental disorders. They can also help patients who have no symptoms or whose symptoms resemble those of another disease state with their diagnostic workup. For instance, LDTs are frequently employed to find excessive levels of heavy metals (e.g., lead, arsenic, cobalt) as a result of exposure in the workplace or environment, or even from joint replacement implants. Since the degree of toxicity of a metal is determined by its chemical form, a precise test methodology is necessary to quantify the metal ion level and provide speciation. While some metals can be tested with IVD, laboratories may opt to use an LDT instead if it can offer extra information that helps with clinical decision-making (e.g., speciation) or if there are concerns about the accuracy of the data produced by the FDA-approved test (e.g., interferences, precision).

Given the potentially dire consequences, toxicology LDTs are especially helpful in validating drug test results that could be used to guide other treatment or social decisions. Examples of these kinds of decisions include postnatal drug test results that are obtained on either the mother or the neonate. Immunoassay results that are falsely negative could put the child in danger, while false positive results could result in the child being wrongfully taken from their parents by child protective services. LDTs also have the benefit of testing biological matrices not typically tested, like meconium, oral fluid, and hair, which can reveal important details regarding the timing of substance exposure. For instance, in neonatal toxicology, the detection of in utero substance exposure during pregnancy can be guided toward the most effective management of the newborn through the use of meconium drug testing and umbilical cord tissue testing. Toxicology LDTs provide the enhanced analytical sensitivity and specificity needed for many of these alternative specimen types, as they contain extremely low concentrations of drugs, drug metabolites, or toxins. FDA-cleared IVDs do not list these specimen types as acceptable, despite their demonstrated clinical utility. It is extremely difficult for IVD assay manufacturers to increase the number of FDA-cleared specimen types due to the wide variations in specimen type and quality, the significant resources needed, and the current regulatory environment. Toxicology LDTs are therefore needed to fill the gap.

1.4.2.4. Emergency Toxicology

To determine whether a drug overdose or toxin is the source of life-threatening symptoms, altered consciousness, or unusual behavior, toxicology testing may be performed in the emergency room. When a patient is poisoned, supportive care usually entails limiting absorption (e.g., charcoal) or increasing excretion (e.g., hemodialysis) pertaining to the material. Quick detection of a particular toxic syndrome (i.e., toxidrome) or toxic agent can be extremely helpful in situations where a particular treatment or counteragent is available, like in the case of an opioid overdose with naloxone or a digoxin overdose with antibody fragments specific to digoxin. Drug testing can also be used to verify the history of drug use provided by the patient, track the efficacy of treatment, and find any possible drug interactions with anesthesia or other medications the patient is prescribed. Because immunoassay tests yield results quickly, it is the most widely used testing methodology for patient management. However, the quantity of compounds that a typical immunoassay workup can identify is limited. The availability of test kits for immunoassay-based LDTs may still lag behind the trend of drug abuse, but they can be useful in extending a standard drug testing workup to include emerging drugs of abuse. The creation and distribution of fentanyl immunoassay kits that are not FDA-cleared is an illustration of how LDTs can function as a temporary solution while FDA clearance is being sought. Because they provide a more thorough assessment for compounds of interest—such as natural toxins, pesticides, novel psychoactive substances, and emerging drugs of abuse—that would otherwise go unnoticed by traditional IVD immunoassay screening methods and for which immunoassays are unlikely to ever be available, MS-based LDTs, both targeted and untargeted, have also shown promise in this context. Even with their potential, it is still difficult to provide STAT MS-based test results for use in the early treatment of poisoning or overdose cases. Potential solutions to this problem include opportunities to enhance testing workflows and lower costs, such as automating mass spectrometers or using off-site expert data review. These developments may also open the door to the wider application of MS-based testing in emergency toxicology.

The data produced can still improve patient care, but the majority of MS-based toxicology testing services are currently unable to provide the turnaround time required for initial patient management in the emergency room. Intensive care unit admission is common for patients with complex emergency medicine cases, such as severe or unexplained toxicity, in order to provide ongoing care. Having access to the results of their MS drug test in a timely manner while they are in the hospital could aid in the detection of unknown drugs or change how the patient is treated. Furthermore, since pediatric toxic exposure cases usually involve household toxins or prescription medications that cannot be detected by an IVD solution, MS-based testing is almost exclusively used in their management. MS toxicology LDTs can also improve public health by acting as an effective instrument for toxicovigilance, or community surveillance.

1.4.3. The Evolving Landscape of LDTs in Clinical Toxicology

Theoretically, a large number of LDTs could be sold as IVD assays for profit. Nonetheless, a number of difficulties have made the use of LDTs in clinical toxicology inevitable. These include the introduction of new illicit and prescription drug types, the regular fluctuations in the availability of drugs for recreational use, and the changes in the patterns of pharmaceutical prescriptions. Because the toxicology landscape is dynamic, readily customizable panels are necessary to take into account regional variations in drug abuse trends and prescribing practices. Because assay design, development, and FDA clearance take a long time, IVD manufacturers are unlikely to provide highly customized panels. Furthermore, compared to LDTs, commercial IVDs are comparatively static and frequently lag rapidly changing drug usage patterns. However, the IVD industry has made significant progress in the last ten years to close the gaps in clinical care that necessitate the use of toxicology LDTs.

While MS LDTs are commonly utilized in clinical toxicology labs, the complexity and necessary resources for development, implementation, and management can be challenging for many healthcare facilities. To make MS testing more accessible, IVD manufacturers have made advancements in automation to simplify sample preparation, increase testing volume, and streamline data analysis, which will alleviate the burden on clinical labs conducting these LDTs. The FDA approval of the first fully automated MS-based analyzer in 2018 showcased these advancements, with other manufacturers expected to follow suit. Furthermore, nearly all major MS manufacturers now offer IVD versions of their analyzers and software, a market shift from previously only offering Research Use Only (RUO) versions not intended for clinical diagnostic use but still commonly used for LDTs.

Over the past ten years, the development of commercial testing kits for various methodologies has advanced clinical toxicology testing and changed the LDT environment. Employing a building block system approach, these kit-based testing solutions frequently provide reagents, calibrators, quality controls, and testing parameters. To make these test kits available in a more clinically relevant timeframe, the rate at which they are being designed, developed, and marketed is accelerating. Many of the kits are non-FDA-cleared and designed to help clinical labs expedite the LDT validation process and enable quick responses to changing drug targets. Some are eventually filed by the manufacturer for FDA clearance, while others continue to be LDTs. Clinical laboratories now have more support than ever, thanks to the prompt production of these kits, vendor application notes for instrument-specific protocols, and sizable drug/toxin libraries. These developments represent encouraging strides in closing the diagnostic testing gap that exists globally between patient requirements and the IVD toxicology tests that are currently accessible. Increasing the number of FDA-cleared tests that better meet clinical needs and making the implementation of high-quality LDTs more manageable for all clinical laboratories, regardless of size or type, will both help to raise the bar for patient care in this area. Although the field of LDTs is still developing, they are still a vital instrument in the clinical laboratory toolbox and a major force behind diagnostic innovation.

A Closer Look

Toxicological Testing and Biomarkers

Toxicological testing and biomarkers play a crucial role in clinical toxicology, offering essential tools for the detection, diagnosis, and monitoring of exposure to toxic substances. Toxicological testing involves a variety of laboratory methods used to identify and quantify toxic substances in biological specimens such as blood, urine, hair, and tissues. These tests can detect a wide range of toxins, including drugs, industrial chemicals, environmental pollutants, and natural toxins. The primary goal of toxicological testing is to provide accurate and timely information that can guide clinical decision-making and treatment strategies in cases of suspected poisoning or overdose.

One of the fundamental aspects of toxicological testing is its ability to provide specific and sensitive detection of toxins. This is achieved through techniques such as gas chromatography-mass spectrometry (GC-MS), high-performance liquid chromatography (HPLC), and immunoassays, among others. These methods allow for the precise identification and quantification of substances at very low concentrations, which is critical for diagnosing acute poisoning and monitoring chronic exposure. For instance, GC-MS is renowned for its high specificity and is often used to confirm the presence of drugs and their metabolites in biological samples.

In addition to detecting toxic substances, toxicological testing also employs biomarkers to assess the biological impact of exposure. Biomarkers are measurable indicators of biological processes, pathogenic processes, or pharmacological responses to a toxic substance. They can be broadly classified into biomarkers of exposure, effect, and susceptibility. Biomarkers of exposure provide direct evidence of the presence of a toxin or its metabolites in the body. For example, blood lead levels are a biomarker of exposure to lead. Biomarkers of effect, on the other hand, indicate a biological response to exposure, such as enzyme levels that reflect liver damage from hepatotoxic substances. Biomarkers of susceptibility help identify individuals at greater risk of adverse effects due to genetic or environmental factors.

The integration of biomarkers into toxicological testing enhances the ability to evaluate the presence of toxins and their physiological and pathological impacts. This holistic approach is particularly important in managing chronic exposures and understanding the long-term health consequences of toxic substances. For instance, monitoring biomarkers such as hemoglobin adducts in individuals exposed to carcinogenic chemicals can provide early warning signs of potential cancer development.

Furthermore, advancements in biomarker research are paving the way for personalized medicine in toxicology. By identifying genetic polymorphisms that affect individual responses to toxins, clinicians can tailor interventions and preventive measures to better protect susceptible populations. This personalized approach is especially relevant in pharmacogenomics, where understanding how genetic variations influence drug metabolism can help prevent adverse drug reactions and optimize therapeutic outcomes.

Summary

- Clinical toxicology is a subspecialty of toxicology dealing with the bedside management of poisoned patients, including definitive toxicological diagnosis, assessment of immediate severity and long-term prognosis, and selection of treatments including antidotes.
- Clinical toxicology involves the research, prevention, and treatment of diseases caused by chemicals, drugs and toxins. Special attention is paid to levels of chemical exposure and to the effects that exposure can have on people.
- Chemical compounds are all around us, from drugs to pollutants, and depending on the compound and the amount or dosage, they have different effects.
- Clinical toxicologists may develop new methods of determining the harmful effects of chemicals and drugs, as well as what dosage causes these effects. Clinical toxicologists also work on studies of specific chemicals and how they can be used safely.
- Chemical exposure lasting longer than 24 h is referred to as acute exposure. a few examples of exposure pathways IP, IV, and subcutaneous injections, oral intubation, and topical application are.
- Drug-drug interactions in the bloodstream are also possible. Because of their high plasma protein binding, anticoagulant rodenticides such as bromadiolone, warfarin or brodifacoum have relatively extended plasma half-lives.
- The establishment of poison control centers was accompanied by the development of poison prevention programs and educational campaigns aimed at raising awareness of common poisons, promoting safe storage, and handling practices, and providing information on poison first aid and emergency response.
- Analytical techniques and instrumentation have played a crucial role in advancing the field of toxicology by enabling the detection, identification, and quantification of toxic substances in various matrices, including biological samples, environmental samples, and forensic specimens.
- Toxicology has grown into a sophisticated discipline, including the study of all types of harmful health consequences that any drug may create. The definitions below are offered to assist the reader in understanding various fundamental concepts.

References

1. Brent, J. (2018). *Pediatric Critical Care Toxicology* (2nd ed.). Springer.
2. Brent, J., & Wallace, K. L. (2018). *Critical Care Toxicology: Diagnosis and Management of The Critically Poisoned Patient* (3rd ed.). Springer.
3. Dart, R. C., & Burkhart, K. K. (2020). *Medical Toxicology* (4th ed.). Lippincott Williams & Wilkins.
4. Flomenbaum, N. E., Goldfrank, L. R., & Hoffman, R. S. (2010). *Principles of Ambulatory Medicine* (7th ed.). Lippincott Williams & Wilkins.

5. Ford, M. D., Delaney, K. A., Ling, L. J., Erickson, T., & Van Der Linden, T. (2018). *Clinical Toxicology* (2nd ed.). Saunders.

6. Forshaw, P. (2015). "Morbo spirituali medicina spiritualis convenit: Paracelsus, madness, and spirits". In S. Schneider (Ed.), *Aisthetics of the Spirits: Spirits in Early Modern Science, Religion, Literature and Music* (pp. 1–20). V&R Press.

7. Goldfrank, L. R., Flomenbaum, N. E., Lewin, N. A., Nelson, L. S., & Hoffman, R. S. (2019). *Goldfrank's Toxicologic Emergencies* (11th ed.). McGraw-Hill Education.

8. Hoffman, R. S., Howland, M. A., Lewin, N. A., Nelson, L. S., & Goldfrank, L. R. (2021). *Goldfrank's Manual of Toxicologic Emergencies* (10th ed.). McGraw-Hill Education.

9. Nelson, L. S., Howland, M. A., & Lewin, N. A. (Eds.). (2020). *Goldfrank's Toxicologic Emergencies* (11th ed.). McGraw-Hill Education.

10. Olson, K. R., & Olson, G. R. (2013). *Poisoning & Drug Overdose* (7th ed.). McGraw-Hill Education.

11. Olson, K. R., Anderson, I. B., Benowitz, N. L., Blanc, P. D., Kearney, T. E., Kim-Katz, S. Y., & Wu, A. H. B. (2018). *Poisoning & Drug Overdose* (8th ed.). McGraw-Hill Education.

Chapter 2

FACTORS AFFECTING TOXICOLOGY

Contents

Introduction

The study of toxicology, which examines the harmful effects of physical, chemical, or biological agents on living things, is impacted by a number of variables that determine the type and degree of toxicity. These variables include traits of the exposed organism, attributes of the toxicant, and environmental circumstances, among many others. Comprehending these variables is essential for efficiently evaluating and reducing toxicological hazards. The toxicity of a toxicant is largely determined by its chemical characteristics. The absorption, distribution, metabolism, and excretion (ADME) of a substance within the body is influenced by various factors, including its chemical structure, concentration, solubility, and reactivity. This process is known as toxicokinetics. For example, substances highly soluble in lipids have a tendency to accumulate in adipose tissues, resulting in prolonged exposure and possible negative consequences. Analogously, substances that undergo metabolism to produce reactive intermediates have the potential to cause harm by attaching themselves to macromolecules in cells and interfering with regular physiological functions. Moreover, the exposure route has a significant effect on a substance's toxicity. Toxins can enter the body through a variety of methods, including ingestion, injection, dermal contact, and inhalation. Each has a different absorption kinetics and target organs. For example, inhalation exposure gives toxicants direct access to the bloodstream and respiratory system, while dermal exposure mainly affects the skin and surrounding tissues. Toxicology is also influenced by exposure frequency and duration; acute exposure usually has immediate effects, but chronic exposure can cause cumulative harm over time.

Moreover, an organism's susceptibility to toxicants is influenced by individual factors such as age, sex, genetics, and underlying medical conditions. For example, due to variations in metabolic capacity, organ function, and behavioral patterns, children and the elderly may be more susceptible to toxic effects. Interindividual variability in toxicity responses can result from genetic polymorphisms in drug-metabolizing enzymes and transporters, which can impact an individual's capacity to detoxify and eliminate xenobiotics. Furthermore, the body's ability to metabolize and excrete toxicants may be compromised by pre-existing medical conditions like liver or kidney disease, which increases the likelihood of unfavorable outcomes. Toxicological responses are also significantly influenced by environmental factors. The distribution and bioavailability of airborne contaminants are influenced by temperature, humidity, altitude, and air flow, which in turn affects the degree of exposure and ensuing toxicity. The fate and behavior of chemicals in soil and water ecosystems can also be influenced by variables like pH, organic matter content, and redox potential, which can ultimately affect the chemicals' capacity for bioaccumulation and ecological harm.

Orientation and Directional Terms:

Term	Definition	Illustration
Molecular modeling	Molecular modeling is an efficient way of studying protein–protein interactions. It provides detailed information about how protein residues interact with each other at the atomic level.	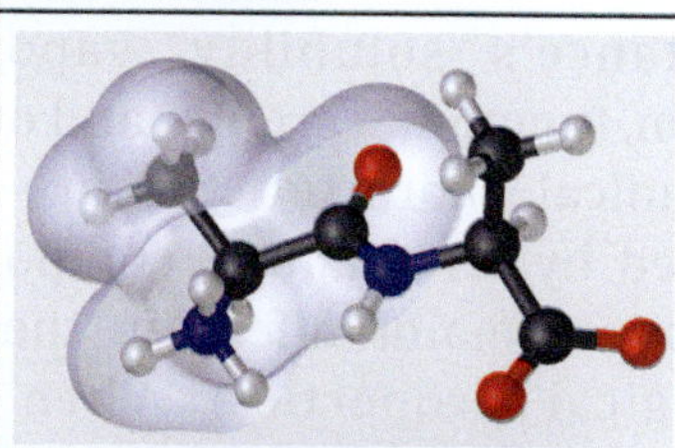
Computational chemistry	Computational chemistry is a type of chemistry that uses computer science to help solve chemical problems.	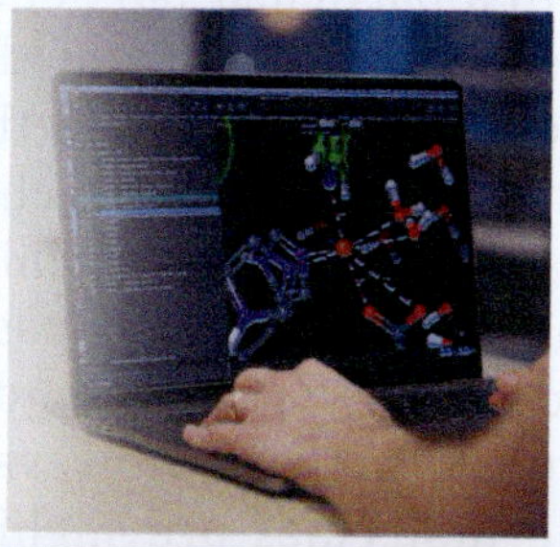
Immune system	The immune system is a complex network of organs, cells and proteins that defends the body against infection, whilst protecting the body's own cells.	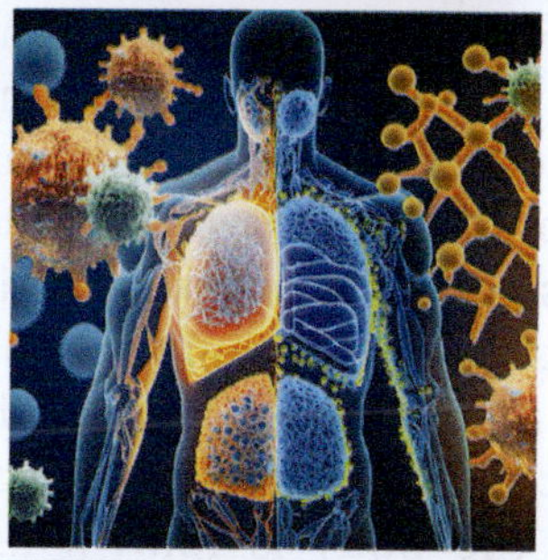
Barbiturates	Barbiturates are a category of sedative-hypnotic medications used for treating seizure disorders, neonatal withdrawal, insomnia, preoperative anxiety, and the induction of coma to address increased intracranial pressure (ICP).	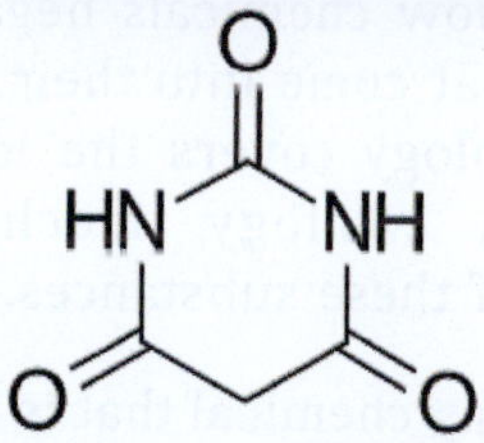
Synthetic drug	Synthetic drugs refer to substances that are artificially modified from naturally-occurring drugs and are capable of exhibiting both therapeutic and psychoactive effects.	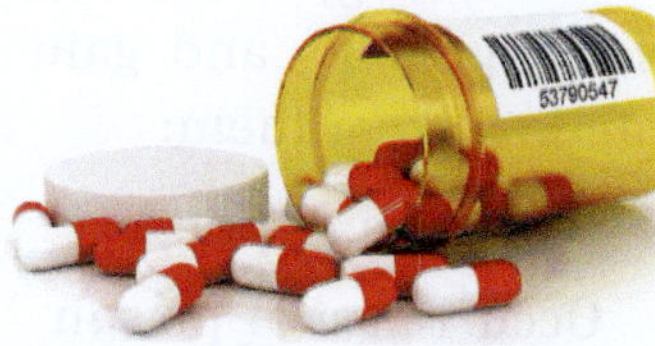

2.1. Chemical Composition in Toxicology

A substance's solubility, vapor pressure, ionization, functional groups, and other physical and chemical characteristics are significantly influenced by its chemical composition. All of these have a major effect on the substance's toxicological properties. When a chemical interacts with a particular part of an organism, toxic reactions take place, and the nature of these reactions is determined by the functional groups of the molecule. It is challenging to dissolve polar or hydrophilic chemicals in lipids. They thus have trouble getting past membrane barriers and getting to the intended locations for the required activity. However, non-polar or lipophilic molecules are highly soluble in organic solvents like lipids, whereas polar chemicals are insoluble in them. They can quickly take effect because they can easily pass through lipoprotein barriers in membranes. A substance's potential for toxicity is influenced by its ionic characteristics, lipid solubility, chemical structure, and type of functional group. The study of chemical characteristics and their effects on the body is known as toxicology. It focuses on how chemicals negatively affect living things that come into their contact. The study of toxicology covers the identification, manifestation, etiology, mechanism, and management of these substances.

Poison is any chemical that is toxic and can cause serious harm to the body. Toxicologists conduct toxicology research and aim to study these poisons and gain the following understanding from them:

- Detection of poison
- Occurrence of poison
- The properties of poison
- The effects of poison
- Treatment options for the poison
- Regulation for the poison

The aim is to protect both the environment and people from toxins and their harmful effects. As the toxic potential to the human body is reduced, research and toxicology testing for different toxic elements will eventually result in a better and more creative set of therapies for treating illnesses.

2.1.1. Chemical Dose or Concentration

A chemical can have negative effects when it binds to the appropriate receptors. The local chemical concentration at the site of action is typically directly proportional to the dose or concentration of the chemical exposed, and effects are proportionate to both. Chemicals that are diluted have less of an effect than those that are diluted more, which may have more obvious effects. Consequently, the correlation between the toxicity of a chemical and its concentration or dose. It was once said by Paracelsus, the father of modern toxicology, that "only the dose is the poison.". The substance's dose plays a crucial role in toxicology since it significantly influences the effects that a person experiences. Because it indicates the amount of the chemical to which the affected individual has been exposed, the dose serves as the main tool for categorizing a chemical's toxicity. All substances combined have the potential to be harmful if used in specific ways and at specific dosages. In toxicology, the term "LD50" is frequently used to describe the dose of a material that exhibits toxicity in that it results in the death of 50% of the test population. Rats or other surrogates are typically used in scientific research to assess toxicity, and human users are then given access to the data. It has long been acknowledged that there is a dose-toxicity relationship, meaning that higher exposure to a chemical can increase the risk of toxicity. It may not be a simple relationship, though, as an endocrine disruptor study has called into question this theory.

2.1.2. Toxicant Translocation

There are two types of toxicants: ones that are systemic in nature, and ones that are local in nature. Effective translocation is essential for the latter. Only when the toxicants are easily delivered to the intended locations can they do damage. Storage depots are specific, relatively dormant tissues that are retained after certain toxicants interact with particular macromolecules in the organisms' bodies during translocation. Effective translocation of toxicants in active forms to the target increases their toxicity, whereas ineffective translocation and storage of toxicants in inactive forms decreases their toxicity. After exposure, toxic substances may relocate within an organism or between various bodily compartments. This phenomenon is known as toxicant translocation. The distribution, metabolism, and excretion of toxicants are all influenced by this process, which in turn affects the toxic effects and bioavailability of the substances. Toxicants can experience multiple mechanisms of translocation within the body after being absorbed through different routes like injection, ingestion, inhalation, or skin contact. Via the bloodstream, toxicants can be transported to distant tissues and organs, which is one frequent route of translocation. Volatile substances, for example, that are inhaled and enter the bloodstream through the lungs can quickly travel to target organs like the brain, liver, or kidneys, where they are toxic.

Additionally, translocation can happen via the lymphatic system, especially for bigger molecules or particles that cannot go straight into the bloodstream. These chemicals are transported by lymphatic vessels to local lymph nodes and then into the bloodstream, enabling systemic distribution. This method is especially important for drugs that are absorbed via the skin or digestive system. Toxicants may go through biotransformation once they are inside the body; this happens most frequently in the liver and other tissues that are involved in metabolism. Toxins undergo a process called biotransformation, which transforms them into metabolites that are more easily absorbed by the body and soluble in water. Although detoxification may be aided by this process, reactive intermediates that may be more hazardous than the parent compound may also form. Toxins can migrate not only throughout the body but also within particular tissues and compartments. For example, lipophilic compounds can build up in adipose tissues, where they can remain for long stretches of time and cause chronic exposure and possible negative effects. Like this, some toxicants have a preference for particular target organs or cellular structures; examples of this include heavy metal buildup in bone and neurotoxins that target the nervous system. The physicochemical characteristics of the toxicant, the route and length of exposure, the metabolic capacity of an organism, and the existence of barriers like the placental or blood-brain barriers all have an impact on the extent and pattern of toxicant translocation. Furthermore, the susceptibility to toxicant translocation and subsequent toxicity can vary among individuals due to factors like age, sex, genetics, and underlying health conditions.

2.1.3. Toxicants Biotransformation

Certain substances are inherently inert. During translocation, these compounds undergo biocatalytic transformation into active form with the help of particular enzymes. That particular chemical consequently becomes more lethal. For example, the potency of AChE antagonists such as organophosphorodithioates and organophosphorodithionates, which both have a P=S group, is only moderate. Thus, inside the bodies of organisms, they are first converted into their highly toxic AChE inhibitors, the potent P=O forms. Thus, the compound's toxicity is increased by xenobiotic biotransformation, which leads to their stimulation. On the other hand, translocation can also entail the transformation of xenobiotics from active to inactive states, which are then frequently stored in nontarget or relatively dormant tissues. The excretion of xenobiotics may be enhanced by biotransformation that turns a substance from a lipophilic to a hydrophilic state. The toxicant is, therefore, unable to harm people at the intended locations. This latter type of biotransformation lessens the toxicity of xenobiotics.

2.1.4. How Can Toxic Substances Harm the Body?

Damage from a toxic substance is referred to as a local effect when it occurs at the site of initial contact with the body. The skin, eyes, nose, throat, and lungs are the most frequent sites where substances come into contact with the body. Moreover, toxic substances have the ability to enter the body and reach internal organs through the bloodstream. Systemic effects are those that arise in this manner. The liver, kidneys, heart, nervous system (including the brain), and reproductive system are the internal organs most frequently impacted. A hazardous substance has the potential to have both systemic and localized effects. For instance, the lining of the respiratory tract (speech, throat, and lungs) becomes quickly irritated if ammonia gas is inhaled. Very little ammonia enters the bloodstream from the lungs. Ammonia is considered to have a local effect since harm is only done at the site of first contact. One material that has local effects on the skin is epoxy resin. However, liquid phenol causes localized skin irritation upon contact and can also be absorbed through the skin, potentially causing systemic effects such as kidney and liver damage. Sometimes, as in the case of phenols, a chemical's localized effects serve as an early warning sign of impending exposure. Then, you receive a warning that the chemical might be entering your body and having systemic effects that are not yet apparent to you. However, some chemicals are extremely dangerous because they give no warning at all. Glycol ethers, or Clozole solvents, for instance, can penetrate the skin and seriously harm internal organs without having any noticeable effects on the skin.

2.1.4.1. Do all Toxic Chemicals Cause Cancer?

Negative. Certain chemicals can lead to cancer, which is the unchecked growth and spread of aberrant cells within the body. Not everything, when consumed in high enough concentrations, causes cancer. Really, regardless of dosage, the majority of substances do not cause cancer. Of the many thousands of chemicals used in modern life, cancer is caused by a comparatively small percentage. Carcinogenicity refers to a chemical's capacity to cause cancer, and carcinogens are substances that can do so. Studies on either humans or animals provide evidence of carcinogenicity. Roughly thirty chemicals have been found to be carcinogenic to humans due to sufficient evidence. Many chemicals, perhaps 200 in number, are probably carcinogens to humans because they have been shown to cause cancer in laboratory animals. The etiology of human cancer is a challenging question. The onset of a carcinogen and the onset of cancer typically occur after a lengthy latency period of 10 to 40 years. So, before enough people are exposed to a substance for an extended period and researchers are able to detect a pattern of increased cancer cases, the substance must be used for many years. Determining whether a rise in cancer cases among people is caused by a specific substance exposure can be challenging as individuals are exposed to numerous substances and exposure to one substance may have happened years ago.

Chemicals are tested for carcinogenicity using laboratory animals because studying cancer in humans is challenging and necessitates exposure to chemicals that may cause cancer. It would take many hundreds of animals to get cancer if animals were exposed to the low levels typical of most human exposure. In order to detect an increase in cancer in a reasonable number of animals, say 25–50, animal cancer tests employ high doses of chemicals to avoid this expense. Animal testing is still costly, takes three years to complete, and frequently yields inconclusive results. If an animal cancer test is positive, it is necessary to try and predict the risk to humans at much lower doses based on the risk to a small number of rats at high doses. If the degree of risk is unknown, chemicals that cause cancer in animals are thought to have a high probability of doing the same in humans. The question of whether a carcinogen has a safe dosage generates debate. Some scientists think that there is some risk associated with any exposure, regardless of how little. On the other hand, the risk—if any—may be so minimal at extremely low exposures that it is equivalent to having no risk at all. The majority of carcinogens seem to need years of exposure or extremely high doses before the risk of cancer from exposure to them becomes a significant worry.

2.1.4.2. Do all Toxic Chemicals Cause Mutations?

Genetic harm can also result from toxic chemicals. Genes are found in chromosomes and make up a the genetic material. The instructions a cell needs to function and proliferate (create new cells) are encoded in its genes and chromosomes. Genes and chromosomes can be altered or damaged by certain substances. Mutations are defined as this type of alteration or damage to a cell. A mutation-causing agent is referred to as a mutagen. The way a cell behaves or divides may be impacted by a mutation. Additionally, the mutations may be transferred to newly formed cells from the damaged ones. This may result in cell populations that are unable to replicate or function in the same ways as the parent cell did prior to the mutation. Certain types of mutation lead to cancer. Mutations are also caused by most chemicals that cause cancer. Not every chemical that results in mutations causes cancer. Assessing a chemical's capacity to induce a mutation is a quick and relatively simple process. Further assessment is warranted if examination reveals a chemical to be mutable.

2.1.4.3. Can Future Generations be Affected?

Chemical exposure may have an impact on the ability to conceive. The incapacity to conceive (infertility or sterility), decreased sex drive, irregular menstruation, spontaneous miscarriages, stillbirths, and birth defects are examples of toxic reproductive effects. Teratogens are substances that directly harm the tissue of the developing fetus while it is inside the mother's womb, resulting in malformations or birth defects. Fetotoxins are additional substances that are harmful to fetuses. The fetus may be harmed if a chemical affects the pregnant woman and her health. A few chemicals have the ability to harm the male reproductive system, leading to aberrant sperm or infertility. The majority of chemicals' toxicity to reproduction is not well understood. Animal tests for the effects of most chemicals on reproduction have not been conducted. Using information from animals to forecast risk in humans is challenging. It is possible that there are safe thresholds for chemical exposure that impact the reproductive system. Finding a safe level, however, is extremely challenging, if not impossible. Researching the effects on human reproduction is even more challenging than researching cancer. As of right now, only a small number of industrial chemicals have been linked to human reproductive problems or birth defects.

2.1.5. Clinical Forms of Toxic Materials

It is possible for toxic materials to exist as liquids, solids, gases, vapors, dusts, fumes, fibers, or mists. The form or physical characteristics of a substance determine how it enters the body and what kind of harm it can do. Different conditions can give rise to different forms of toxic materials, and each of these forms may carry a unique set of hazards. For instance, solid lead solder poses no risk since it is unlikely to enter the body. However, soldering transforms the lead into a liquid that could spill or come into touch with the skin. The spilled liquid may resolidify into dust, which is small particles that can be swallowed or inhaled and absorbed. Lead can produce a fume when heated to extremely high temperatures, such as when it is welded. The fume is made up of minuscule particles that are highly dangerous to breathe in or absorb. Thus, it is critical to understand the form (or forms) that a particular substance takes in the workplace. Below is a breakdown of every form.

- **Solid.** A solid is a material that retains its form, like stone. Most solids are generally not hazardous since they are not likely to be absorbed into the body, unless present as small particles such as dust.
- **Liquid.** Anything that flows freely is called a liquid, such as water. At room temperature, a lot of dangerous substances are liquid. Certain liquids can harm the epidermis. Certain substances may or may not cause skin damage as they pass through the skin and enter the body. Additionally, liquids can evaporate (give off vapors) and form inhaled gases.
- **Gas.** A gas is made up of separate chemical molecules, such as oxygen, that are dispersed throughout air at standard pressure and temperature. Certain gases are poisonous, combustible, or explosive. If a gas is present but does not immediately cause irritation and has no color or odor, it may be difficult to detect. Certain gases, such as carbon monoxide, can still be extremely dangerous.
- **Vapor.** When a substance is mostly a liquid at room temperature and pressure, it takes the form of a vapor. Vapors are produced when most organic solvents evaporate. Vapors have the potential to irritate the eyes, skin, or respiratory system in addition to being inhaled into the lungs. Some are poisonous, combustible, or explosive. The tendency of various liquids to evaporate is denoted by the terms vapor pressure or evaporation rate.
- **Dust.** Tiny solid particles in the atmosphere make up dust. Dust can be produced by grinding or pulverizing solids, as well as by powder (settled dust) going airborne. Due to their potential for respiratory tract inhalation, dusts may be dangerous. Respirable dust can enter the lungs and cause damage, but larger dust particles are typically trapped in the nose and windpipe (trachea), where they can be expelled. Some may then pass through the lungs and enter the bloodstream, such as lead dust. When they get to high concentrations in the air, some organic dusts, like grain dust, can blow up.
- **Fume.** When solid chemicals—often metals—are heated to extremely high temperatures, they evaporate into vapor, then eventually solidify again, creating fumes, which are made up of minuscule, fine solid particles in the atmosphere. Metal

fumes are produced when metal is brazed or welded, for example. Due to their ease of inhalation, fumes are dangerous. Numerous metal fumes can result in metal fume fever, a condition that includes fever, chills, and flu-like aches. Lead fumes, for example, can cause poisoning when inhaled but do not result in metal fume fever.

- **Fiber.** A solid particle that is at least three times longer than it is wide is called a fiber. The size of the fiber determines the level of danger. Smaller fibers, like asbestos, have the potential to seriously damage the lungs. Bigger fibers get stuck in the respiratory system and are released before they can enter the lungs.
- **Mist.** Liquids are agitated or sprayed to create mists, which are made up of liquid particles of different sizes. When mists are sprayed on the skin or breathed in, they can be dangerous. Two common uses for mists are the application of pesticides and the machining of metal with metal working fluids.

2.2. Factors Related to Exposure

Toxicological testing and research aim to determine the harmful effects of various toxicants. The routes of exposure and the dose—that is, the concentration of exposure—are the two primary determinants of the negative effects.

The factors that affect chemical toxicity are as follows:

- Dosage: acute exposure (large single exposures) and chronic exposure (small and continuous exposures)
- Route of Exposure: ingestion, skin absorption or inhalation
- Species
- Age
- Sex
- Health
- Environment
- Individual characteristics

2.2.1. Means of Exposure

The toxin enters the organism's body through intraperitoneal (IP), intramuscular, subcutaneous, and oral interactions in addition to IV, IP, and subcutaneous injections. The routes of exposure have a major impact on a chemical's toxicity. Because a chemical is injected intravenously, its active form is directly delivered to the desired location, resulting in larger and faster effects. The other routes of exposure are inhalation, IP, subcutaneous, intramuscular, oral, and topical, listed in decreasing order of toxicity. Longer exposure times to toxins result in a decrease in the LC50 or LD50 number. Compared to short-term exposure values, long-term exposure values are evaluated at substantially lower levels. It has been shown that exposure to a toxicant at the same dose or concentration for varying lengths of time can cause effects of varying grades. Long-term effects outweigh those of short-term exposures. This only demonstrates that the toxicity of a material increases with prolonged contact times. Normally, exposure happens by ingestion, skin or eye contact, and inhalation.

- **Inhalation.** Inhaling a chemical into your lungs is the most frequent way to be exposed. The lungs are made up of a network of branching airways called bronchi, which are terminated at each end by clusters of microscopic air sacs called alveoli. The bloodstream receives oxygen and other chemicals from the alveoli. Certain chemicals are allergens that can irritate the throat or nose. Inhaling them and allowing them to come into contact with the bronchi can also result in discomfort, coughing, or chest pain (chemical bronchitis). Certain chemicals can still be harmful even if they don't produce these warning signs when inhaled. There are instances when a chemical is in the air in the form of dust or mist. Depending on their size, some of these particles might end up in the alveoli or bronchi. While some of them might be coughed out, others might lodge in the lungs and harm the lungs. Certain particles have the potential to dissolve, enter the bloodstream, and exert their effects on different parts of the body.

- **Skin Contact.** The skin acts as a barrier to protect the body from outside substances. Certain substances, though, are readily absorbed through the skin and into the bloodstream. Chemicals can more readily pass through cut or cracked skin. Strong acids and alkalis are examples of caustic substances that can also chemically burn skin. Others may cause skin irritation. The oils in the skin are dissolved by many chemicals, especially organic solvents, leaving the skin dry, cracked, and vulnerable to infection and chemical absorption.
- **Eye Contact.** Certain chemicals can cause eye irritation or burns. On rare occasions, they might enter the bloodstream by passing through the eye. Chemicals can easily damage the eyes, so any contact with the eyes should be treated seriously.
- **Ingestion.** The least frequent way for workers to be exposed to chemicals is through ingestion. When chemicals inadvertently contaminate food, beverages, or cigarettes, or are left on hands, clothing, or the beard, they can be consumed. Dust-borne chemicals found in the workplace, such as metal dusts like cadmium or lead, are easily consumed.

2.2.2. Exposure Protocol

Toxicants may be exposed using a range of exposure methods. Toxicants are introduced to organisms in aquatic environments using a variety of exposure methods, such as:

- The static system, in which the toxicant is mixed with the water and the organisms are introduced to it in still water.
- A recirculatory device in which specific pumps are used to circulate the toxicant solution.
- A renewal mechanism, in which the toxicant substance is replaced every so often.
- Flow through system: the toxicant solution intermittently or constantly moves into and out of the test chamber.

These various exposure systems majorly impact how toxic the substances are to organisms. For the aquatic medium, the surrounding medium factors that impact chemical toxicity have been thoroughly investigated. The water's physicochemical properties, which have an impact on chemical toxicity, are medium-related factors.

2.2.3. Water Temperature

The temperature of the water is expected to have a major impact on xenobiotic toxicity. Rising water temperatures not only alter the chemical forms of some compounds and increase their solubility, but they also regulate the amount of dissolved oxygen in the water. Various researchers' studies show that the relationship between chemical toxicity to aquatic organisms and temperature is not constant. Depending on the substance, species, response, and technique employed, temperature changes can have a positive, negative, or no effect on a substance's toxicity. Aquatic organisms rely heavily on chronic chemical thresholds, which may be largely insensitive to fluctuations in water temperature. Certain pesticides have been reported to be more toxic at higher temperatures, and more lethal at lower temperatures.

When 22 chemicals' toxicity levels are compared to different temperatures in relation to cladocerans, it is found that lower temperatures have a more lethal effect. The findings were particularly helpful in the case of DDT toxicity. It was discovered that the toxicity of DDT tripled between 10 and 27º C. Similar findings for fish species, mollusks, and insect larvae have also been reported in relation to pesticides and various other chemicals.

2.2.4. Dissolved Oxygen

At 0°C, freshwater can absorb 14.6 mg/L of oxygen; at 20°C, this number gradually decreases to 9.1 mg/L, and at 30°C, it reaches 7.5 mg/L. Consequently, it follows that as temperature rises, the amount of dissolved oxygen in the water decreases. Essentially, breathing requires the presence of oxygen.

The content of the toxicant at the gill membrane and, consequently, the toxicity of the chemical can be changed by any physiological alteration that impacts the respiratory flow rate of aquatic organisms. Therefore, it makes sense that stressing aquatic life would increase the toxicity of any chemical present in the water by reducing the amount of dissolved oxygen in the water. As dissolved oxygen levels in waterfall, chemicals become more harmful to aquatic life. Nonetheless, most of the findings show that the toxicity of chemicals only differs by a factor of two or less when tests are conducted at high and low dissolved oxygen levels, suggesting that it is not a substantial moderating factor.

2.2.5. pH

When pH is low, chemicals that ionize are potentially more hazardous. Chemicals are usually more toxic to living things in their undissociated forms because they can easily cross cell membranes. For example, the majority of pesticides are lipophilic, meaning they can permeate cell membranes' lipoprotein bimolecular layer and cause toxicity there. They also don't dissociate easily. Therefore, pH does not seem to have a significant effect on the toxicity of these substances (Figure 2.1).

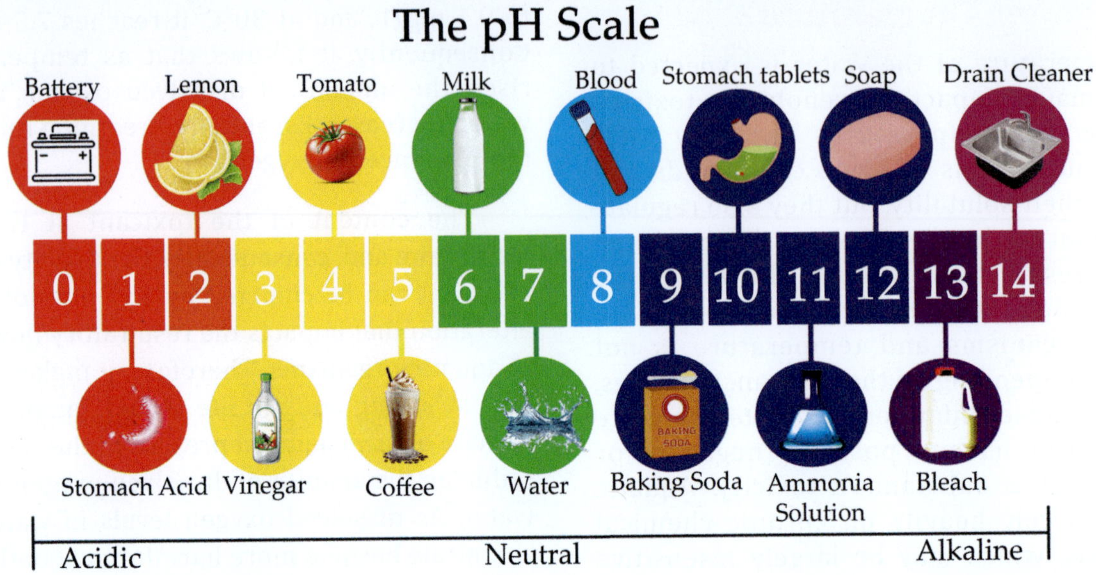

Figure 2.1. *Image of pH scale.*

Source: https://media.licdn.com/dms/image/C4D12AQFkjEuHr1A2QA/article-cover_image-shrink_600_2000/0/1579683606371?e=2147483647&v=beta&t=Rcp1Z3PnSaGvETcajFBLNkB5YMQ8IiUX7isxLcPtQ94.

Ammonia toxicity is known to be significantly influenced by the pH of the water. Consequently, the impact of pH on ammonia toxicity can be used as an example. Unionized ammonia (NH3), which is highly toxic to fish, has a toxic range of 0–7 mg/1) for salmonids, which is relatively low. In contrast, the toxicity of ionized ammonia (NH4+) is negligible or nonexistent. A substance's toxicity increases by a factor of six for each pH unit above the middle range, which is typically where ammonia (NH3) concentrations are found. Another example of how pH influences a chemical's toxicity is cyanide toxicity. The ionic cyanide (CN-) form is more prevalent at pH 8 than the molecular form (HCN), which is more prevalent at pH levels lower and higher, respectively. In its undissociated form, cyanide is twice as toxic as it is in its ionic form. Thus, changes in water pH may have a major effect on cyanide toxicity (Figure 2.2).

Most metal-containing compounds behave differently. The ionization of metals in the presence of pH variations greatly influences their toxicity. Ionic forms of metals are more toxic to living organisms than are their undissociated or molecular forms. Therefore, any kind of pH change can have an impact on the ionic proportion and, consequently, the toxicity of metallic compounds (Franklin et al., 2000).

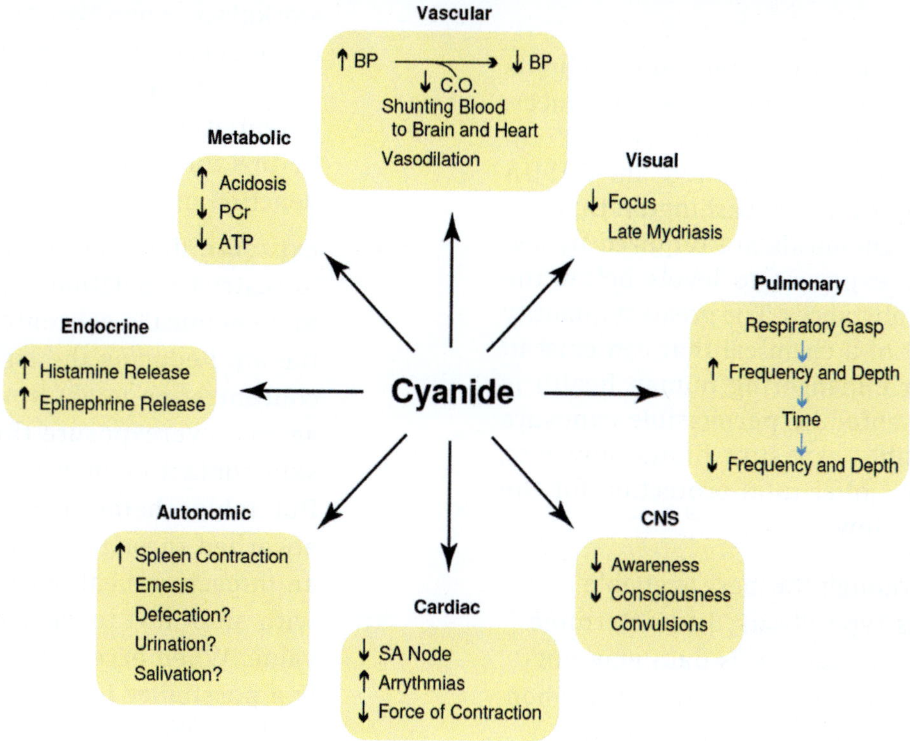

Figure 2.2. *Illustration of cyanide poison.*

Source: https://d3i71xaburhd42.cloudfront.net/c0f07a469429a0f40d587535966826974e4c5692/7-Figure10–2-1.png.

2.2.6. Salinity

The greatest chemical differences between freshwater and saltwater probably have a big effect on the toxicity of a substance. These differences, however, have no appreciable impact on how hazardous substances are. Freshwater and marine species are almost equally tolerant when subjected to stress in their native environments. Consequently, it seems that salt has minimal impact on xenobiotic toxicity. However, some species may be more affected by changes in the water's salinity. When salinity approaches their isosmotic threshold, which is approximately one-third of seawater (i.e., water with a salinity of between 30 and 40%), euryhaline organisms are typically more hardy. However, when the salinity of the water significantly drops, marine life usually becomes less tolerant. Therefore, it is reasonable to conclude that when the salinity of the surrounding medium noticeably decreases, the toxicity of xenobiotics may increase. Herbert and colleagues studied the effects of salinity on the toxicity of various chemical pollutants to rainbow trout and Atlantic salmon in 1964 and 1965. They came to the conclusion that their isosmotic concentration increased with increasing salinity (from pure water to water with a salinity of 30–40%), which in turn increased the toxicity of zinc and ammonium chloride. A similar relationship was found after naphthalene's toxicity to the euryhaline mummichog was investigated. Mummichog mortality rates are lower in low salinities than in high salinities, and this difference has been linked to osmoregulatory failure and naphthalene uptake.

2.2.7. Exposure Limits

Health and safety authorities set exposure limits to regulate exposure to dangerous substances. "Permissible Exposure Limits (PELs)" in Washington State are outlined in WISHA regulations. Employers in Washington that use these restricted chemicals are required by law to limit worker exposure to levels below the PELs for these substances. The greatest quantity (concentration) of a chemical that can exist in the air without endangering human health is typically represented by permissible exposure limits. Permissible exposure limits, however, might not always offer total protection for the reasons listed below.

- Even though the best available data is typically used to determine exposure limits, this data may not always be complete, especially when it comes to chronic (long-term) health effects. Frequently, workers are exposed to chemicals for many years before we learn about the long-term health effects. As new information becomes available, exposure limits are adjusted accordingly.
- The majority of workers are protected by exposure limits. Nonetheless, some employees might be impacted by a chemical at concentrations lower than these upper bounds (refer to Sensitivity). Workers putting in a lot of physical effort may inhale more air and chemicals, which could lead to an excessive amount of absorption.
- Chemical interactions are not taken into account when setting exposure limits. Industrial hygienists use a mathematical formula to modify the exposure limits for chemicals in the workplace when two or more of those substances have similar health effects. Chemicals with synergistic or potentiating effects are not covered by this formula; instead, refer to Reaction and Interaction.
- Exposure limits are typically set to restrict inhalation exposure to a chemical's concentration in the air. Reducing the airborne concentration might not shield against overexposure through skin contact or ingestion. In the PEL table, chemicals that could be absorbed through the skin and have an impact on health are designated with an S next to their numerical value. When excessive skin exposure is a possibility for workers exposed to these chemicals, protective clothing must be provided. Certain chemicals, such as dust-borne lead and cadmium, can enter the body through contact with hands, hair, clothing, food, and cigarettes.

2.2.8. How Can Exposure be Measured and Monitored?

The exposure to toxic chemicals at work can be quantified by measuring the amount of a particular chemical in the air and the length of time you were exposed to it. This measurement, known as air or environmental monitoring or sampling, is typically carried out with a variety of instruments by industrial hygienists. In order to precisely reflect the concentration you are inhaling, the air is drawn from your breathing zone, which is the area around your mouth and nose. The Permissible Exposure Limit (PEL) for that chemical can then be compared to the exposure levels determined by this monitoring. To ascertain your exposure to the majority of chemicals, environmental monitoring is the most reliable method. Air monitoring, however, may understate the quantity of chemicals you absorb if you absorb them through methods other than inhalation, such as through the skin or food. Blood, urine, or exhaled air can occasionally be used to measure the levels of these and some other chemicals, or the breakdown products of these chemicals, in the body. Biological monitoring is the term for this type of testing, and the outcomes may provide an estimate of the actual dose absorbed by the body. When results of air monitoring exceed a certain threshold, biological monitoring for one substance, lead, is mandated by law. For a select few chemicals, the American Conference of Governmental Industrial Hygienists (ACGIH) has recommended exposure limits for biological monitoring. These are published with TLVs and are referred to as Biological Exposure Indices (BEIs).

2.2.9. Practical Clues to Exposure

- **Odor.** Chemicals are inhaled when they are smelled. Finding an odor does not necessarily indicate that you are breathing in dangerous quantities of a chemical, though, as certain substances have odors that are detectable at much lower concentrations. However, even if a chemical is not detectable, it might still be there. Even at dangerous concentrations, certain chemicals are odorless. The odor threshold is the lowest concentration of a chemical that most people are able to detect. Good warning properties are attributed to a chemical if its odor threshold is less than the amount that is considered hazardous. Ammonia is one such. Most people detect it at 5 ppm, which is less than the 25 ppm PEL. It is crucial to bear in mind that individual differences exist in odor thresholds for the majority of chemicals. Furthermore, some chemicals, such as hydrogen sulfide, cause olfactory fatigue, which is the rapid loss of smell. Remembering these warnings, the odor threshold of a chemical can be used as a rough indicator of your exposure level. Odor is not a reliable indicator. Keep in mind that your sense of smell may be superior to or inferior to average, that certain chemicals—like carbon monoxide—have no smell at all, while other chemicals—like mercaptans added to natural gas—have strong smells but cause olfactory fatigue.
- **Taste.** If you inhale or ingest a chemical, it may leave a taste in your mouth. Some chemicals have a particular taste, which may be mentioned in an MSDS.
- **Particles in Nose or Throat and Settled Dust or Mist.** You have inhaled a chemical particle if you cough up mucus (sputum or phlegm) that contains particles or if you blow your nose and notice particles on your handkerchief. Sadly, most particles that enter the lungs through inhalation are too small to see.
- **Immediate Symptoms.** You may have been overexposed if you or your coworkers exhibit symptoms that are known to be brought on by a chemical during or soon after its use. Tears in the eyes, burning in the skin, nose, or throat, coughing, headaches, or dizziness are possible symptoms.

2.3. Factors Related to Organisms

Chemical toxicity is assessed in relation to a specific creature or a collection of organisms. Because of this, it is crucial to consider organism-related variables when studying the toxicity of xenobiotics. The following list of crucial organism-related influencing factors:

2.3.1. Test Species

Test organism variation greatly affects the toxicity of xenobiotics, just as varying groups of organisms have different chemical tolerances. Within the same group, different organisms have different levels of toxicity from one another based on their species. Due to differences in susceptibility brought on by particular genetic factors, chemical toxicity varies even among different members of the same species. This means that while some members of a species may be immune to a chemical, others may be vulnerable to it. Due to these variances, it is often advised that a chemical be tested on one plant (perhaps an algae), one or two invertebrates, and at least one vertebrate to obtain a clear picture of its toxicity. This means that a chemical can be tested in an aquatic environment against a range of algae, a fish, and an aquatic insect or crustacean. In general, toxins tend to affect invertebrates more than they do mammals. Fish species may differ in how sensitive they are to a given substance. Salmonids and minnows are approximately 15 times more susceptible to copper toxicity than sunfish. There are significant species-to-species differences in the toxicity of pesticides containing organophosphorus (OP). Between sensitive (bluegills and guppies) and tolerant species, there were differences in pesticide susceptibility ranging from 6 to 900 fold. Fish with fat heads and goldfish.

2.3.2. Sex

Men and women react to substances differently due to differences in hormones and metabolism, which causes differences in chemical toxicity. It's not always the case, but in certain species, males biotransform chemicals more quickly than females do. Toxic effects of aldrin, an organochlorine pesticide, for instance, affect male rats much more than female rats. The more lethal epoxide form of dieldrin is produced by the male rats' biocatalytic conversion of aldrin. On the other hand, the female rat bioconverts parathion more quickly than the male, and the resultant poisonous substance is called paraoxon. Rats are therefore more susceptible to parathion in their female than in their male form. There are distinct excretion pathways in addition to sex-specific metabolic differences, which could influence vulnerability. Glycuronide conjugate excretion through the kidneys is preferred by females, whereas biliary elimination is generally preferred by men. For example, tumors caused by dinitrotoluene are more common in men due to different excretion routes. Another example of how vulnerability varies based on hormonal and metabolic factors is the kidney damage that rodents experience from exposure to chloroform. Given that testosterone, a hormone linked to sex, is assumed to affect the way microsomal enzymes biotransform chloroform, male rodents are more susceptible to the negative effects of chloroform.

2.3.3. Age

Most often, young mammals are more susceptible to the effects of xenobiotics. The vulnerability of young people to most chemicals is between 1.5 and 10 times greater than that of adults. Due to a lack of resilience and deficiencies in their biotransformation enzyme systems, young children may be particularly vulnerable. The enzyme systems required to catalyze biotransformation processes are absent in newborns, as was previously mentioned. After reaching a peak, these enzyme systems grow steadily before beginning to decline. In response to biotransformation reactions involving the detoxication of xenobiotics, organism susceptibility may change simultaneously. Not every drug, though, is more dangerous for kids than another. Children are less likely to be harmed by one class of CNS stimulants: DDT.

2.3.4. Life-Stage

Toxin levels in chemicals vary as they go through their life cycles. Early or immature life stages are typically more susceptible to the negative effects of toxicants than are adult or late life stages. The fry and fingerling stages of fish development are the most delicate. Omkar also reported that juvenile freshwater prawns were found to be more susceptible to pesticide exposure than adult specimens (1980–81, private data). For some organisms or groups of organisms, exposure to toxins during a specific stage of their life cycle can have a substantial effect on the creatures' fate. Molting is a particularly vulnerable time for aquatic arthropods. prawns that had been exposed to pesticides molting; these molted prawns eventually died, but other prawns from the same batch survived the tests.

2.3.5. Size

The toxicity of chemicals is also influenced by the size of the organisms. It has been noted that larger individuals are typically more toxicant resistant, and this is also the case for certain fish species. As rainbow trout get bigger, they eventually develop a greater tolerance to copper, according to Hearth and Sprague (1978). On the other hand, they concluded that a fish's lethal tolerance to copper may or may not depend on its size after researching the toxicity of copper to fish. Compared to larger species, smaller species are more susceptible to pesticides. Using a freshwater shrimp as a test subject, it was discovered that smaller members of the same species were more susceptible to some pesticides than larger members.

2.3.6. Health and Nutrition

The toxicity of substances to organisms is influenced by their nutritional and health status. Healthy individuals are typically more resistant to toxins than sick ones. It has been observed that sick and parasitized individuals are more susceptible than healthy individuals to some toxins. For example, it has been observed that sick fish are more susceptible to the organophosphate insecticide guthion and sodium chloride. Chemical toxicity is influenced by the organisms' dietary needs as well. It has been demonstrated that wild populations of marine copepods are more resistant to copper when there is a sufficient food source. Diet has a major impact on an organism's sensitivity to pesticides. When protein-rich diets are offered, rainbow trout's tolerance to lethal concentrations of the organochlorine pesticide chlordane is increased by six times.

Fish exposed to toxaphene use vitamin C to flush their bodies of the toxic material. Thus, increasing your diet's vitamin C intake supports your body's natural detoxification processes. It has been demonstrated that adding vitamin C to the diet can lessen the toxicity of pesticides to fish. However, either an excess or a lack of vitamin C has no bearing on the symptoms of lead intoxication.

2.3.7. Acclimation

Depending on the toxicant's mode of action and the sorts of detoxifying mechanisms present in the animals, those exposed to sublethal doses of a toxin may develop greater tolerance or less resistance. For instance, the threshold of LC50 was elevated by a factor of 1.5 when trout were exposed to sublethal (0.22 mg/1) levels of arsenic for three weeks. Fish became one-third more sensitive in the first week after acclimating to a level of cyanide that was one-third of the deadly limit. After three weeks, the tolerance returned to its prior level.

2.4. Absorption, Distribution, and Excretion of Toxicants

The three main processes of toxicants' absorption, distribution, and excretion influence the fate and effects of different substances and chemicals in the body. The subcategories of these processes are excretion, distribution, and absorption. Prioritizing comprehension of the procedures entails assessing the possible risks and hazards associated with exposure to toxic compounds. According to Lehman (2008), there are several ways for toxins to enter the body, but the most common ones are through ingestion, inhalation, and skin contact. After being absorbed, they can circulate throughout the body via the bloodstream and gather in different tissues and organs, where they may have a detrimental effect on a person's health. When assessing a poison's potential for harm and toxicity, it's also important to take into account how quickly it leaves the body. Toxicants' absorption, distribution, and excretion, as well as the variables influencing these processes and the consequences for environmental safety and public health (Figure 2.3).

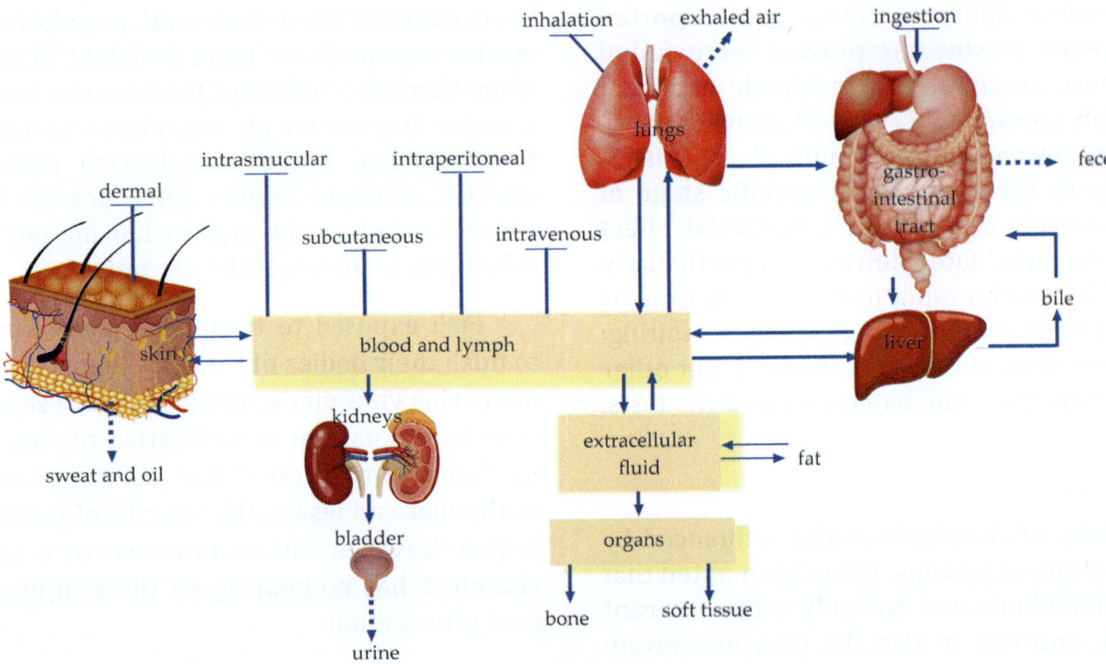

Figure 2.3. *Illustration of toxicants absorption, distribution, and excretion.*

Source: https://cdn.britannica.com/48/3548-004-1D127145/Routes-absorption-excretion-distribution-toxicants-human-body.jpg.

2.4.1. Translocation of Xenobiotics across Membranes

Translocation can occur via simple diffusion, specialized transport, filtration that may receive active assistance, or pinocytosis. The main ways that harmful chemical exposure occurs are through oral, respiratory, and dermal exposure. Because the epithelia lining the respiratory, GI, and cutaneous systems have close cell connections or, in the case of the skin, continuous lipid layers, they serve as significant barriers to the entry of foreign particles. Transporter proteins cross cell membranes to form functional epithelial barriers that either actively block the entry of foreign substances or make it easier for specific substrates to cross the barrier. Thus, a substance's capacity to directly permeate lipid cell membranes and interact with transporter proteins to cause toxic effects that dictate when a substance becomes toxic and how strong its effects are. Dermal penetration is unusual because outer epithelial cellular layers (corneocytes) lack transporter proteins and are not living cells. Therefore, in this case, absorption is contingent upon the toxicants' ability to cross the lipid matrix separating the corneocytes. Toxins usually pass through a variety of cell types, including the stratified epithelium of the skin, the thin cell layers of the GI tract or lungs, the capillary endothelium, and finally the cells of the target organ. The plasma membranes of these cells are remarkably similar to one another (Riederer, 2004) (Figure 2.4).

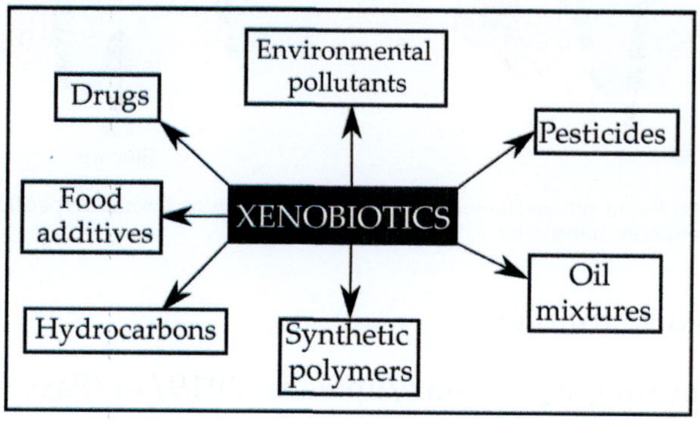

Figure 2.4. *Schematic of xenobiotics.*

Source: https://biomolecules101.wordpress.com/wp-content/uploads/2018/11/xenobiotics-1.png.

2.4.1.1. Membrane Permeability

As was previously said, a chemical substance must overcome several obstacles to reach a sufficient concentration of cells capable of performing the desired effect. There are three primary types of membranes in succession:

- Those consisting of several cell types in layers, similar to skin;
- Those made up of a single layer of cells, like intestinal epithelium; and
- Those with a cell thickness of less than one, like a single cell's membrane.

The cell membrane, also known as the plasma membrane, is a crucial component of biological cells. It has a thickness of approximately 100 A°, and the pores within the membrane range in size from 4 to 40 A°. Lipid-soluble compounds can easily pass through the lipid layer of the cell membrane. Current theories suggest that the cell membrane is a lipid-based biomolecular layer that is surrounded on both sides by a protein layer. The structure of the plasma membrane indicates that the key physio-chemical characteristics of any xenobiotic that influence its ability to cross the membrane are its size, level of ionization, shape, and lipid solubility in both its nonionized and ionized forms.

2.4.1.2. Chemical Transfer's Mechanism

The mechanism by which chemical agents may cross membrane can be classified into two main categories: inert passive transfer and active specialized transport, where the membrane actively contributes to the transfer of chemical agents across membranes. There is an alternative mechanism called pinocytosis (Figure 2.5).

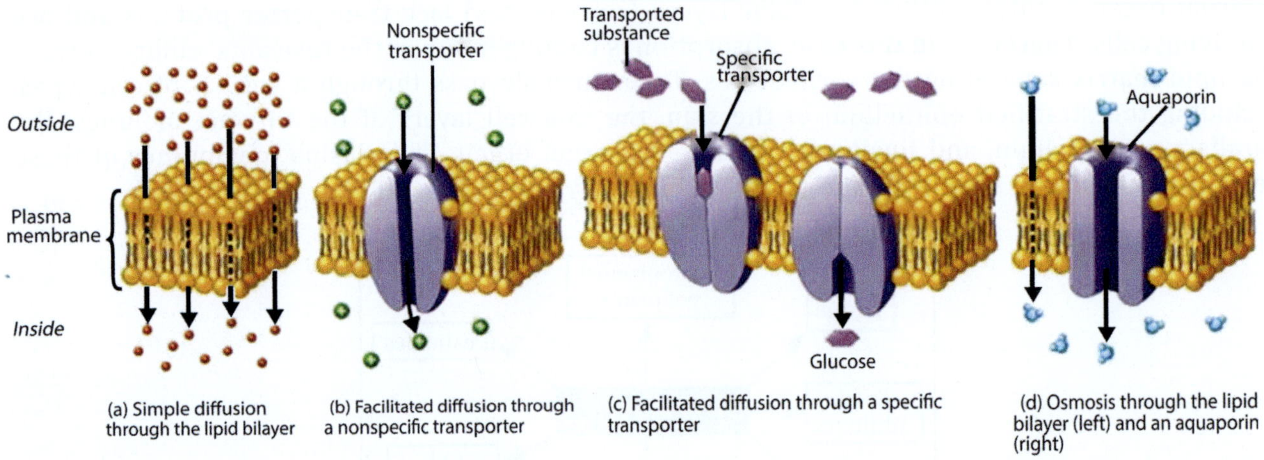

Figure 2.5. *Schematic of passive transfer.*

Source: https://microbenotes.com/wp-content/uploads/2019/11/Passive-Transport.jpg.

2.4.2. Absorption

Absorption is the process of transferring an unaltered material from its site of exposure or delivery to the bloodstream. Most toxic chemicals interact with one or more internal organs to manifest their harmful effects in the systemic circulation, with the exception of those that cause local reactions at the exposure site. During absorption, toxic chemicals from the external environment get past cellular barriers and into the body. Absorption of xenobiotics is dependent on a number of factors. Numerous variables, such as chemical solubility and concentration, circulation, absorbing location, absorbing surface area, and delivery route, affect how well xenobiotics are absorbed. Skin, lungs, and gastrointestinal tract are possible entry points for xenobiotics into the body. Still, a variety of parenteral methods are regularly used in experiments with dangerous materials. The most common of these are intravenous (IV), subcutaneous (SC), and intraperitoneal (IP).

2.4.2.1. Gastrointestinal Absorption

Xenobiotics can either directly or indirectly enter the body system through the mouth as environmental contaminants. Because absorption happens throughout the entire length of a xenobiotic, its chemical properties determine whether it will be absorbed in an almost neutral intestine or in a very acidic stomach. The mechanisms governing the passage of substances across biological membranes and their absorption from the GI tract are the same, as was previously mentioned. The sublingual route of administration is important in medicine because certain drugs, such as nitroglycerin, are better absorbed in this manner. Non-ionic diffusion across the lipid layer of the GI epithelial membrane is responsible for the majority of chemical absorption through the GI tract. Amino acids, carbohydrates, pyrimidines, and a variety of organic and inorganic ions are transported by specialized active mechanisms. Weak acidic compounds mainly ionize at the pH of gastric juice, absorb through the intestinal mucosa primarily, and gastric mucosa only weakly (Figure 2.6).

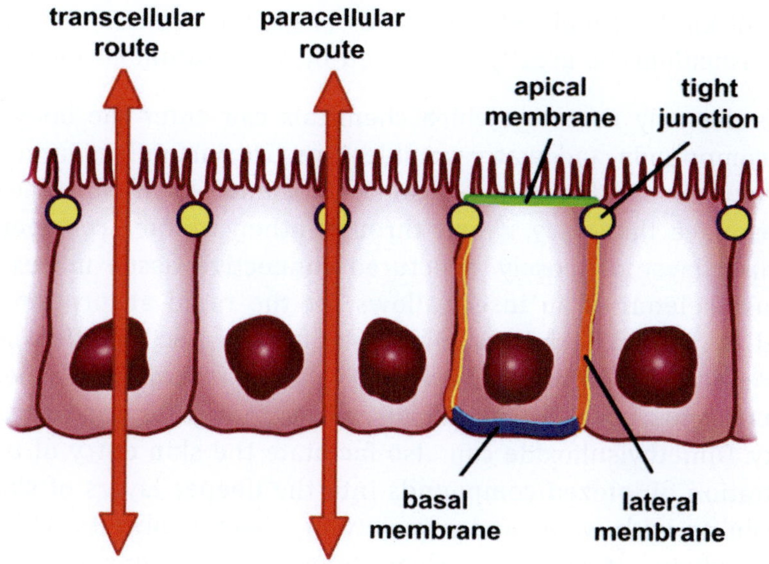

Figure 2.6. *Illustration of GI epithelial membrane.*

Source: https://upload.wikimedia.org/wikipedia/commons/thumb/1/1d/Selective_permeability_routes_in_epithelium.png/800px-Selective_permeability_routes_in_epithelium.png.

If the stomach's contents become alkaline, acid chemicals become more ionized and are less easily absorbed. Conversely, basic materials absorb better and become less ionized. Food can influence how well chemicals are absorbed. Weak acids are less easily absorbed and bases are more easily absorbed in the intestine than in the stomach, which has a pH of approximately 5. For instance, prolonged fasting has been shown to reduce the absorption of various substances, most likely as a result of negative effects on the intestinal epithelium. If a chemical is unstable in GI fluid or binds to food or other GI contents, its absorption from the GI tract may be limited or decreased. The compounds can be altered by acids, enzymes, or intestinal flora to produce a new chemical different from the parent component in terms of toxicity. For example, it is less dangerous when taken orally rather than intravenously because the digestive enzymes in the GI tract break down the venom of snakes.

2.4.2.2. Skin Absorption

The skin is the tissue that is most frequently exposed to various substances. Thankfully, the skin stops water evaporation and diffusion, except for the sweat glands. Even though the epidermis is only 0.2 mm thick, it significantly reduces absorption. The stratum corneum, sometimes referred to as the horny outer layer, is a continuous sheet of keratin-tightly packed, flattened cells that acts as a barrier to the entry of chemicals that dissolve in water. However, some substances can affect the entire body when absorbed through the skin. For example, when organic solvents like carbon tetrachloride penetrate the epidermis in this way, the results can be dangerous. Agricultural workers have been killed by nicotine insecticides and pesticides (parathion, malathion) through percutaneous absorption. Skin contact readily absorbs mustard gas chlorovinylarsine dichloride (Lewisite). Skin penetration of xenobiotics can occur at different rates and intensities in different body parts. The abrasion or loss of the stratum corneum results in a rapid rise in the permeability of the epidermis for all kinds of molecules, small or large, lipid-soluble or water-soluble. This is because cutaneous permeability is greatly influenced by the stratum corneum.

The epidermis is the only route by which chemicals can enter the body, slowing down the process. The polar compounds and water-soluble ions are virtually eliminated, and the rates are largely dictated by their lipid/water partition coefficients. Even substances soluble in lipids penetrate at a slower pace than they would through other, thinner cell membranes. An easily permeable, vascularized layer of loosely structured connective tissue makes up the underlying dermis. The chitinous skeleton of an insect allows for the rapid absorption of substances that are poorly absorbed by the epidermis of mammals, hence species differences are important. For example, DDT is much less harmful to mammals than it is to insects when applied topically. Numerous detrimental agents, such as acids, alkalis, or mustard gases, can damage barrier cells and enhance permeability. Dimethylsulfoxide can also facilitate the skin entry of toxins into the body. The enhanced penetration of ionized compounds into the deeper layers of skin is made possible by this liquid's miscibility with water and a variety of organic solvents. These compounds may have applications in medicine. It remains unclear, though, if any safe solvents could be employed for the percutaneous delivery of systemic medication.

2.4.2.3. Lungs Absorption

Numerous foreign substances that are inhaled as gases or aerosols pass through alveolar membranes and enter the bloodstream. In alveolar capillaries, substances with small atomic or molecular radii or comparatively high lipid/water partition coefficients quickly acclimate to blood. Particulate matter, irritants, and toxins are a few of the substances that can cause illness or poisoning. These substances may originate from occupational diseases such as silicosis or from the general environment. Here, the alveolar epithelium's rate of material absorption is greatly influenced by the size of the particles. This is probably due to the fact that smaller particles have more surface area available for solubilization. For example, kidney damage results from the absorption of uranium dioxide particles smaller than 3μ into the bloodstream. However, there was no negative impact upon the introduction of larger particles. If a particle's size is larger than 10 μ, it can become impacted in the throat or nasal cavity, preventing it from entering the alveolar region. Smaller particles can spread throughout alveoli, but larger particles (between 1 and 5 μ) often settle in the bronchiolar region of the lung. Water solubilities, also known as blood/partition coefficients, play a major role in the principles that control the absorption and excretion of toxic gases and vapors as well as the rates at which toxic effects begin and diminish. Any given chemical's concentration in blood can vary from that in plasma or water based on the hazardous agent's ability to bind to specific proteins and dissolve in plasma lipids. The degree to which a toxic gas dissolves in tissue more readily than in blood determines how much farther it diffuses in tissues.

The particles may also be eliminated by the bronchi before they enter the GI system. The movement of the fluid surface coating lining an alveoli and the availability of recruitable macrophages are prerequisites for this method's effectiveness. This pathway is especially important because it makes it possible to remove 80% of a chemical's lung contents. The lymphatic system is an additional means of eliminating toxins from the alveoli. The lung's interstitial tissue allows particles, both free and phagocytized, to flow through the lymphatic system. Certain particles remain in the alveolus and may form an alveolar dust plaque or module.

2.4.2.4. Parenteral Administration

Chemicals can be injected subcutaneously (SC), intramuscularly (IM), intraperitoneally (IP), or intravenously (IV) in experimental settings. There is no denying that the IV approach has the advantage of introducing a chemical into circulation with the least amount of delay (directly in the bloodstream). This technique is used when information regarding studies on metabolism and excretion or toxicants is needed because absorption is prevented. Toxins are absorbed rapidly through the IP route because of the strong blood flow to the peritoneal cavity (large surface area). The absorption of substances administered by SC and IM routes usually occurs gradually. It is possible to administer substances that do not irritate tissue through the SC route; if not, sloughing might happen. Some irritants can only be injected through the SC route using the IM method.

2.4.3. Distribution

"Distribution" refers to how xenobiotics move through the body and land in tissues and extracellular fluid, where they take effect. The toxin will normally enter the bloodstream after first entering the lymph, then the interstitial fluid at the site of absorption. Ingested materials are primarily transported to different organs and body tissues by the swift flow of blood through the cardiovascular circulation system. The circulatory system of the heart is to blame for this. Prior to being distributed throughout the body by the circulatory system, a hazardous substance must first cross capillary endothelium. The target organ's cells must then be penetrated by it via interstitial fluid. Certain barriers, like the blood-brain, blood tests, and blood placenta barriers, restrict the entry of xenobiotics into specific tissues by forming tight-fitting, continuous cellular layers that prevent toxicants from entering through passive diffusion through intercellular spaces. Toxins can enter these protected tissues directly through lipid cell membrane penetration or indirectly through active or assisted transmembrane transporter protein transport.

Hence, a compound's rate and range of distribution depend on a variety of factors:

- Lipophilicity
- Blood flow and organ size
- Plasma protein and tissue binding
- Molecular size (i.e., physicochemical properties of a compound)
- Availability of special transport system
- Disease state
- Special compartmental and barriers (e.g., BBS, placental barrier, blood-cerebrospinal barrier, and other barriers)
- The capability of transmembrane transporter proteins to interact
- Chemicals enter the various fluid compartments after entering the bloodstream:
- Plasma;
- Interstitial fluid;
- Transcellular fluid; and
- Cellular fluids.

The most absorbent nonionized fractions are soluble/lipid-based. Most tissues experience chemical equilibration fairly quickly, so chemical activity isn't restricted by the rate of chemical penetration. However, there are a few outliers.

For example, the fatty and bone tissues receive relatively little blood flow, which makes it take longer for these tissues to reach equilibrium. Additionally, due to binding or because of their affinity for fat, some molecules may accumulate in various locations. Either at the chemical's site of action or someplace else could see the buildup. In the latter scenario, the buildup may serve as a chemical storage facility. Even though the chemical in the storage depot isn't active in this case, it is still in equilibrium with other chemicals, which keeps the chemical's effective concentration at the site of action. However, there may be an uneven distribution of substances throughout the body because of affinities for specific environments, such as fat for highly lipophilic compounds or bone for compounds that bind to Ca[21]. Rein et al., (2013) have reported that prolonged storage of the substance in the depot sites may lead to accumulation and incredibly low concentrations in blood plasma..

2.4.3.1. Tissue Permeability Barriers

For biological complexity and specialization, concentration gradients must be able to form and persist across permeability barriers. This makes it impossible for most tissues, including the testes, to have continuous membrane barriers, and it increases the likelihood that diffusion will occur through the extracellular spaces surrounding membranes. In endothelia and epithelia, extracellular diffusion takes place via microscopic openings in the membranes of nearby cells. This particular intercellular space is known as the zona occluded, or tight junction. Permeability barriers with effective tight junctions are located at the capillary endothelium level (e.g., placenta, brain, and thymus barriers). The term "blood-organ barriers" describes them. Through blood bile barriers, the hepatocyte membranes are directly accessible to the blood. At this point, the physical barrier separating blood and bile is composed of close connections formed by nearby hepatocytes. There are "blood-organ barriers" that don't even require blood. Tight junctions, for example, are located near the luminal surface of bladder epithelial cells in the blood-urine barrier and inside the seminiferous tubules of the blood-testes barrier. As a result, the blood-testes barrier is more like the blood-urine barrier than the blood-brain barrier (BBS), which is occasionally contrasted. A few notable challenges are covered here.

- Blood-Brain Barrier

The BBS divides the extracellular space of the brain from its plasma and is located in the glial field that surrounds brain capillaries or capillary endothelial cells. The blood-cerebrospinal fluid barrier is located in the choroid plexus. These are not complete barriers to the passage of substances into the central nervous system; rather, they characterize a site that is less permeable than most other parts of the body. Substances enter the body through various cells and enter the brain primarily via similar mechanisms. These materials are able to freely enter the brain because plasma proteins are unable to bind to them. As was previously mentioned, nonionized substances can readily enter the brain at a rate proportionate to their lipid water partition coefficient, whereas ionized compounds are unable to do so. Chemicals exit cerebrospinal fluid by bulk fluid flow through the villi of arachnoids, which differs from how they enter. Additionally, some compounds may be extracted from the cerebrospinal fluid using specialized active transport mechanisms that function similarly to those that are present for organic ions in tubules.

- Placental Barrier

The principles governing chemical transfer through the placenta must be thoroughly understood because many xenobiotics can cross the placenta and negatively impact the fetus. They may result in fetal fatalities and congenital defects. Chemicals are primarily transported across placental membranes by simple diffusion; carrier-mediated transport is usually restricted to endogenous substrates. The lipid water partition coefficient, in particular, is crucial for placental transport, and these same elements are important for it. The concentration of chemicals in the various tissues of the fetus will be influenced by the ability of each tissue to concentrate chemicals, which may depend on the concentration of plasma proteins and the binding affinity for distinct chemicals.

- Blood-Test Barrier

Like the other barriers, the blood-testes barrier is an odd construction made of cell tight junctions that are positioned between blood and another discrete fluid compartment, either directly or indirectly. It is found in the voids between Sertoli cells in the seminiferous epithelium. Many parallel lines of fused membranes make up the tight junction of the complex Sertoli cell junctional complex. The barrier serves as a vital defense mechanism for germ line cells against external and internal biological threats. The barriers also help shield meiotic cells from environmental mutagens and prevent autoimmune orchitis.

2.4.3.2. Transfer across Other Membranes

The general mechanisms also affect other body membranes, such as those controlling ocular fluid, salivary glands, and mammary glands, as well as those involved in the passage of xenobiotics. Since mechanisms of substance transport across these membranes are still poorly understood, only a few general principles may be important determinants for these fluids.

2.4.3.3. Redistribution

Chemicals may be initially distributed throughout the body, but they may later be redistributed to tissues and areas with reduced blood flow as more binding sites become available. For example, immediately upon absorption, inorganic lead concentrates in the liver, kidney, and erythrocytes. Later, the lead is transferred to the bone and takes the place of calcium in the crystal lattice. According to Chillingstone and Hardman (2017), the bones contain 90% of the lead that is still in the body one month later.

2.4.4. Excretion

Toxins and their metabolites are transferred irreversibly from the body to the external environment by excretion. Therefore, excretion serves as a primary means of shielding the body from the damaging effects of toxicants by eliminating them from the body. Substances that are eliminated quickly are less likely to accumulate in tissues and damage essential cells. Although the terms excretion and elimination are sometimes used synonymously, the former term refers to any processes, such as biotransformation, that lower the body's concentration of the parent chemical. Major organ excretion is referred to as renal excretion by organs other than the kidneys is referred to as extrarenal or nonrenal excretion.

2.4.4.1. Biliary Excretion

The liver is the first organ the blood from the GI tract passes through before it enters the main circulation. The chemicals can be removed from the blood by the liver, preventing them from entering other bodily parts. The molecule and its metabolites can be removed in the bile without going back into the bloodstream to be removed by the kidneys because the majority of chemicals are metabolized in the liver. A substance that is released by liver cells into bile can subsequently pass through to the small intestine. If the properties or metabolites of chemicals are suitable for intestinal reabsorption, an enterohepatic cycle may occur whereby biliary secretion and intestinal reabsorption continue until renal excretion eventually removes substances from the body. The biliary pathway primarily excretes anions, cations, and nonionized compounds with both lipophilic and polar groups. During these processes, the substances most often enter the bile by active secretion. The lipid-soluble material may enter the bile from the parenchymal cells and then be reabsorbed by the intestine. Another possible entry point is simple diffusion, but this doesn't seem to be very important.

The model for the organic anions' transport mechanism is called bromosulfalein (BSP). This has long been the method used to assess liver function. BSP elimination decreases following liver damage and returns to normal as liver function improves. There is a particular mechanism for the biliary excretion of organic cations. One notable example is the quaternary procaine amide derivative ETHOBROMIDE. Benzomethamine, oxyphenonium, mepiperphenidol, and NO-methyl-nicotinamide are among the quaternary ammonium compounds that compete with this drug's secretion to decrease it; these drugs are secreted into the bile. Furthermore, the liver has a channel for removing nonionized substances that have polar and lipophilic groups. Together with these three organic molecule transport systems, the liver most likely contains an extra transport pathway for the excretion of metals. For example, there is an apparent biliary transit maximum and lead is discharged into the bile despite the high bile/plasma concentration ratio. Whether other metals have a similar process is still unknown.

Different species excrete differing amounts of foreign materials in bile, but it is usually the highest in dogs and rats. Biliary excretion is influenced by compound molecular weight as well as molecular size. When the molecular weight increases, there is a corresponding decrease in excretion in the urine and an increase in biliary excretion. A great example of this are the substituted fluorescein dyes. Because an infant's hepatic excretory system is still developing, some substances are more dangerous to them than they are to adults. If this is the reason why certain chemicals are more toxic to babies, more research is required.

2.4.4.2. Gastrointestinal Tract

Numerous substances are present in the feces. The agent or substance may be expelled because the GI tract eliminated it. It was not absorbed after oral administration, or it was excreted into the bile. Certain ionized foreign substances in the blood may be expelled into the gut if the concentration gradient is favorable; the relationship to the pKa value is a decisive factor. Their elimination seems to occur through passive diffusion. Organic acids and very weak bases (pKa 0.3), which would only be weakly ionized at a pH of l, are not present in gastric juice.

2.4.4.3. Expired Air

The body expels a lot of volatile substances in the expired air without changing them. Among the chemicals expelled via this route are volatile substances, carbon monoxide, fluorobenzene, and some alcohols. Their elimination is dependent on the solubility of blood gases and is probably achieved by simple diffusion for each of them. Gases rapidly expelled, such as nitrous oxide and benzene, have low blood/gas solubility. On the other hand, substances like ethanol or bromobenzene that have a high solubility in gas or blood are gradually removed by expired air.

2.4.4.4. Sweat

Very small amounts of substances are usually expelled in sweat. However, diethyl di-thiol-iso-phthalate, the majority of the drug used to treat leprosy in human subjects, is excreted through perspiration. The compounds that were least ionized at a pH of 7.4 had the highest concentration ratios of different sulphonamides excreted in sweat following oral treatment to human subjects; this suggests that the sweat gland epithelium is only readily permeable to unionized molecules (Pearlmutter et al., 2020).

2.4.4.5. Saliva

Some sulfonamides are released by humans in their parotid saliva. Ruminants' alkaline parotid saliva contains higher concentrations of excreted pentobarbitone and other acidic or other medications. If this pathway is involved in the secretion of other foreign chemicals from animal or human systems, more investigation is required.

2.4.4.6. Milk

Several foreign substances and their metabolites are partly eliminated in the milk of nursing mammals. Since plasma has a pH of 6.56, milk has a higher pH 7, simple diffusion is used to remove the compounds. The presence of basic substances may be higher than that of acidic compounds, on the other hand. It has been reported that milk contains erythromycin, tetracycline, thiouracil, and DDT.

2.4.4.7. Vaginal Secretions

It is unclear what function chemical excretion through vaginal secretions serves. However, hippuric acid, a benzoic acid glycine conjugate, has been discovered in bovine estrus secretions. More knowledge is needed regarding the expulsion of other foreign substances through vaginal secretions.

2.4.4.8. Other Routes

For the additional elimination pathways, including tracheobronchial secretions, intestinal fluid, lachrymal fluid, and others, only a very small amount of knowledge accessible.

A Closer Look

Dose-Response Relationship

Understanding how different doses of a substance affect the severity and type of response is a foundational concept in toxicology known as the dose-response relationship. This relationship describes how the magnitude and nature of a toxic effect are related to the amount of exposure to a substance. The central tenet is that the severity of the response increases with the dose, which can be depicted graphically through a dose-response curve. This curve typically plots the dose of the substance on the x-axis and the observed effect on the y-axis. The shape of the curve helps toxicologists determine the threshold dose, which is the minimum amount of the substance required to elicit a detectable response. Below this threshold, the substance may have no observable effect.

A crucial aspect of the dose-response relationship is the concept of the threshold level. At doses below the threshold, the body's defense mechanisms can manage the exposure without significant adverse effects. However, once the threshold is surpassed, toxic effects start to manifest, and the severity of these effects generally increases with higher doses. The threshold concept is vital for setting safety standards and regulatory limits for exposure to various substances. For example, regulatory agencies use this information to establish permissible exposure limits for chemicals in the workplace or acceptable daily intakes for food additives and contaminants.

The dose-response relationship also includes key measures such as the lethal dose 50 (LD50) and the effective dose 50 (ED50). The LD50 is the dose required to kill 50% of a test population, often used in animal studies to gauge the acute toxicity of a substance. The ED50, on the other hand, is the dose that produces a therapeutic or desired effect in 50% of the population, commonly used in pharmacology to determine effective drug dosages. These measures help in comparing the relative toxicity or efficacy of different substances and are critical in risk assessment and drug development.

Additionally, the dose-response relationship can illustrate different types of effects, such as beneficial, toxic, or lethal, depending on the substance and its dose. For instance, certain chemicals might have therapeutic effects at low doses but become toxic at higher doses—a phenomenon known as hormesis. This underscores the importance of dose in determining whether a substance acts as a poison or a remedy.

Understanding this relationship is not just about identifying harmful levels but also about recognizing safe and beneficial levels. For example, essential nutrients and vitamins have dose-response relationships where both deficiency and excessive intake can lead to adverse health effects. Therefore, establishing the optimal dose is crucial for maintaining health and preventing toxicity.

Summary

- Toxicology, the study of the adverse effects of chemical, physical, or biological agents on living organisms, is influenced by various factors that dictate the extent and nature of toxicity.
- The chemical makeup of a substance heavily influences its physical and chemical properties, including its solubility, vapor pressure, ionization, functional groups, etc. The substance's toxicological qualities are significantly impacted by all of these factors.
- Toxicology includes the study of chemical properties and how they affect the body. It focuses on the adverse effects of chemicals in living organisms that come in contact with them. Toxicology includes the detection, symptoms, pathogenesis, mechanism, and treatment of these chemicals.
- A conventional relationship between dose and toxicity has traditionally been accepted, in that greater exposure to a chemical can lead to higher risk of toxicity. However, this concept has been challenged by a study of endocrine disruptors and, therefore, may not be a straightforward relationship.
- Toxicants come in two varieties: those that have local effects and those that have systemic effects. For the second, efficient translocation is crucial. The toxicants cannot cause harm unless they are easily transported to the targeted areas.
- Toxicant translocation refers to the movement of toxic substances within an organism or between different compartments of the body following exposure.
- Toxic chemicals can also cause genetic damage. The genes, which exist in chromosomes, make the genetic material of the cell. Genes and chromosomes contain the information that tells the cell how to function and how to reproduce (form new cells). Some chemicals may change or damage the genes or chromosomes.
- Exposure to chemical substances may affect your children or your ability to have children. Toxic reproductive effects include the inability to conceive children (infertility or sterility), lowered sex drive, menstrual disturbances, spontaneous abortions (miscarriages), stillbirths, and defects in children that are apparent at birth or later in the child's development.
- Toxic materials can take the form of solid, liquid, gases, vapor, dust, fumes, fiber, and mist. How a substance gets into the body and what damage it causes depends on the form or the physical properties of the substance.
- The goal of toxicology research and toxicology testing is to identify the adverse effects of different toxicants. The adverse effects depend on two main factors, which are the routes of exposure and the dose, which is the concentration of the exposure.
- The toxicity of xenobiotics is predicted to be significantly influenced by the water's temperature. In addition to changing some compounds' chemical forms and increasing their solubility, rising water temperatures also control the amount of dissolved oxygen in the water.

References

1. Ahamed, M., & Siddiqui, M. K. J. (2007). Environmental lead toxicity and nutritional factors. *Clinical Nutrition, 26*(4), 400–408.
2. Balco, G., Stone, J. O., Lifton, N. A., & Dunai, T. J. (2008). A complete and easily accessible means of calculating surface exposure ages or erosion rates from 10Be and 26Al measurements. *Quaternary Geochronology, 3*(3), 174–195.
3. Bechmann, I., Galea, I., & Perry, V. H. (2007). What is the blood–brain barrier (not)? *Trends in Immunology, 28*(1), 5–11.
4. Braunbeck, T., Böttcher, M., Hollert, H., Kosmehl, T., Lammer, E., Leist, E., & Seitz, N. (2005). Towards an alternative for the acute fish LC50 test in chemical assessment: The fish embryo toxicity test goes multi-species-an update. *ALTEX-Alternatives to Animal Experimentation, 22*(2), 87–102.
5. Chillistone, S., & Hardman, J. G. (2017). Factors affecting drug absorption and distribution. *Anaesthesia & Intensive Care Medicine, 18*(7), 335–339.
6. Choi, O., & Hu, Z. (2008). Size dependent and reactive oxygen species related nanosilver toxicity to nitrifying bacteria. *Environmental Science & Technology, 42*(12), 4583–4588.
7. Collos, Y., & Harrison, P. J. (2014). Acclimation and toxicity of high ammonium concentrations to unicellular algae. *Marine Pollution Bulletin, 80*(1–2), 8–23.
8. Croom, E. (2012). Metabolism of xenobiotics of human environments. *Progress in Molecular Biology and Translational Science, 112*, 31–88.
9. Cuhra, M., Traavik, T., & Bøhn, T. (2013). Clone-and age-dependent toxicity of a glyphosate commercial formulation and its active ingredient in *Daphnia magna*. *Ecotoxicology, 22*, 251–262.
10. Franklin, N. M., Stauber, J. L., Markich, S. J., & Lim, R. P. (2000). pH-dependent toxicity of copper and uranium to a tropical freshwater alga (*Chlorella* sp.). *Aquatic Toxicology, 48*(2–3), 275–289.
11. Genuis, S. J. (2011). Elimination of persistent toxicants from the human body. *Human & Experimental Toxicology, 30*(1), 3–18.
12. Ghibellini, G., Leslie, E. M., & Brouwer, K. L. (2006). Methods to evaluate biliary excretion of drugs in humans: An updated review. *Molecular Pharmaceutics, 3*(3), 198–211.
13. Glass, D. C., & Gray, C. N. (2001). Estimating mean exposures from censored data: Exposure to benzene in the Australian petroleum industry. *Annals of Occupational Hygiene, 45*(4), 275–282.
14. Herzog, C. (2014). Influence of parenteral administration routes and additional factors on vaccine safety and immunogenicity: A review of recent literature. *Expert Review of Vaccines, 13*(3), 399–415.
15. Ibla, J. C., & Khoury, J. (2006). Methods to assess tissue permeability. In *Cell-Cell Interactions: Methods and Protocols* (pp. 111–117).
16. Lehman-McKeeman, L. D. (2008). Absorption, distribution, and excretion of toxicants. In *Casarett and Doull's Toxicology: The Basic Science of Poisons* (Vol. 1, No. 1, pp. 131–159). McGraw-Hill.

17. Liu, Y., Luo, J., Chen, X., Liu, W., & Chen, T. (2019). Cell membrane coating technology: A promising strategy for biomedical applications. *Nano-Micro Letters, 11*, 1–46.

18. Lloyd, J. B. (2000). Lysosome membrane permeability: Implications for drug delivery. *Advanced Drug Delivery Reviews, 41*(2), 189–200.

19. Lotte, C., Patouillet, C., Zanini, M., Messager, A., & Roguet, R. (2002). Permeation and skin absorption: Reproducibility of various industrial reconstructed human skin models. *Skin Pharmacology and Physiology, 15*(Suppl. 1), 18–30.

20. Lu, Q., Luo, Q., Li, J., Wang, X., Ban, C., Qin, J., & Chen, X. (2022). Evaluation of the chemical composition, bioactive substance, gas production, and rumen fermentation parameters of four types of distiller's grains. *Molecules, 27*(18), 6134.

21. Maibach, H. I. (2021). Cutaneous metabolism of xenobiotics. In *Percutaneous Absorption* (Vol. 1, No. 1, pp. 447–458). CRC Press.

22. Marques, M. R., Loebenberg, R., & Almukainzi, M. (2011). Simulated biological fluids with possible application in dissolution testing. *Dissolution Technology, 18*(3), 15–28.

23. Mruk, D. D., & Cheng, C. Y. (2015). The mammalian blood-testis barrier: Its biology and regulation. *Endocrine Reviews, 36*(5), 564–591.

24. Paredi, P., Kharitonov, S. A., & Barnes, P. J. (2002). Analysis of expired air for oxidation products. *American Journal of Respiratory and Critical Care Medicine, 166*(supplement_1), S31–S37.

25. Parkinson, A., & Ogilvie, B. W. (2008). Biotransformation of xenobiotics. In *Casarett and Doull's Toxicology: The Basic Science of Poisons* (Vol. 7, pp. 161–304).

26. Patra, R. W., Chapman, J. C., Lim, R. P., Gehrke, P. C., & Sunderam, R. M. (2015). Interactions between water temperature and contaminant toxicity to freshwater fish. *Environmental Toxicology and Chemistry, 34*(8), 1809–1817.

27. Pearlmutter, P., DeRose, G., Samson, C., Linehan, N., Cen, Y., Begdache, L., & Koh, A. (2020). Sweat and saliva cortisol response to stress and nutrition factors. *Scientific Reports, 10*(1), 19050.

28. Pflederer, T., Rudofsky, L., Ropers, D., Bachmann, S., Marwan, M., Daniel, W. G., & Achenbach, S. (2009). Image quality in a low radiation exposure protocol for retrospectively ECG-gated coronary CT angiography. *American Journal of Roentgenology, 192*(4), 1045–1050.

29. Raies, A. B., & Bajic, V. B. (2016). In silico toxicology: Computational methods for the prediction of chemical toxicity. *Wiley Interdisciplinary Reviews: Computational Molecular Science, 6*(2), 147–172.

30. Rein, M. J., Renouf, M., Cruz-Hernandez, C., Actis-Goretta, L., Thakkar, S. K., & Da Silva, P. M. (2013). Bioavailability of bioactive food compounds: A challenging journey to bioefficacy. *British Journal of Clinical Pharmacology, 75*(3), 588–602.

31. Rendal, C., Kusk, K. O., & Trapp, S. (2011). Optimal choice of pH for toxicity and bioaccumulation studies of ionizing organic chemicals. *Environmental Toxicology and Chemistry, 30*(11), 2395–2406.

32. Riederer, M. (2004). Uptake and transport of xenobiotics. In *Plant Toxicology* (Vol. 1, No. 1, pp. 145–164). CRC Press.

33. Rotter, S., Sans-Piché, F., Streck, G., Altenburger, R., & Schmitt-Jansen, M. (2011). Active bio-monitoring of contamination in aquatic systems—An in-situ translocation experiment applying the PICT concept. *Aquatic Toxicology, 101*(1), 228–236.

34. Singh, S., Parulekar, W., Murray, N., Feld, R., Evans, W. K., Tu, D., & Shepherd, F. A. (2005). Influence of sex on toxicity and treatment outcome in small-cell lung cancer. *Journal of Clinical Oncology, 23*(4), 850–856.

35. Slitt, A. L. (2019). Absorption, distribution, and excretion of toxicants. In *Casarett & Doull's Toxicology: The Basic Science of Poisons* (9th ed., Vol. 1, No. 1, pp. 159–192). McGraw-Hill Education.

36. Tetro, N., Moushaev, S., Rubinchik-Stern, M., & Eyal, S. (2018). The placental barrier: The gate and the fate in drug distribution. *Pharmaceutical Research, 35*, 1–16.

37. Vähäkangas, K., & Myllynen, P. (2009). Drug transporters in the human blood-placental barrier. *British Journal of Pharmacology, 158*(3), 665–678.

38. Villiger, M., Stoop, R., Vetsch, T., Hohenauer, E., Pini, M., Clarys, P., & Clijsen, R. (2018). Evaluation and review of body fluids saliva, sweat and tear compared to biochemical hydration assessment markers within blood and urine. *European Journal of Clinical Nutrition, 72*(1), 69–76.

Chapter

3

PRINCIPLES OF POISON MANAGEMENT

Contents

Introduction

The methodical process of preventing, identifying, and treating toxic exposures in order to ensure the well-being and safety of those who have been harmed is known as "poison management.". A few essential elements make up effective poison management, starting with preventing poisoning through public awareness campaigns and safety precautions. To reduce the frequency of poisoning, public health campaigns and laws governing the safe use and storage of household products, medications, and chemicals are essential. When assessing a poisoning incident, it is crucial to act quickly and accurately. To do this, a thorough history of the exposure must be obtained, including the kind of poison, its dosage, when it was exposed, and how it entered the body (by ingestion, inhalation, skin, etc.). The symptoms and severity of the poisoning, which can range from minor irritation to life-threatening conditions, must be promptly determined by healthcare professionals. To assess the degree of the toxic exposure, a clinical evaluation may involve laboratory testing, monitoring vital signs, and physical examination.

Stabilizing the patient's condition is the next stage in the management of poisoning. This usually entails doing basic life support procedures like keeping the airway closed, making sure the patient is breathing sufficiently, and sustaining circulation. Advanced life support procedures might be required in extreme circumstances. Certain treatment plans can be put into action after the patient has stabilized. To stop the poison from being absorbed further, decontamination techniques like gastric lavage, the administration of activated charcoal, or whole bowel irrigation may be used. The kind and quantity of poison consumed, along with the amount of time that has passed since exposure, all influence the method for the selection of decontamination. Another essential component of poison management is antidotes. Certain antidotes can counteract the toxic effects of some poisons or help the body eliminate them more effectively. Naloxone, for instance, is used to stop opioid overdoses, and activated charcoal can absorb a variety of ingested toxins and stop them from entering the bloodstream. Proper antidote administration in a timely manner can greatly enhance patient outcomes.

Throughout the entire management process, supportive care is crucial. This includes keeping an eye on and preserving critical bodily processes, controlling symptoms, and averting complications. Depending on the poisoning and the patient's condition, intravenous fluids, blood pressure support drugs, and treatments for seizures or cardiac arrhythmias may be required. Furthermore, in severe cases, continuous hospital monitoring may be necessary to watch for long-term effects and guarantee recovery. Poison control centers are essential to poison management because they offer quick, professional advice to the general public as well as medical professionals. These centers provide round-the-clock support, directing the initial response to poisoning incidents and suggesting suitable treatment plans. Additionally, they gather information on poisoning incidents, which is useful for monitoring and preventing public health issues. A multidisciplinary strategy involving emergency medical services, physicians, toxicologists, and poison control centers is necessary for effective poison management. To improve outcomes, healthcare professionals must receive education and training in identifying and treating poisoning. Preventive measures and public awareness are equally important in lowering the rate of poisoning. Poison management seeks to reduce the effects of toxic exposures and safeguard the public's health by fusing immediate medical attention with continued preventative and educational initiatives.

Orientation and Directional Terms:

Term	Definition	Illustration
Pharmacokinetics	Branch of pharmacology dedicated to describing how the body affects a specific substance after administration. The substances of interest include any chemical xenobiotic such as pharmaceutical drugs, pesticides, food additives, cosmetics, etc.	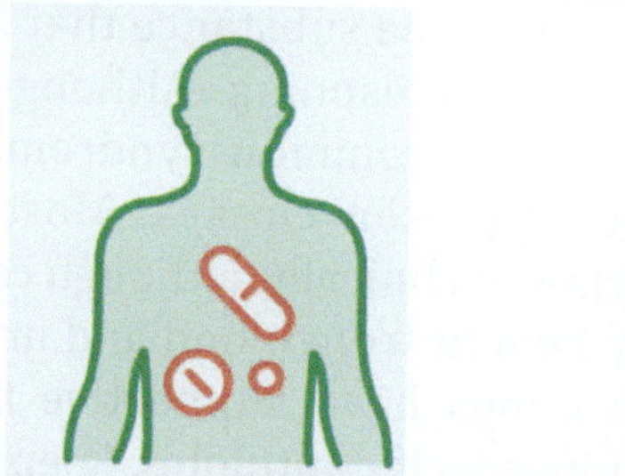
Pharmacodynamics	The study of the biochemical and physiologic effects of drugs. The effects can include those manifested within animals, microorganisms, or combinations of organisms.	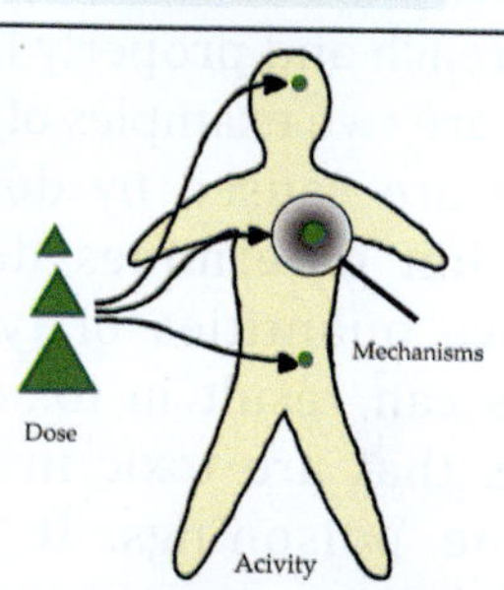
Drug metabolism	The metabolic breakdown of drugs by living organisms, usually through specialized enzymatic systems.	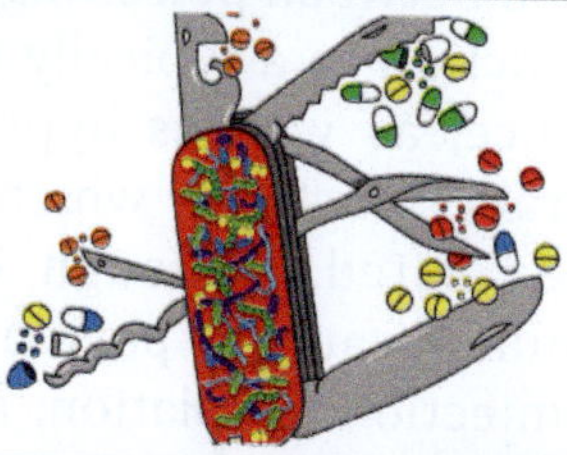
Nuclear chemistry	The sub-field of chemistry dealing with radioactivity, nuclear processes, and transformations in the nuclei of atoms, such as nuclear transmutation and nuclear properties.	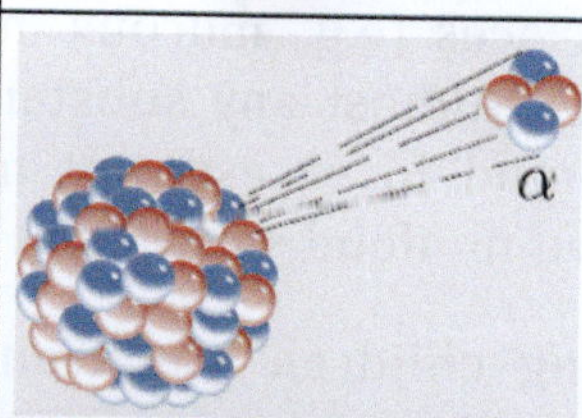
Chemotherapy	A type of cancer treatment that uses one or more anti-cancer drugs as part of a standardized chemotherapy regimen. Chemotherapy may be given with a curative intent or it may aim to prolong life or to reduce symptoms.	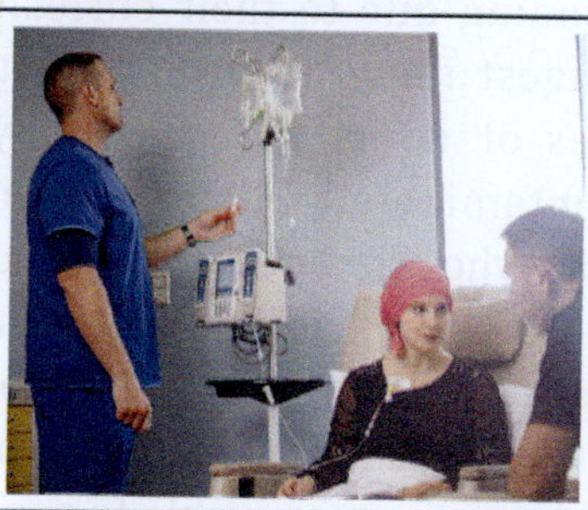

3.1. General Principles of Poisoning

Contact with a substance that causes toxicity is known as poisoning. Although symptoms can vary, some common syndromes may point to specific poison classes. Most poisonings are diagnosed clinically, although certain poisonings may benefit from blood and urine testing. Most poisonings have supportive treatment; some require specific antidotes. Keeping poisons out of children's reach and properly labeling medicine containers are two examples of prevention. Most poisonings are caused by dosage. Over time, concentration determines dosage. Exposure to excessive quantities of typically nontoxic substances can result in toxicity. Exposure to substances that are toxic in any amount can cause some poisonings. It is important to distinguish between poisoning and intolerance, a toxic reaction to a typically nontoxic dose of a substance, as well as hypersensitivity and idiosyncratic reactions, which are erratic and not dose-related. Although ingestion is the most common cause of poisoning, other causes include injection, inhalation, and contact with body surfaces (e.g., mucous membranes, skin, and eyes). Almost any substance can be toxic if consumed in excess, but many commonly consumed nonfood substances are usually safe.

Young children are prone to accidental poisoning due to their curiosity and tendency to ingest items regardless of their unpleasant tastes or odors; typically, only one substance is contaminated. Older children, teenagers, and adults who attempt suicide frequently experience poisoning; various drugs, such as alcohol, acetaminophen, and other over-the-counter (OTC) medications, may be used. Older adults may be more susceptible to accidental poisoning due to confusion, poor vision, mental illness, or multiple prescriptions for the same medication from various doctors. Sometimes, someone who wants to murder or maim a person will poison them (e.g., to rob them or rape them). Drugs that cause disability (e.g., benzodiazepines, gamma-hydroxybutyrate, scopolamine, and others) frequently have sedative, amnestic, or both effects. In rare cases, parents with some medical background poison their kids for unclear psychological reasons or to make them sick so they can get help (a condition known as factitious disorder imposed on another, formerly known as Munchausen syndrome by proxy). The majority of poisons undergo metabolism, travel through the gastrointestinal (GI) tract, or are eliminated after being exposed, ingested, and absorbed. Sometimes, tablets (e.g., large concretions or bezoars) in the GI tract, where they often stay and continue to be absorbed, causing toxicity (aspirin, iron, and enteric-coated drugs, for example).

3.1.1. Symptoms and Signs of Poisoning

Depending on the substance, different poisoning symptoms and signs exist. Furthermore, different patients who have been poisoned by the same substance may exhibit remarkably different symptoms. Nonetheless, six symptom clusters known as toxic syndromes, or toxidromes, are frequently encountered and may indicate specific chemical classes. Individuals who consume more than one substance are less likely to exhibit symptoms specific to that substance. In most cases, symptoms appear shortly after contact; however, in some cases, they take longer. The reason for the delay could be that, instead of the parent substance being toxic, only a metabolite is (e.g., hepatotoxins, methanol, and ethylene glycol). Consuming hepatotoxins (e.g., amanita phalloides mushrooms, acetaminophen, iron, and others) may result in acute liver failure, which manifests one to several days later. When exposed to metals or hydrocarbon solvents over an extended period, symptoms usually take hold. Toxins that are ingested and absorbed typically result in systemic symptoms. The mucous membranes of the gastrointestinal (GI) tract are primarily damaged by caustics and corrosive liquids, which can result in perforation, enteritis, or stomatitis. Certain pollutants (e.g., hydrocarbons, alcohol) that give off distinct breath odors. Toxin contact on the skin can result in a range of acute cutaneous symptoms (e.g., blistering, rashes, and pain); prolonged exposure can result in dermatitis.

If toxins are water-soluble when inhaled, they may result in upper airway injury symptoms (e.g., ammonia, and chlorine) and signs of noncardiogenic pulmonary edema and lower airway injury if they are less soluble in water (e.g., phosgene). Gas inhalation that contains hydrogen sulfide, cyanide, or carbon monoxide can result in cardiac or respiratory arrest as well as organ ischemia. Toxins, whether solid, liquid, or vapor, can harm the cornea, sclera, and lens of the eye, resulting in pain, redness, and vision loss. Certain substances (e.g., drugs: cocaine, phencyclidine, amphetamine) can lead to extreme agitation, which increases the risk of acidosis, rhabdomyolysis, and hyperthermia.

3.1.2. Diagnosis of Poisoning

- Consideration of poisoning in patients with altered consciousness or unexplained symptoms
- History from all available sources
- Selective, directed testing

The initial step in diagnosing poisoning involves assessing the patient's overall condition. In cases of severe poisoning, immediate intervention may be necessary to address airway obstruction or cardiac arrest. Poisoning can often be identified based on the symptoms present, particularly if there is a change in consciousness ranging from restlessness to unconsciousness. In cases of intentional poisoning in adults, it is important to consider the possibility of multiple substances being involved. Obtaining a thorough patient history is essential in diagnosing poisoning. Since some individuals may not be able to provide accurate information due to various reasons, it is important to also gather information from friends, family members, and first responders. Patients may also provide inaccurate details about the substance ingested. Examining the patient's living environment for evidence, such as pill containers or notes, can also provide valuable insights. Medical and pharmacy records may offer additional helpful information. In cases of suspected workplace poisoning, it is important to interview colleagues and superiors. In such incidents, the material safety data sheet (MSDS) for any industrial chemicals involved should be readily accessible, as it contains information on toxicity and treatment recommendations.

Poison control centers can provide information about industrial and household chemicals in many parts of the world. Because ingredients, first aid instructions, and antidotes printed on product containers are sometimes erroneous or out of date, consultation with the centers is strongly advised. Furthermore, there is a chance that the package was tampered with or the container was changed. Based solely on appearance, poison control centers might be able to assist in identifying unknown pills. Toxicologists are readily available to the centers. The phone number of the closest center can be found in the front of the local phone book, among other emergency numbers. Physical examination may occasionally reveal indications of specific drug classes (e.g., toxidromes, breath odor, topical drug use, needle marks or tracks indicating injection drug use, and stigma associated with long-term alcohol consumption). Changes in consciousness may be brought on by other factors (e.g., even if a patient is known to have been poisoned). (e.g., encephalopathy, Wernicke encephalopathy, hypoglycemia, stroke, central nervous system infection, and head trauma), which should also be considered. After consuming drugs, older children, adolescents, and adults should always be evaluated for attempted suicide. Furthermore, kids frequently share drugs and other materials they find, so it is important to conduct thorough investigations to find any more playmates or siblings who might be poisoned.

3.1.2.1. Testing

Laboratory testing is usually not very helpful. Commonly referred to as toxic screens, these easily accessible, standard tests are qualitative rather than quantitative in order to identify common drugs of abuse. These tests only look for a small number of substances, and they may yield false-positive or false-negative results. Furthermore, the presence of a drug of abuse does not always mean that the patient's symptoms or signs were brought on by the drug (for example, a patient who recently took an opioid may actually be obtunded due to encephalitis rather than the drug). The most common method of drug testing is urine, however it is not very effective and typically only finds drug classes or metabolites rather than individual drugs. An opioid urine immunoassay test, for instance, reacts to very small amounts of morphine or codeine analogues but is unable to detect fentanyl or methadone. Instead of detecting cocaine itself, the test used to identify cocaine finds a metabolite. Blood levels for the majority of substances are either difficult to measure or do not inform treatment decisions. Certain substances (e.g., blood levels) of certain medications (acetaminophen, aspirin, digoxin, ethylene glycol, carbon monoxide, iron, lithium, methanol, phenobarbital, phenytoin, theophylline), may be used to guide treatment decisions. Due to the fact that acetaminophen ingestion is frequent, frequently asymptomatic in the early stages, and can result in serious delayed toxicity that can be avoided with an antidote, many authorities advise measuring the levels of the drug in all patients with mixed ingestions. With certain drugs, additional blood tests (e.g., Methemoglobin levels for specific drugs, PT [prothrombin time] for warfarin overdose, and other factors) aid in directing treatment.

Serum electrolytes, blood urea nitrogen (BUN), creatinine, serum osmolality, glucose, coagulation studies, and arterial blood gases should all be tested in patients with altered consciousness, abnormal vital signs, or who have consumed certain substances. Additional assessments e.g., certain suspected poisons or in specific clinical circumstances, such as brain CT scans, methemoglobin levels, and carbon monoxide levels, may be recommended. Regarding specific poisonings e.g., Plain abdominal x-rays can reveal the presence and location of ingested substances, owing to various factors such as iron, lead, arsenic, and other metals, or to packets of cocaine or other illicit drugs consumed by individuals referred to as body packers. For poisonings involving drugs with cardiovascular effects or unknown substances, electrocardiography (ECG) and cardiac monitoring are recommended. If toxicity symptoms or blood levels of a substance increase after first declining or last an abnormally long period, a bezoar, a sustained-release preparation, or re-exposure (i.e., suspecting repeated covert exposure to a drug used recreationally.

3.1.3. Treatment of Poisoning

- Supportive care
- Activated charcoal for serious oral poisonings
- Occasional use of specific antidotes or dialysis
- Only rare use of gastric emptying

Seriously poisoned patients may require assisted ventilation or treatment of cardiovascular collapse. Patients with impaired consciousness may require continuous monitoring or restraints. The discussion of treatment for specific poisonings. Consultation with a poison control center is recommended for any poisonings except the mildest and most routine.

3.1.3.1. Initial Stabilization

- Maintain airway, breathing, and circulation
- IV naloxone
- IV dextrose and thiamine
- IV fluids, sometimes vasopressors

Patients who are suspected of having a systemic poisoning need to have their airway, breathing, and circulation maintained. Patients in need of emergency cardiopulmonary resuscitation have no blood pressure or pulse. Patients who suffer from apnea or have compromised airways (e.g., a decreased gag reflex, foreign material in the oropharynx), an endotracheal tube should be placed (see Tracheal Intubation). Mechanical ventilation or additional oxygen should be given to patients who exhibit respiratory depression or hypoxia as needed.

Patients with apnea or severe respiratory depression should be treated with IV naloxone (2 mg in adults; 0–1 mg/kg in children; doses as high as 10 mg may be necessary in some cases) while keeping airway support. Naloxone may hasten the withdrawal process in opioid addicts, but withdrawal is preferable to severe respiratory depression. Naloxone treatment alone won't cure respiratory depression; continuous mechanical ventilation and endotracheal intubation are needed instead. Patients should be closely watched if naloxone alleviates respiratory depression. If the condition returns, they should receive mechanical ventilation, endotracheal intubation, or another IV naloxone bolus. While it has been suggested that respiratory drive can be maintained without triggering withdrawal by using a low-dose continuous naloxone infusion, this can actually be very challenging to achieve.

Patients with altered consciousness or central nervous system (CNS) depression should receive IV dextrose (50 mL of a 50% solution for adults; 2 to 4 mL/kg of a 25% solution for children), unless hypoglycemia has been ruled out by an immediate bedside blood glucose test.

Thiamine (100 mg IV) is given with or before glucose to adults with suspected thiamine deficiency (e.g., alcoholics, undernourished patients).

Hypotension is treated with intravenous fluids. Vasopressor and fluid therapy may need to be guided by invasive hemodynamic monitoring if fluids prove ineffective. For the majority of poison-induced hypotension, norepinephrine 0.5 to 1 mg/min IV infusion is the first-choice vasopressor.

3.1.3.2. Topical Decontamination

Any part of the body exposed to a toxin, including the eyes, should be thoroughly rinsed with water or saline. Jewelry and all contaminated apparel, including socks and shoes, should be taken off. Transdermal delivery systems and topical patches are eliminated.

3.1.3.3. Activated Charcoal

Charcoal is typically administered, especially in cases where several or unidentified substances have been consumed. The use of charcoal has not been shown to lower overall morbidity or mortality, but it does not increase risk (unless patients are at risk of aspiration or vomiting). Charcoal is administered as soon as feasible after usage. Because of its large surface area and molecular configuration, activated charcoal is able to adsorb most toxins. Activated charcoal in multiple doses may be useful for drugs that are subject to enterohepatic recirculation (e.g., theophylline, and phenobarbital) as well as for preparations with prolonged release. If bowel sounds are hypoactive, charcoal may be administered every 4 to 6 h for serious poisoning with such substances. Alcohols, simple ions (e.g., caustics), and charcoal are ineffective when used. g. iron, lithium, cyanide, and other metals). Five to ten times the amount of the suspected toxin consumed is the recommended dosage. However, the usual dose is 1 to 2 g/kg, or roughly 10 to 25 g for children under 5 years old and 50 to 100 g for older children and adults, because the amount of toxin ingested is usually unknown. Charcoal is administered as a slurry in soft drinks or water. Up to 30% of patients report vomiting as a result of it being unpalatable. Administration through a gastric tube may be explored, but care should be taken to avoid trauma from tube insertion or charcoal aspiration; advantages must exceed disadvantages. It is probably best to use activated charcoal without sorbitol or other cathartics, as they have no discernible advantages and may lead to electrolyte imbalances and dehydration.

3.1.4. Effects of Poisoning

The effects of poisoning range from mild to severe. Some cases are fatal. How poisoning affects you depends on many factors, including:

- **The amount that enters your body.** Too much of anything can be poisonous. Even oxygen, in high concentrations, can make you sick. The more toxic something is, the less it takes to make you sick or harm you. Poisons are generally more dangerous in larger quantities.
- **The type of poison.** Certain types of poison cause mild symptoms that go away with at-home care. Other substances are more likely to cause severe illness.
- **How it enters your body.** Poisons can enter your body through your skin, mouth, nose or eyes. Swallowing a toxic substance (like a household cleaner) often causes more harm than touching it with your skin.
- **How long you are exposed to it.** A poisoning can be either acute or chronic. An acute exposure might just be seconds or minutes. A chronic exposure involves long-term exposure to a poison. Chronic exposures often happen on the job, especially in mining, factory settings or agriculture.
- **How soon you get treatment.** Quick treatment may limit or stop the effects of poisoning entirely.
- **Factors unrelated to the poison itself, like your age and overall health.** Poisons affect children differently than adults. Children are smaller, so a dose that wouldn't harm you could be deadly to them. People with underlying medical conditions might also get sicker from poisons or have a harder time recovering.

Depending on these factors, healthcare providers may be able to treat poisoning and prevent lasting effects. More serious cases may lead to hospitalization, long-term treatment or permanent disabilities or injuries.

3.1.5. Gastric Emptying

Despite its intuitive benefits and former widespread acceptance, gastric emptying should not be performed on a regular basis. It carries hazards and does not demonstrably lower overall morbidity or mortality. If a potentially fatal ingestion can be completed within an hour, gastric emptying is taken into consideration.

Nevertheless, a lot of poisonings appear too late, and it's not always obvious if a poisoning poses a threat to life. Gastric emptying is, therefore, rarely recommended and should not be done if a caustic substance has been consumed. Gastric lavage is the recommended technique if gastric emptying is used. Aspiration, epistaxis, and infrequently oropharyngeal or esophageal injury are among the complications that can arise from gastric lavage. Ipecac syrup is not always effective, frequently results in prolonged vomiting, and may not effectively clear the stomach of significant amounts of poison. Ipecac syrup might be necessary if the ingested substance is extremely toxic and the emergency department's transport time is exceptionally long, but this is not common in the US. A tube is used to inject and remove tap water from the stomach during gastric lavage. Tablet fragments are retrieved using the largest tube that is practical (typically 24 French for children, > 36 French for adults). To avoid aspiration, tracheal intubation should be performed prior to lavage in patients with altered consciousness or a weak gag reflex. The tube is inserted orally, and patients are positioned in the left lateral decubitus position to prevent aspiration. Stomach contents should be aspirated and a 25-g dose of charcoal should be instilled through the tube right away after insertion because lavage can occasionally push substances further into the gastrointestinal (GI) tract. The stomach contents are then removed using a syringe or gravity after aliquots of tap water (roughly 3 mL/kg) are injected. 500 to 3000 mL of fluid must typically be infused during lavage, which continues until the withdrawn fluids seem free of the material. A second dose of 25 g of charcoal is injected after lavage.

3.1.5.1. Whole-Bowel Irrigation

This procedure flushes the GI tract and theoretically decreases GI transit time for pills and tablets. Irrigation has not been proved to reduce morbidity or mortality. Irrigation is indicated for any of the following:

- Some serious poisonings due to sustained-release preparations or substances that are not adsorbed by charcoal (e.g., heavy metals)
- Drug packets (e.g., latex-coated packets of heroin or cocaine ingested by body packers)
- A suspected bezoar

A commercially prepared solution of polyethylene glycol (which is nonabsorbable) and electrolytes, as sometimes used to cleanse the bowel for colonoscopy, is given at a rate of 1 to 2 L per h for adults or at 25 to 40 mL/kg/h for children until the rectal effluent is clear; this process may require many h or even days. The solution is usually given via a gastric tube, although some motivated patients can drink these large volumes.

3.1.5.2. Alkaline Diuresis

Weak acids are better eliminated by alkaline diuresis (e.g., such as phenobarbital, salicylates). One-liter (5% D/W) of a solution containing three 50-mEq (50 mmol/L) sodium bicarbonate ampules and 20–40 mEq (20–40 mmol/L) potassium can be administered at a rate of 250 mL/h for adults and 2–3 mL/kg/h for children. Potassium needs to be replenished and urine pH is maintained above 8. Although they are rarely dangerous, hypernatremia, alkalemia, and fluid overload can happen. However, individuals with renal insufficiency should not undergo alkaline diuresis.

3.1.5.3. Dialysis

Common toxins that may require dialysis or hemoperfusion include

- Ethylene glycol
- Lithium
- Methanol

- Salicylates
- Theophylline

These treatments are not as effective when the poison is a big, charged (polar) molecule, when it is heavily bound to tissue protein, or when it has a large volume of distribution (fatty tissue, for example). Examples of such substances include digoxin, phencyclidine, phenothiazines, and tricyclic antidepressants. Clinical status and laboratory results are typically used to determine the need for dialysis. Dialysis techniques include hemoperfusion, which more quickly and effectively eliminates some toxins from the body, hemodialysis, peritoneal dialysis, and lipid dialysis, which eliminates lipid-soluble materials from the blood (see Renal Replacement Therapy).

3.1.5.4. Specific Antidotes

In rare cases, heavy metal poisoning can be treated with chelating medications in addition to other medications. Treatments for various cardiac toxins, such as verapamil and bupivacaine, have included the use of high-dose insulin therapy and IV fat emulsions at concentrations of 10% and 20% (Tables 3.1 and 3.2).

Table 3.1. *Common Specific Antidotes*

Toxin	**Antidote**
Acetaminophen	*N*-Acetylcysteine
Anticholinergics	Physostigmine*
Anticoagulants, oral factor Xa inhibitors (apixaban, edoxaban, rivaroxaban)	Andexanet alfa
Benzodiazepines	Flumazenil*
Black widow spider bite	Lactrodectus antivenom
Botulism	Botulinum antitoxin
Beta-blockers	Glucagon IV lipid emulsion
Calcium channel blockers	Calcium IV insulin in high doses with IV glucose IV lipid emulsion
Carbamates	Atropine Pralidoxime chloride
Crotaline snake bites (US)	Crotalinae polyvalent immune Fab (ovine)
Cyanide	Hydroxocobalamin Cyanide antidote kit (includes amyl nitrate, sodium nitrite, and sodium thiosulfate)
Dabigatran	Idarucizumab

Digitalis glycosides (e.g., digoxin, digitoxin, oleander, foxglove)	Digoxin-specific Fab fragments
Ethylene glycol	Fomepizole Ethanol
Heavy metals	Chelating drugs (see table Guidelines for Chelation Therapy)
Ionizing radiation	Potassium iodide
Iron	Deferoxamine
Isoniazid	Pyridoxine (vitamin B6)
Methanol	Fomepizole Ethanol
Methemoglobin-forming agents (e.g., aniline dyes, some local anesthetics, nitrates, nitrites, phenacetin, sulfonamides)	Methylene blue
Methotrexate	Leucovorin (folinic acid) Glucarpidase (carboxypeptidase-G2)
Opioids	Naloxone
Organophosphates	Atropine Pralidoxime
Scorpion envenomation (*Centruroides* sp)	Centruroides immune F(ab')2
Sulfonylurea	Octreotide
Thallium	Prussian blue
Tricyclic antidepressants	Sodium bicarbonate
Unfractionated heparin	Protamine
Valproic acid	L-Carnitine†
Warfarin	Vitamin K Fresh frozen plasma Prothrombin complex concentrate (PCC)
** Use is controversial.*	
† There is limited evidence for the efficacy of L-carnitine as a general antidote for acute valproic acid overdose. However, L-carnitine is likely to be safe and it is reasonable to consider using it in patients with decreased level of consciousness.	
Fab = fractionated antibodies.	

Source: https://www.msdmanuals.com/professional/injuries-poisoning/poisoning/general-principles-of-poisoning#Treatment_v1118317.

Table 3.2. Guidelines for Chelation Therapy

Chelating Drug*	Metal	Dosage†
Deferasirox/deferiprone/deferoxamine	Iron	
Dimercaprol, 10% in oil	Antimony Arsenic Bismuth Copper salts Gold Lead Mercury Thallium*	3–4 mg/kg via deep IM injection every 4 h on day 1; 2 mg/kg IM every 4 h on day 2; 3 mg/kg IM every 6 h on day 3; then 3 mg/kg IM every 12 h for 7–10 days until recovery
Edetate calcium disodium (calcium disodium edathamil) diluted to ≤ 3%	Cobalt Lead Zinc Zinc salts	25–35 mg/kg via deep IM injection or IV slowly (over 1 h) every 12 h for 5–7 days, followed by 7 days without the drug; then repeated
Penicillamine	Arsenic Copper salts Gold Lead	5–7.5 mg/kg orally 4 times a day (the usual starting dose is 250 mg 4 times a day) to a maximum adult dose of 2 g/day
Succimer	Arsenic (occupational exposure in adults) Cadmium salts Lead if children have blood lead levels > 45 mcg/dL (> 2.15 micromol/L) Lead (occupational exposure in adults) Mercury (occupational exposure in adults)	10 mg/kg orally every 8 h for 5 days, then 10 mg/kg orally every 12 h for 14 days

Triethylenetetramine	Copper	Dosing for Wilson disease only‡ 13 years and older: 750 –1250 mg, orally, in divided doses given 2, 3, or 4 times daily; maximum dose: 2000 mg daily 12 and under: 500–750 mg, orally, in divided doses given 2, 3, or 4 times daily; maximum dose: 1500 mg daily
** Thallium salts are chelated with varying success by this drug (see thallium salts in table Symptoms and Treatment of Specific Poisons).*		
† Dosages depend on type and severity of poisoning.		
‡ This chelating agent was approved in 2018 for the treatment of Wilson disease; it was not approved for use in the treatment of exogenous copper intoxication.		

Source: https://www.msdmanuals.com/professional/injuries-poisoning/poisoning/general-principles-of-poisoning#Treatment_v1118317.

3.1.6. Ongoing Supportive Measures

Most signs and symptoms, such as. G. treatments include the standard supportive measures for conditions like agitation, sedation, coma, cerebral edema, hypertension, arrhythmias, renal failure, and hypoglycemia. The standard drug treatments may not be effective in treating drug-induced hypotension and arrhythmias. Extracorporeal circulatory support, an intra-aortic balloon pump, dopamine, epinephrine, and other vasopressors may be considered for refractory hypotension. Cardiac pacing might be required for refractory arrhythmias. Torsades de pointes can frequently be managed with titrated isoproterenol infusion, overdrive pacing, or 2 to 4 g of magnesium sulfate intravenously. First, benzodiazepines are used to treat seizures. When benzodiazepines are not working, phenobarbital and propofol have been used. It is necessary to manage severe agitation; high doses of benzodiazepines, other strong sedatives (e.g., propofol), or, in severe situations, the need for mechanical ventilation and paralysis induction. Instead of using antipyretics to treat hyperthermia, physical cooling techniques, and strong sedation are used. Liver or kidney transplantation may eventually be necessary due to organ failure.

3.1.6.1. Hospital Admission

Predicted delayed toxicity, persistently abnormal vital signs, and altered consciousness are general indications for hospital admission. For instance, patients who have consumed sustained-release preparations—especially those containing medications with potentially dangerous side effects—are given consideration for admission (e.g., cardiovascular medications). Most patients can be released if there are no additional reasons for admission, if the results of any indicated laboratory tests are normal, and if the symptoms go away after the patient has been monitored for 4 to 6 h. If ingestion was deliberate, patients need to be evaluated psychiatrically.

3.1.7. Prevention of Poisoning

The number of poisoning deaths in children under five years old has significantly decreased in the US thanks to the widespread use of child-resistant containers with safety caps. The severity of poisonings can be decreased by limiting the quantity of OTC analgesics in a single container and getting rid of redundant and confusing formulations, especially when it comes to acetaminophen, aspirin, or ibuprofen.

Other preventive measures include

- Clearly labeling household products and prescription drugs
- Storing drugs and toxic substances in cabinets that are locked and inaccessible to children
- Promptly disposing of expired drugs by mixing them in cat litter or some other non-tempting substance and putting them in a trash container that is inaccessible to children
- Using carbon monoxide detectors
- Refraining from prescribing opioids and using nonopioid treatments whenever possible

Public education campaigns to promote keeping drugs in their original containers (e.g., not putting pesticides in drinking containers) are crucial. Patients, pharmacists, and medical professionals can avoid confusion and mistakes by using imprint identifications on solid medications.

3.1.8. Acetaminophen Poisoning

Hepatotoxicity can develop one to three days after ingestion of acetaminophen poisoning, and gastroenteritis can occur within hours. Serum acetaminophen levels indicate the severity of hepatotoxicity following a single acute overdose. To avoid or reduce hepatotoxicity, N-acetylcysteine is the recommended treatment. More than 100 OTC medications contain acetaminophen, also known as N-acetyl-para-aminophenol or APAP. Many liquid, tablet, and capsule formulations for children as well as numerous cough and cold remedies are among the products. Acetaminophen is also a common ingredient in prescription drugs, which means that overdosing on acetaminophen is frequent.

3.1.8.1. Pathophysiology of Acetaminophen Poisoning

The hepatic cytochrome P-450 enzyme system produces the main toxic metabolite of acetaminophen, N-acetyl-p-benzoquinone imine (NAPQI), which is detoxified by the liver's glutathione stores. The liver's glutathione stores are depleted during an acute overdose. Consequently, NAPQI builds up, leading to hepatocellular necrosis and potentially harming other organs (e.g., pancreas, kidneys, etc.). Theoretically, hepatic enzyme preconditioning may increase the formation of NAPQI, and undernutrition—which is also common in alcoholics—reduces hepatic glutathione stores, which could increase the risk of toxicity. Therapeutic acetaminophen dosages in alcoholics, however, are not linked to liver damage. To cause toxicity, an acute oral overdose must total ≥ 150 mg/kg (about 7.5 g in adults) within 24 h.

- *IV acetaminophen:* A hospital-grade IV acetaminophen formulation intended for use in patients older than two years old has been linked to several hundred reports of overdoses, including a number of fatalities, including several in children. Because the medication is dosed in milligrams but dispensed in milliliters, the majority of these adverse events were the consequence of dosing errors. Since these overdoses are iatrogenic, trustworthy data on the duration and total dosage is accessible. Thus, the Rumack-Matthew nomogram has proven to be an effective tool for toxicity prediction. Toxic effects are unlikely to occur from overdoses of <150 mg/kg. It has not yet been determined how to treat an IV acetaminophen overdose, but speaking with a toxicologist or a poison control center is advised.

3.1.8.2. Symptoms and Signs of Acetaminophen Poisoning

Acute acetaminophen poisoning symptoms are typically mild until 48 h after ingestion, and mild poisoning may not cause any at all. There are four stages to acute acetaminophen poisoning symptoms, which include anorexia, nausea, vomiting, and abdominal pain in the right upper quadrant. Pancreatitis and renal failure can happen, sometimes even in the absence of liver failure. Hepatotoxicity resolves or advances to multiple organ failure, which can be lethal, after more than 5 days (Table 3.3.).

Table 3.3. Stages of Acute Acetaminophen Poisoning

Stage	Time Post Ingestion	Description
I	0–24 h	Anorexia, nausea, vomiting
II	24–72 h	Right upper quadrant abdominal pain (common)
		AST, ALT, and, if poisoning is severe, bilirubin and PT (usually reported as the INR) sometimes elevated
III	72–96 h	Vomiting and symptoms of liver failure
		Peaking of AST, ALT, bilirubin, and INR
		Sometimes renal failure and pancreatitis
IV	> 5 days	Resolution of hepatotoxicity or progression to multiple organ failure (sometimes fatal)
AST = aspartate aminotransferase; ALT = alanine aminotransferase; INR = international normalized ratio; PT = prothrombin time.		

Source: https://www.msdmanuals.com/professional/injuries-poisoning/poisoning/acetaminophen-poisoning#Symptoms-and-Signs_v8343411.

3.1.8.3. Diagnosis of Acetaminophen Poisoning

- Serum acetaminophen levels
- Rumack-Matthew nomogram

All patients with non-accidental ingestions of acetaminophen that might be suicide attempts, as well as children who have ingested the drug, should be evaluated for acetaminophen overdose because these overdoses often involve formulations containing the drug and are not reported. Additionally, acetaminophen ingestion should be taken into consideration for all patients who have inadvertently consumed the drug because it frequently exhibits minimal symptoms in the early stages and is both treatable and potentially fatal. Acetaminophen levels in the serum or, more precisely, the amount consumed can be used to predict the likelihood and severity of hepatotoxicity resulting from an acute ingestion. The Rumack-Matthew nomogram is used to estimate the likelihood of hepatotoxicity if the time of acute ingestion is known; if the time of acute ingestion is unknown, the nomogram cannot be used. The levels of a single acute overdose of either traditional or rapid-relief acetaminophen (which is absorbed seven to eight minutes faster) are measured and plotted on the nomogram no later than 4 h after ingestion. The absence of toxic symptoms and a level ≤ 150 mcg/mL (≤ 990 micromol/L) suggest a very low likelihood of hepatotoxicity. Elevated concentrations may suggest hepatotoxicity. Acetaminophen levels are measured 4 h after ingestion and 4 h later for a single acute overdose with extended-relief acetaminophen (which has two peak serum levels approximately 4 h apart); if either level is above the Rumack-Matthew line of toxicity, treatment is necessary. In order to determine risk, the worst-case scenario is used if the precise moment of a single ingestion cannot be verified. Put another way, the Rumack-Matthew nomogram is used to plot the earliest possible time of ingestion. For instance, 6 PM is used as the time of ingestion (worst case) if a patient reports that the overdose was taken between 6 and 9 PM. Similarly, an acetaminophen level drawn at presentation would be interpreted as a 24-h level if the child resided in a home without acetaminophen products but had spent the previous 24 h visiting a relative whose home did have such products. In real life, determining worst-case estimates is often challenging.

Further testing is recommended if poisoning is proven or highly suspected, or if the exact time of ingestion is uncertain. Prothrombin time is measured when there is a suspicion of severe poisoning, and liver tests are performed. The stages of acute acetaminophen poisoning are indicated in the table by the results of aspartate aminotransferase (AST) and alanine aminotransferase (ALT). Acetaminophen poisoning is more likely to cause AST levels greater than 1000 IU/L than chronic hepatitis or alcoholic liver disease. Severe poisoning may result in elevated bilirubin and the international normalized ratio. Elevations of low-level transaminase (e.g., adults receiving therapeutic doses of acetaminophen for days or weeks may experience side effects (up to two or three times the upper limit of normal). Even with continued acetaminophen use, these elevations seem to be temporary, resolve or diminish within a few days, are typically clinically asymptomatic, and are most likely insignificant. New biomarkers for acetaminophen-induced hepatotoxicity have been developed and marketed: acetaminophen/cysteine protein adducts. The biomarkers may show acetaminophen exposure, but they do not prove that acetaminophen causes hepatotoxicity. While they are being studied, additional biomarkers like keratin-18, high-mobility group box-1 (HMGB-1), and microRNA are not considered conventional diagnostic instruments.

3.1.8.4. Prognosis for Acetaminophen Poisoning

With appropriate treatment, mortality is uncommon.

Poor prognostic indicators at 24 to 48 h postingestion include all of the following:

- pH < 7.3 after adequate resuscitation
- International normalized ratio (INR) > 3
- Serum creatinine > 2.6
- Hepatic encephalopathy grade III (confusion and somnolence) or grade IV (stupor and coma)
- Hypoglycemia

- Thrombocytopenia

Acute acetaminophen toxicity does not predispose patients to cirrhosis.

3.1.8.5. Treatment of Acetaminophen Poisoning

- Oral or IV N-acetylcysteine
- Possibly activated charcoal

If acetaminophen is likely to remain in the gastrointestinal (GI) tract, activated charcoal may be administered. Acetaminophen poisoning has an antidote in the form of N-acetylcysteine. This medication, a glutathione precursor, increases hepatic glutathione stores and may have additional mechanisms of action to reduce acetaminophen toxicity. It helps prevent hepatic toxicity by deactivating the harmful acetaminophen metabolite NAPQI (N-acetyl-p-benzoquinone imine) before it can harm liver cells. It does not, however, repair liver cell damage that has already taken place. If the dose or serum level of acetaminophen indicates a high likelihood of hepatotoxicity, N-acetylcysteine is administered for acute poisoning. The medication works best when taken within 8 h of acetaminophen consumption. Even though the antidote's effectiveness is questionable after 24 h, it should still be administered. Acetylcysteine should be administered until toxicity is ruled out if the degree of toxicity is unknown. Giving N-acetylcysteine intravenously (IV) or orally has no effect. An IV infusion is administered continuously. Following a loading dose of 150 mg/kg in 200 mL of 5% D/W administered over 15 min, maintenance doses of 50 mg/kg in 500 mL of 5% D/W administered over 4 h and 100 mg/kg in 1000 mL of 5% D/W administered over 16 h are administered. In order to reduce the overall amount of fluid given to children, dosage adjustments may be necessary; speaking with a poison control center is advised.

N-acetylcysteine has an oral loading dose of 140 mg/kg. Seventeen additional doses of 70 mg/kg are administered every 4 h after this one. Even when taken in a diluted 1:4 ratio in fruit juice or carbonated drinks, oral acetylcysteine is not pleasant and can still induce vomiting. An antiemetic can be used if vomiting happens within an hour after taking a dose, the dose should be repeated. On the other hand, vomiting could be prolonged and restrict oral use. Although uncommon, allergic reactions have happened when using IV and oral medications. Supportive care is given for liver failure. Individuals who suffer from advanced liver failure might need to have a liver transplant. Patients who consume more than 50 grams of acetaminophen in a single dose may exhibit severe metabolic acidosis, fatigue, unconsciousness, and hyperglycemia 4 h after consumption. The precise process is not known. Case studies detail effective therapy using an N-acetylcysteine infusion that is continued until there is no longer any acetaminophen in the patient's serum. It has been reported that both continuous venovenous hemodialysis and intermittent hemodialysis can effectively treat massive acetaminophen ingestion. It is advised to speak with a toxicologist or poison control center.

3.1.8.6. Chronic Acetaminophen Poisoning

Hepatotoxicity is caused in a small number of patients by repeated overdoses or chronic excessive use. Chronic overdoses are typically the result of taking excessively high doses of medication to treat pain rather than an attempt at self-harm. The symptoms could be any of the ones associated with an acute overdose, or they could be nonexistent.

1. Diagnosis

- Serum levels of AST, ALT, and acetaminophen levels

- The Rumack-Matthew nomogram cannot be used, but the likelihood of clinically significant hepatotoxicity can be estimated based on AST, ALT, and serum acetaminophen levels.
- If AST and ALT levels are normal (< 50 IU/L [0.83 microkat/L]), and the acetaminophen level is < 10 mcg/mL (< 66 micromol/L), significant hepatotoxicity is very unlikely.
- If AST and ALT levels are normal but the acetaminophen level is ≥ 10 mcg/mL (≥ 66 micromol/L), significant hepatotoxicity is possible; AST and ALT levels are remeasured after 24 h. If repeat AST and ALT levels are normal, significant hepatotoxicity is unlikely; if the levels are high, significant hepatotoxicity is assumed.
- If initial AST and ALT levels are high, regardless of the acetaminophen level, significant hepatotoxicity is assumed.

2. Treatment

- Sometimes *N*-acetylcysteine

Uncertainty surrounds the use of N-acetylcysteine in the management of acute hepatotoxicity or chronic acetaminophen toxicity. Theoretically, if residual (unmetabolized) acetaminophen is present, administering the antidote more than 24 h after ingestion may be beneficial. The following approach has not been proven effective but may be used:

- When acetaminophen is initially elevated and AST and ALT levels are normal, hepatotoxicity may occur. In these cases, N-acetylcysteine is administered orally as a loading dose of 140 mg/kg and then every 4 h for the first 24 h. N-acetylcysteine is discontinued if repeat AST and ALT levels (after 24 h) are normal; if repeat levels are high, they are remeasured every day, and acetylcysteine is continued until levels are normal.
- If hepatotoxicity is likely (especially if initial AST and ALT levels are high), a full course of acetylcysteine is given (i.e., loading dose as above, then 70 mg/kg every 4 h for 17 doses).

Prognostic factors are similar to those in acute acetaminophen poisoning.

3.2. Clinical Approach to Poisoned Patients

Like a Rod of Asclepius, the concepts of medical toxicology and critical care medicine are entwined. This evidence dates back to the Middle Ages, as documented in Moses Maimonides' Treatise on Poison and Their Antidotes, written in the late 12th century. When treating patients who have been poisoned, intensive care doctors should use a methodical approach to assessment and treatment. A wide range of symptoms and clinical findings can result from accidental or deliberate poisoning from both legal and illegal substances. Therefore, identifying the patient who has been poisoned greatly depends on their history and physical examination. Acute stabilization and supportive care should be the main goals of initial management until the right substance is found. The management strategy calls for the provision of supportive care, the avoidance of poison absorption, the use of antidotes when necessary, and the improvement of elimination methods.

3.2.1. Initial Assessment

Resuscitation is the first priority in treating an unstable or critically ill patient (ABC:

airway, breathing, circulation). Apart from performing resuscitation, intensivists need to take into account two vital concerns that might surface in cases of patients with severe poisoning: maintaining the ability to operate and guaranteeing the security of medical personnel. Diagnostic testing and treatment interventions are frequently started at the same time in poisoned patients.

3.2.1.1. Risk Assessment

After the initial stabilization and resuscitation, a risk assessment is carried out to forecast the patient's course, the necessary interventions, and the course of clinical toxicity. Results from ancillary tests, the examination, and the history are used to formulate it. By collecting data based on substances or systems, the likelihood of a patient being poisoned can be evaluated. Toxic syndromes are distinct sets of symptoms and indicators caused by substances that belong to a specific class of toxin (toxidromes). The physical examination focused on toxidrome may provide important information about the type of toxin in question. Table 3.4 provides a summary of the main toxidromes and the research findings related to them.

Table 3.4. Common Toxidromes

Toxidromes	***Mental status***	***Pupils***	***Vitals***	***Other manifestations***	***Examples of toxic agents***
Sympathomimetic	Hyper alert, agitation, hallucination, paranoia	Mydriasis	Hyperthermia, tachycardia, hypertension, widened pulse pressure	Diaphoresis, tremors, hyperreflexia, seizures	Cocaine, amphetamines, ephedrine, theophylline, caffeine
Anticholinergic	Agitation, hallucinations, delirium, coma	Mydriasis	Hyperthermia, tachycardia, hypertension, tachypnea	Dry flush skin, dry mucous membranes, decreased bowel sounds, urinary retention, myoclonus	Antihistamines, TCA, anti-Parkinsonism agents, atropine, antispasmodics
Hallucinogenic	Hallucinations, perceptual distortions, depersonalization, agitation	Mydriasis (usually)	Hyperthermia, tachycardia, hypertension, tachypnea	Nystagmus	Phencyclidine, MDMA, MDEA
Opioid	CNS depression, coma	Miosis	Bradypnea, apnea	Hyporeflexia, pulmonary edema, needle marks	Heroin, morphine, methadone, diphenoxylate
Sedative-hypnotic	CNS depression, confusion, stupor, coma	Variable	Often normal; hypothermia, bradycardia, hypotension, bradypnea, apnea	Hyporeflexia	Benzodiazepines, barbiturates, alcohols, zolpidem

Cholinergic	Confusion, coma	Miosis	Bradycardia, hypertension, tachypnea, hypotension, bradypnea	Salivation, urinary and fecal incontinence, diarrhea, emesis, diaphoresis, lacrimation, GI cramps, bronchoconstriction, muscle fasciculations and weakness, seizures	Organophosphate and carbamate insecticides, nerve agents, nicotine, physostigmine, edrophonium
Serotonin syndrome	Confusion, agitation, coma	Mydriasis	Hyperthermia, tachycardia, hypertension, tachypnea	Tremors, myoclonus, hyperreflexia, clonus, diaphoresis, flushing, trismus, rigidity, diarrhea	MAOIs, SSRIs, meperidine, dextromethorphan, TCA

TCA, tricyclic antidepressant; MDMA, 3,4-methylenedioxymethamphetamine; MDEA, methylenedioxymethamphetamine; CNS, central nervous system; GI, gastrointestinal; MAOI, monoamine oxidase inhibitor; SSRI, selective serotonin reuptake inhibitor

Source: https://www.ncbi.nlm.nih.gov/pmc/articles/PMC6996652/#:~:text=The%20first%20step%20is%20to,exact%20poison%20agent%20is%20known.

3.2.1.2. Diagnostic Testing

Though toxidromes are created to assist diagnosis, a particular patient may not have all the symptoms associated with a given toxidrome; always some discrepancies are noted after the examination of a poisoned patient. History may be inaccurate and hence, the following laboratory tests should usually be obtained:

- Complete blood count
- Basic serum electrolytes, BUN, and creatinine
- Liver function test
- Serum lactate
- Arterial blood gas
- Electrocardiogram
- Urine pregnancy test in all women of childbearing age

Measurement of drug or toxin concentrations in body fluids is not required in most poisonings, but in some exposures, it does influence management. The list of drug concentrations that may assist patient assessment and management is shown in Table 3.5.

Table 3.5. *Commonly Measured Drug Concentrations*

Acetaminophen	Methanol
Carbamazepine	Methotrexate
Carbon monoxide	Organophosphorus
Digoxin	Paraquat
Ethanol	Phenobarbital

Ethylene glycol	Phenytoin
Iron	Salicylate
Lithium	Theophylline
Methemoglobin	Valproic acid

Source: https://www.ncbi.nlm.nih.gov/pmc/articles/PMC6996652/#:~:text=The%20first%20step%20is%20to,exact%20poison%20agent%20is%20known.

Commercially available toxicology screening assays often do not directly impact patient management and come with their own set of limitations. Most tests utilize enzyme immunoassays which can detect only common drugs within a particular class. The timing of these screenings is a significant concern as drugs may take some time to show up in the results, potentially leading to a discrepancy between the test outcome and the patient's clinical status. Cross-reactivity among different drug groups is common, and a negative test result does not necessarily rule out an exposure. Sampling error is also a major issue. Despite these limitations, toxicology screenings can be useful for medicolegal purposes. More comprehensive qualitative toxic screenings, using liquid and gas chromatography and mass spectrometry, offer a more thorough analysis of urine, blood, and other bodily fluids.

3.2.2. Supportive Care

3.2.2.1. Airway Management

The need to secure the airway is determined by the absence of reflexes that protect the airway, as well as by concerns about aspiration or respiratory failure. The best way to secure the airway is to use rapid sequence intubation (RSI) along with preoxygenation and neuromuscular blockade, unless the patient is in a moribund state. The procedure that should be used is tracheal intubation. However, alternatives to RSI should be taken into consideration, either because preoxygenation cannot be provided to the patient sufficiently or because there are worries that the patient might be difficult to intubate. An alternative to rapid sequence intubation (RSI) is delayed sequence intubation (DSI). It involves giving sedatives that don't impair breathing reflexes, waiting a short while to preoxygenate, and then giving paralytics. For numerous reasons, orotracheal intubation is favored over nasotracheal intubation whenever it is feasible. Technically more challenging than orotracheal intubation, nasopharyngeal intubation raises the risk of sinusitis, purulent and serous otitis, and ventilator-associated pneumonia. There needs to be an emergency plan in place for maintaining the airway as well as a way to create a surgical airway (cricothyrotomy) if needed.

3.2.2.2. Respiratory Support

Numerous toxins obstruct ventilation and oxygenation. Therefore, as soon as the airway is secured, the adequacy of respiration needs to be evaluated. It is important to use a lung protective strategy when choosing the ventilator settings. Lung protective techniques stop oxygen toxicity and barotrauma from causing ARDS. Although frequently employed in the intensive care unit, these tactics have not been examined in patients who have been poisoned.

3.2.2.3. Circulation and Hemodynamics

Assessing the circulatory status comes first, followed by opening the airway and sustaining respiratory function. Cardiovascular abnormalities such as hypertension, hypotension, cardiac arrhythmias, or conduction disturbances are frequently observed in poisoned patients. The poisoned patient may or may not have elevated blood pressure as a result of exposure to any one of several substances. Of these, the most frequent causes of high blood pressure are benzodiazepine or ethanol withdrawal, stopping a medicine that has been therapeutically prescribed and causing rebound hypertension, and untreated or insufficiently treated underlying hypertension. The underlying cause of hypertension dictates how it should be treated. Direct vasodilators like phentolamine or nitroprusside should be taken into consideration when hypertension is brought on by overdosing on medications with direct adrenergic activity, such as amphetamines, ephedrine, or pseudoephedrine. 16 Benzodiazepines should be used for sedation when drugs with indirect adrenergic activity or drug abuse withdrawal are the cause of hypertension. Hemoglobin abnormalities (i.e., methemoglobin, sulfhemoglobin, or carboxyhemoglobin) and poisons that interfere with the electron transport chain within the mitochondria (e.g., sodium azide, hydrogen sulfide, or cyanide) inhibit the molecule's ability to use oxygen, causing histotoxic hypoxia and shock. One common indicator of these toxicities is elevated plasma lactate concentration, which occurs in conjunction with a metabolic acidosis. 21Impaired cardiac contractility can result in shock due to myocardial depression, dysrhythmias, and conduction abnormalities. All poisoned patients should have an ECG to check for any cardiac abnormalities (Table 3.6), as these could provide information about the poison, the degree of poisoning, and the course of treatment.

Table 3.6. Toxins Causing Dysrhythmias

Heart rate	*Narrow QRS*	*Wide QRS*
Tachycardia	Amphetamines	Antihistamines
	Anticholinergic agents	Cocaine
	Theophylline	Propoxyphene
		Sodium channel blockers
		Tricyclic antidepressants
Bradycardia	α-Adrenergic lytic agents	β-Adrenergic blocking agents
	β-Adrenergic blocking agents	Calcium channel antagonists
	Calcium channel antagonists	
	Cardiac glycosides	
	Class Ia antiarrhythmics	
	Sodium channel blockers	

Source: https://www.ncbi.nlm.nih.gov/pmc/articles/PMC6996652/#:~:text=The%20first%20step%20is%20to,exact%20poison%20agent%20is%20known.

The patient who has been poisoned requires customized fluid resuscitation. When necessary, intravenous crystalloid fluid is administered as part of the initial resuscitation process. Vasopressor infusion should begin as soon as feasible. It is more appropriate to administer vasopressors or inotropes (noradrenaline) in a distributive shock or cardiogenic shock rather than just fluids. In order to better direct resuscitation, bedside sonography can be used to assess cardiac contractility and determine volume responsiveness. The best vasopressor drugs for poisoned patients are not well understood. Because of this, the choice of vasopressor needs to be based on the clinical and patient profiles. Calcium channel antagonists and β-adrenergic blocking agents can cause shock, but nonadrenergic vasoactive medications are a useful treatment. The pancreatic alpha cells secrete the peptide hormone glucagon, which activates adenyl cyclase. This process raises intracellular cyclic adenosine monophosphate (cAMP) via a nonadrenergic pathway. Positive chronotropic and inotropic effects result from an increase in intracellular calcium brought on by this rise in cAMP. Glucagon has been shown in numerous case reports and laboratory studies to be effective in reversing hypotension brought on by overdosing on β-adrenergic blocking agents and calcium channel antagonists. A glucagon infusion (3–15 mg/h) should come after an intravenous dose of 5–10 mg of glucagon given over a 10-minute period. Glucagon should be given with an antiemetic since it lowers esophageal tone, which results in emesis. Recently, the toxicity of calcium channel antagonists and β-adrenergic blocking agents has been treated with high-dose insulin euglycemia (HIE) therapy. The reduction in insulin release from pancreatic β-cells, which results in insulin resistance in the heart, and modifications in myocyte metabolism from fatty acids to carbohydrates are the pathophysiology of calcium channel antagonist toxicity. Increased cardiac contractility and improved perfusion are the results of high-dose insulin euglycemia therapy, which also enhances myocyte utilization of carbohydrates as an energy source.

One of the most recent developments in the treatment of critically ill poisoned patients is lipid emulsion therapy (LET). Patients with local anesthetic toxicity received treatment with it. It has also been applied to the control of toxicity resulting from different poisonings. LET has been shown in numerous reports to reverse the toxicity of anticonvulsants, benzodiazepines, calcium channel antagonists, tricyclic antidepressants, and β-adrenergic blocking agents. When traditional treatment is ineffective for poisoned patients in refractory shock, extracorporeal membrane oxygenation (ECMO) may be necessary. When a patient is poisoned, ECMO acts as a stopgap measure until the toxins are broken down or removed, at which point their heart should return to normal. Even though ECMO is more expensive and has more side effects, recent technological advancements have made it a more sensible option for patients experiencing refractory shock.

3.2.3. Decontamination

3.2.3.1. Gastrointestinal Decontamination

Once a cornerstone in the treatment of the poisoning, gastrointestinal (GI) decontamination is no longer advised. When a patient presents very early (less than an hour after ingestion) or after taking a very large or dangerous overdose for which there is no known antidote, it is typically taken into consideration. Although GI decontamination should ideally reduce the absorption of numerous ingested toxins, its application is not linked to better results (e.g., death, duration of stay). In the emergency department, GI decontamination should be attempted as soon as possible. If decontamination is initiated in the ICU, there is very little chance that the patient will benefit from it.

3.2.3.2. Activated Charcoal

One decontaminant that is frequently used is activated charcoal. It is made in two steps:

first, different carbonaceous materials are pyrolyzed, and then, at high temperatures, oxidizing agents like steam or carbon dioxide are added to "activate" the material and boost its adsorptive capacity. Toxins in the GI lumen are limited in their absorption by being adsorbed onto activated charcoal and transported through the GI tract. Alcohols, corrosives, and metals are not effectively absorbed by it. Giving activated charcoal to a patient is not a routine management decision; rather, it necessitates a risk assessment for each individual patient.

3.2.3.3. Whole Bowel Irrigation

Another method of decontamination is whole bowel irrigation (WBI), which increases the flow of toxins through the digestive tract. A nasogastric or orogastric tube can be inserted, and large doses of osmotically balanced polyethylene glycol solution (PEG) can be given hourly—1–2 L—until the patient passes at least two clear, liquid stools. WBI can be initiated or continued in the ICU, in contrast to other GI decontamination methods. WBI is the conventional treatment for body packers. Those who consume large quantities of illicit drug packets in order to transport them illegally are known as body packers. Lethal dosages of the medication may unintentionally leak into the body packers' system, posing a serious risk to their lives. Given the potentially fatal risk involved in even one packet leak, WBI should therefore be started in order to eliminate the packets as soon as possible. Patients with an ileus, obstruction, or GI tract injury are considered contraindications.

3.2.4. Elimination

3.2.4.1. Multidose Activated Charcoal

Activated charcoal with multiple doses (MDAC) is used to improve the removal of different ingested toxins. Patients who are susceptible to delayed absorption as a result of consuming delayed-release products may find benefit from multidose activated charcoal. MDAC may also be beneficial for patients who consume toxins that circulate through the enteroenteric or enterohepatic pathways. A chemical that has been absorbed is secreted into the bile, the small intestine, and finally back into the body during enterohepatic circulation. Absorbable materials are secreted into the intestine during enteroenteric circulation and then reabsorbed. Charcoal can help with elimination by adsorbing toxins secreted into the intestine that aren't reabsorbed by giving MDAC. After the first standard dose of charcoal, multidose activated charcoal is typically given at a dose of 0.5 g/kg.

3.2.4.2. Urine Alkalinization

Acidotic drugs are more likely to ionize in alkaline urine, which enhances urine elimination by blocking the drug's resorption through the renal tubular epithelium. Strong acids such as salicylate and phenobarbital toxicities respond best to urine alkalinization. Urine alkalinization is contraindicated in patients with fluid overload, hypokalemia, and renal impairment.

- Correct any existing hypokalemia.
- Administer 1–2 mEq/kg IV sodium bicarbonate bolus.
- Infuse 100 mEq of sodium bicarbonate mixed with 1 L of D5W at 250 mL/h.
- A total of 20 mEq of potassium chloride may be added to maintain normokalemia.
- Check urine pH (every 15–30 minutes), aiming for a pH of 7.5–8.5.
- A further IV bolus of sodium bicarbonate may be warranted if sufficient alkalinization of the urine is not reached.

3.2.4.3. Extracorporeal Removal

Hemodialysis, hemofiltration, and continuous renal replacement therapies are examples of extracorporeal removal techniques with limited applications in poisoning patients. In order for an extracorporeal method to remove a toxin effectively, it needs to have a low molecular weight, low volume of distribution (VD < 1 L/kg), low protein-binding capacity, and low endogenous clearance. Figure 3.1 depicts the choice to employ the extracorporeal technique.

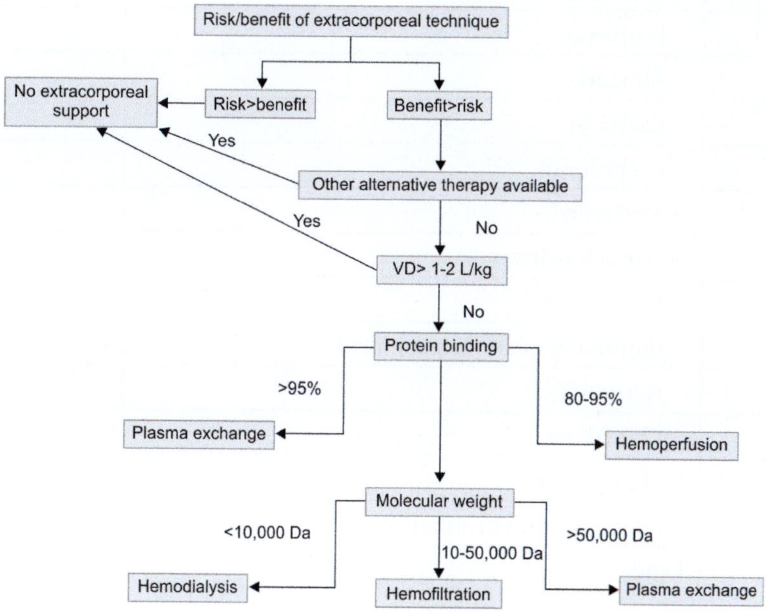

Figure 3.1. *Decision tree for usage of extracorporeal removal of toxins.*

Source: https://www.ncbi.nlm.nih.gov/pmc/articles/PMC6996652/bin/ijccm-23-S234-g001.jpg.

3.2.5. Antidotes

Most poisoned patients can be treated with standard supportive care. But in a few circumstances, specific therapy or antidotes are required. The list of antidotes of common poisonings given in the National Poisons Information Centre (NPIC), which is an integral part of National Poison Control Programme, is shown in Table 3.7.

Table 3.7. *Antidotes for Some Poisons*

Group	*Poisons*	*Antidote*
Agricultural pesticides	Organophosphates	
	Malathion	
	Acephate	
	Dichlorvos	
	Dimethoate	

	Fenitrothion	Atropine sulfate
	Monocrotophos	
	Phorate	
	Quinalphos	Pralidoxime
	Carbamates	
	Propoxur	
	Aldicarb	
	Carbaryl	
	Carbofuran	
	Methomyl	
	Organochlorines	
	Endosulfan	
	Gamma benzene hexachloride	Cholestyramine
	Heptachlor	
	Chlordane	
	Rodenticides	
	Cholestyramine bromadiolone	Vitamin K
Industrial chemicals	Lead	Dimercaprol
		D-Penicillamine
		Calcium disodium edetate
	Mercury	Dimercaprol
		Dimercaptosuccinic acid
		D-Penicillamine
	Arsenic	Dimercaprol
		D-Penicillamine
	Methyl alcohol	Ethanol
		Folic acid/folinic acid
	Ethylene glycol	Ethanol
		Pyridoxine hydrochloride
		Folic acid
		Thiamine
	Cyanide	Amyl nitrite, sodium nitrite

		Sodium thiosulfate(cyanide antidote kit)
		Hydroxocobalamin
		Dicobalt edetate
	Methemoglobinemia producing agents (nitrites, nitrates, dapsone, copper, aniline, chlorates, naphthalene)	Methylene blue
Drugs	Acetaminophen	*N*-Acetylcysteine
	Iron	Deferoxamine
	Benzodiazepines	Flumazenil
	Opioids	Naloxone
	Isoniazid	Pyridoxine
	Digoxin	Digoxin-specific antibodies
Environmental toxins	Datura	Physostigmine
	Snake bites	Anti-snake venom
	Dog bite	Anti-rabies vaccine
	Botulism	Botulinum antitoxin

Source: https://www.ncbi.nlm.nih.gov/pmc/articles/PMC6996652/#:~:text=The%20first%20step%20is%20to,exact%20poison%20agent%20is%20known.

3.2.6. Ancillary Support

Critically ill poisoned patients are at increased risk of GI bleeding. In the ICU, 75% of the poisoned patients have endoscopic evidence of gastric mucosal injury by 18 h after admission, with 5% of patients developing overt bleeding. Gastrointestinal bleeding prophylaxis should be started on admission to the ICU and can be achieved best through the use of histamine 2-receptor antagonists or proton-pump inhibitors.

Poisoned ICU patients are at risk for venous thromboembolic disease if they have a prolonged course requiring them to remain in bed. Approximately 33% of all ICU patients develop ultrasonographically detectable deep venous thrombosis (DVT) despite receiving prophylaxis. Meta-analyses show that the use of heparin or pneumatic compression stockings decreases the incidence of DVT by at least 50%. DVT prophylaxis should be initiated with unfractionated heparin, low-molecular-weight heparin, or compression devices as soon as the patient is admitted to the ICU if a prolonged stay is anticipated.

The goal of nutritional support is to meet the patient's nutritional needs without overfeeding. Overfeeding should be avoided because excess carbohydrates can lead to increased carbon dioxide production. Enteral feedings, which help maintain the integrity of the gut mucosal barrier, are preferred over the parenteral route.

3.3. Management of Poisoning and Intoxications

Any number of substances, including medications, can cause poisoning, which can be extremely toxic and even fatal. The nephrologist may be involved in targeted treatments and poisonings that result in kidney disease. The initial acute resuscitation and a risk assessment are the two main steps in treating a poisoned patient. During the risk assessment, the patient's condition, potential treatments, and the expected severity of the exposure are all considered. Interventions that must be completed quickly, like gastrointestinal decontamination (e.g., Antidotes (e.g., activated charcoal) are given when necessary. When methods of improving elimination, like urine alkalinization or extracorporeal therapies, are needed, a nephrologist is typically involved. The amount of data available to inform decisions about extracorporeal treatments for poisoned patients is growing. Clinical indicators, such as whether severe toxicity is present, expected, or will persist, and whether the extracorporeal treatment will significantly remove the poison, are principles to consider. For low-molecular-weight medications that have low endogenous clearance and volume of distribution, as well as minimal protein binding (<80%), extracorporeal clearance is optimized. Dosages of certain antidotes (e.g., ethanol, fomepizole, and N-acetylcysteine) should be increased to maintain therapeutic concentrations after the start of extracorporeal treatment. Blood and effluent flows should be optimized, the filter with the largest surface area should be chosen, and the duration should be adjusted to remove enough poison to minimize toxicity to maximize the benefit of an extracorporeal treatment. The most effective extracorporeal treatment is intermittent hemodialysis, which is advised in the majority of cases. If intermittent hemodialysis is not easily accessible, continuous kidney replacement therapy may be prescribed.

Across the globe, poisonings are a leading cause of morbidity and mortality. Many exposures can result in poisoning, such as medications, chemicals (e.g., pesticides, industrial, home, or natural poisons) derived from animals (e.g., spiders, snakes, or vegetation). Moreover, poisoning can result from acute, chronic, or acute-on-chronic exposures and can be purposeful or unintentional (including occupational). Every scenario may present differently, which calls for various management strategies. Over 2 million toxic exposures were reported to US poison control centers in 2020.1 Drug overdoses are estimated to be the leading cause of death for young adults, accounting for 100,000 of the estimated fatalities. 2 Although clinical/medical toxicologists and critical care physicians typically handle poisonings, nephrologists play a vital role in some cases. This has to do with the fact that kidney disease may increase the risk of certain poisonings and/or the use of methods for elimination enhancement in toxicological treatment.

Administering prompt and suitable treatment at the onset can decrease the severity and length of poisoning. The standard procedure for a poisoned patient involves immediate resuscitation and stabilization, as well as thorough clinical and laboratory assessments. Time-sensitive interventions, including antidotes, decontamination of the gastrointestinal tract, and methods to enhance elimination, may be necessary. These decisions are typically tailored to the individual case, taking into account the type of exposure, the patient's condition, and any symptoms present. Treatment recommendations are often based on limited evidence, such as case studies or theoretical reasoning. Fortunately, there are now more clinical guidelines informed by data and expert consensus to aid in decision-making processes.

3.3.1. Resuscitation and Supportive Care

All poisonings should be taken seriously, particularly those that are acute, deliberate, and have a rapid progression rate. A thorough evaluation of the patient's breathing, circulation, airway, and neurological function is the first step in the management process. Standard indications are followed when implementing initial interventions, which may include ventilatory support, fluid, inotrope, or vasopressor administration, as well as endotracheal intubation. Volume replacement plays a crucial role in managing volume depletion as it enhances hemodynamics, optimizes kidney function, and facilitates the elimination of certain medications (, digoxin, baclofen, lithium, and dabigatran). Titrated benzodiazepine doses are used to treat agitation and seizures. Admission to the intensive care unit and ongoing cardiac monitoring are frequently necessary in cases of severe poisoning. This is advised until recovery and the anticipated peak effects (which could make it difficult to determine whether the poison is still being absorbed). Following a minimum observation period, the patient's medical clearance may be taken into consideration if there is no clinical toxicity. Intentional poisonings frequently call for mental health services.

3.3.2. Risk Assessment

The clinician uses a cognitive process called toxicological risk assessment to forecast the course of a patient's illness after a particular exposure. It is used in conjunction with resuscitation and supportive care to direct patient triaging and therapy initiation. Identifying the poison (what?), the exposure (how much?), the duration (how long?), the patient factors (who?), and the timing (when?) are the three components of the risk assessment. Certain poisonings present with a common set of clinical features, called a toxidrome (e.g., serotonin toxicity, sympathomimetic, cholinergic, opioid, and anticholinergic), and in situations where clinical data is scarce, they could aid in the identification of a poison. The toxicological risk assessment requires several investigations, including an ECG, blood gas, routine blood chemistry, including renal function, and drug assays when necessary.

Considering the poisoning that is being treated, this information is interpreted. For instance, poisoning typically manifests quickly (e.g., within 2–4 h) following acute deliberate poisoning; however, there are some exceptions, such as if a sustained-release xenobiotic or one that is converted into a more toxic substance is consumed (e.g., methanol, acetaminophen) or poisons that injure cells (e.g., salicylate, 2,4-dinitrophenol, bromoxynil). There are some acute exposures that are linked to more serious consequences. In this case, risk can be estimated using the dose (e.g., More than 400 mg/kg of valproic acid5), signs (e.g., coma in cases of poisoning with carbamazepine), blood or plasma concentration (e.g., concentration of salicylate >100 mg/dl or >7.2 mmol/L7), or additional laboratory testing (e.g., lactate concentration in metformin poisoning greater than 15 mmol/L8). Persistent poisoning (e.g., weeks) may be linked to ongoing toxicity as a result of concurrent AKI illness or drug-drug interactions that build up a therapeutic drug over time. Clinical toxicity may be quite high in this case (e.g., neurotoxicity (such as lithium-induced confusion and seizures or digoxin-induced total heart block) despite comparatively lower plasma concentrations than those seen following acute poisoning. The risk assessment is modified in light of new data from the past, current research, and/or clinical development. In most cases, it is highly recommended to seek advice from a Poison Control Center or a clinical/medical toxicologist.

3.3.3. Gastrointestinal Decontamination

By lowering the quantity of poison that is absorbed, intestinal decontamination is a crucial intervention that can potentially shorten the duration and lessen the severity of poisoning. Activated charcoal is most frequently used—usually in adult dosages of 50 g—for gastrointestinal decontamination. The recommended timing for using activated charcoal is 2 h after consumption; however, there are some notable exceptions, such as medications with extended release (e.g., theophylline, diltiazem) and enteric-coated medications (e.g., valproic acid). In the event of significant exposures, a second dose of activated charcoal may be administered 2–4 h later, especially if the drug concentration is observed to rise following the initial dose (e.g., salicylates, acetaminophen, and valproic acid). When it comes to acids or alkali, alcohols (such as methanol and ethylene glycol), ions, or metals like iron and lithium, activated charcoal is ineffective. In order to perform whole bowel irrigation, a large volume (1 L/h) of an isotonic solution, such as macrogol (polyethylene glycol), is administered enterally until the rectal effluent is clear. Extended-release formulations, "body packers," exposures that are insensitive to activated charcoal, and extremely toxic exposures are among the indications.

3.3.4. Antidotes

Antidotes counteract the effects of poisons either directly or indirectly, for example, by acting on a receptor (e.g., naloxone for opioids), metabolic inhibitors (e.g., binding for inactivation, fomepizole for methanol). Depending on the poison, there are different indications, but generally speaking, medication is only given when there is evidence of toxicity and/or a high drug concentration (e.g., acetaminophen with N-acetylcysteine). The antidote dosage is titrated based on clinical response or the findings of investigations and varies according to the poisoning exposure. Table 3.8 provides a list of the antidotes that are more frequently used.

Table 3.8. Examples of Poisons for which Antidotes are Recommended

Poison	**Antidote**
Acetaminophen (paracetamol)	N-acetylcysteine[a]
Anticholinergic drugs	Physostigmine for significant delirium
Anticholinesterase insecticides	Atropine and possibly pralidoxime or obidoxime
Benzodiazepines	Flumazenil (rarely required)
β-adrenergic antagonists	Adrenaline, insulin-dextrose infusion
Calcium channel blockers	Calcium, insulin-dextrose infusion
Carbon monoxide	Oxygen
Cyanide	Hydroxocobalamin and/or thiosulfate
Dabigatran	Idarucizumab
Digoxin	Digoxin Fab antitoxin, atropine
Envenomation (*e.g.*, snake, spider)	Antivenom
Ethylene glycol/methanol	Ethanol or fomepizole[a]
Iron	Deferoxamine
Isoniazid	Pyridoxine[a]
Lead	Ca,Na_2-EDTA or succimer (DMSA)
Methotrexate	Folinic acid, glucarpidase

Opioids	Naloxone
Poison-induced methemoglobinemia (*e.g.*, dapsone, alkyl nitrite)	Methylene blue
Salicylates	Bicarbonate
Sulfonylureas	Octreotide, glucose
Tricyclic antidepressants	Bicarbonate
Valproic acid	L-carnitine[a]
Warfarin	Vitamin K

DMSA, dimercaptosuccinic acid.

[a]The dose of the antidote must be adjusted during extracorporeal treatment.

Source: https://journals.lww.com/cjasn/fulltext/2023/09000/management_of_poisonings_and_intoxications.17.aspx

When prescribing antidotes, nephrologists should take certain factors into account. Among these are extracorporeal therapies that eliminate antidotes, causing dose up-titration (e.g., ethanol or fomepizole), antidote buildup in individuals with severe renal illness, causing a reduction in dosage (e.g., EDTA), as well as chronic or recurrent toxicity in individuals with severe renal illness who need to take antidote doses repeatedly (e.g., digoxin and dabigatran).

3.3.5. Enhanced Elimination

The two types of elimination enhancement modalities are extracorporeal, which calls for an artificial device outside the body, and corporeal, which improves physiological processes. The use of urine alkalinization and extracorporeal treatments is growing (Figure 3.2). At this point, nephrologists are often consulted for advice.

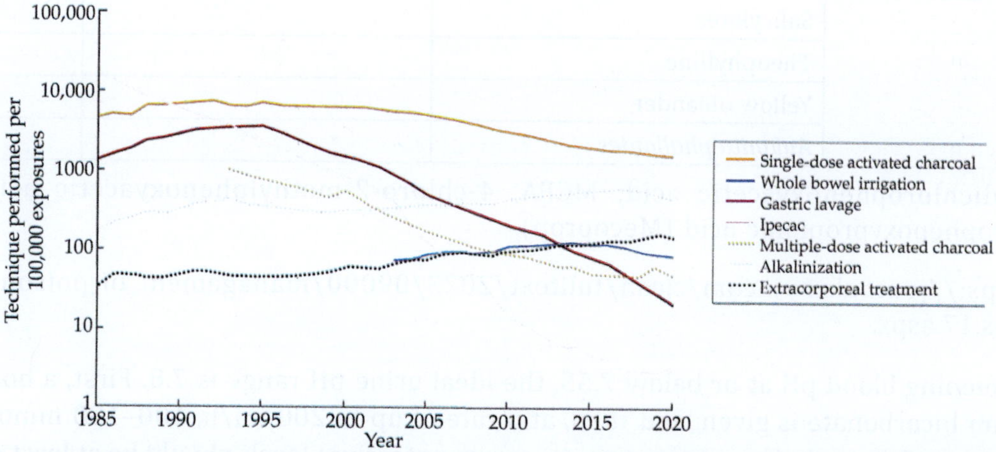

Figure 3.2. *Trends in the use of elimination enhancement techniques in the United States.*

Source: https://images.journals.lww.com/cjasn/Original.01277230-202309000-00017.fig1.jpeg.

3.3.5.1. Corporeal Treatments

- Urine Alkalinization

Urine pH can be raised to increase the amount of a weak acid that is ionized or the solubility of the poison. Ionized poisons are more easily excreted in urine and less easily reabsorbed through kidney tubules. The amount that kidney clearance contributes to the overall body clearance of the poison determines how effective urine alkalinization is; i.e., even a ten-fold increase in kidney elimination won't have a clinically significant impact if less than 1% of the ingested poison is eliminated unaltered in the urine. Twelve factors determine whether a poison can be alkalinized in urine: (1) it must be excreted by the kidneys unaltered; (2) it must have a lower volume of distribution (VD; see below); (3) it must have lower protein binding; and (4) it must have a weak acid (pKa between 3 and 7). Urine alkalinization can be used for herbicides (e.g., chlorpropamide, phenobarbital, and salicylates) as well as other substances (e.g., methotrexate, fluoride, 4-chloro-2-methylphenoxyacetic acid, mecoprop) and 2,4-dichlorophenoxyacetic acid [2,4-D] (Table 3.9).

Table 3.9. Poisons Whose Elimination May be Enhanced by Corporeal Techniques

Urine Alkalinization	Multiple-Dose Activated Charcoal	Sodium Polystyrene Sulfonate	Prussian Blue
Chlorophenoxy herbicides	Carbamazepine	Lithium	Radiocesium
(*2,4-D, MCPA, MCPP*)	Colchicine	Potassium	Thallium
Chlorpropamide	Dapsone		
Diflusinal	Digoxin		
Fluoride	Phenobarbital		
Methotrexate	Phenytoin		
Phenobarbital	Quinine		
Salicylates	Salicylates		
	Theophylline		
	Yellow oleander		
	Amanita phalloides		

2,4-D, 2,4-dichlorophenoxyacetic acid; MCPA, 4-chloro-2-methylphenoxyacetic acid; MCPP, methylchlorophenoxypropionic acid (Mecoprop).

Source: https://journals.lww.com/cjasn/fulltext/2023/09000/management_of_poisonings_and_intoxications.17.aspx.

While keeping blood pH at or below 7.55, the ideal urine pH range is 7.8. First, a bolus of 100 mmol sodium bicarbonate is given, and then, at a rate of up to 200 ml/h, 100–150 mmol/L in 5% dextrose in water. Prior to buffer administration, serum potassium levels should be at least 4 mmol/L. Urine cannot be easily alkalinized when hypokalemia is present because potassium is reabsorbed in the collecting duct in exchange for a proton. Moreover, kaliuresis brought on by alkalinization can result in dangerous hypokalemia and subsequent dysrhythmias. Ionized calcium and serum potassium levels need to be regularly checked and adjusted as needed. Pulmonary, cerebral, and hypernatremia edema are further possible side effects. Because they can worsen metabolic acidemia and exacerbate toxicity, such as in the case of a salicylate poisoning where acidemia can accelerate salicylate entry in the central nervous system, carbonic anhydrase inhibitors are contraindicated for urine alkalinization of poisons.

3.3.6. Fecal Elimination Enhancement

Activated charcoal (MDAC) in multiple doses improves the excretion of some poisons by blocking their enterohepatic circulation or by encouraging passive back diffusion (also known as gut dialysis) from the intestinal capillaries to the gut lumen. 25 g of activated charcoal is typically taken every 2 h until the desired clinical or biochemical results are reached. According to current guidelines, MDAC is advised in cases of quinine, theophylline, carbamazepine, dapsone, and phenobarbital poisoning. Furthermore, MDAC might help treat poisonings from phenytoin, salicylates, cardiac glycosides, *Asmanita phalloides*, or colchicine. Poisons from the gut capillaries may be absorbed by ion exchange resins and enter the lumen. Lithium half-life reduction is possible with sodium polystyrene sulfonate, which has been used historically to treat hyperkalemia. In the intestinal lumen, prussian blue binds radiocesium and thallium, improving their fecal elimination (Table 3.9).

3.3.7. Forced Diuresis

Administration of large volumes of isotonic fluids with or without loop diuretics is rarely used today to enhance elimination of poisons due to low efficacy and the risk of complications, including pulmonary edema and electrolyte abnormalities.

A Closer Look

Chronic poisoning

Chronic poisoning refers to the gradual accumulation of a toxic substance in the body over an extended period, leading to progressive and often subtle adverse health effects. Unlike acute poisoning, which occurs from a single or short-term exposure and has immediate symptoms, chronic poisoning results from continuous or repeated exposure to low levels of a toxin. This type of poisoning can be particularly insidious because symptoms may develop slowly and be non-specific, making diagnosis challenging.

One common example of chronic poisoning is lead poisoning, which historically affected many children exposed to lead-based paints and contaminated water supplies. Lead accumulates in the bones and soft tissues, affecting neurological development and causing cognitive impairments, behavioral problems, and physical health issues such as anemia and hypertension. Another well-known example is mercury poisoning, often resulting from the consumption of contaminated fish. Chronic mercury exposure can lead to neurological symptoms like tremors, memory problems, and mood disturbances, as well as kidney damage.

Occupational exposure is a significant source of chronic poisoning. Workers in industries such as manufacturing, mining, and agriculture may be exposed to hazardous substances like asbestos, benzene, or pesticides over long periods. Asbestos exposure, for instance, can lead to chronic respiratory diseases like asbestosis and mesothelioma, a type of lung cancer. Benzene, a solvent used in various industrial processes, is a known carcinogen linked to leukemia and other blood disorders. Pesticides, depending on their chemical nature, can cause a range of chronic health issues, from neurological disorders to endocrine disruption and cancer.

Environmental pollutants also contribute to chronic poisoning. Persistent organic pollutants (POPs) such as polychlorinated biphenyls (PCBs) and dioxins can remain in the environment for long periods and accumulate in the food chain, leading to chronic exposure in humans. These substances are associated with various health problems, including immune system suppression, reproductive disorders, and increased cancer risk.

The diagnosis of chronic poisoning requires a high index of suspicion, detailed exposure history, and appropriate laboratory tests. Biomonitoring, which involves measuring the levels of toxins or their metabolites in biological samples such as blood or urine, is crucial for confirming exposure. For instance, blood lead levels can be measured to diagnose lead poisoning, while urine tests can detect mercury exposure. Additionally, biomarkers of effect, such as liver enzymes for hepatotoxic chemicals or neurological tests for neurotoxins, help assess the extent of organ damage.

Management of chronic poisoning involves several strategies. The primary approach is to eliminate or reduce exposure to the toxic substance. This may involve workplace interventions, such as improving ventilation or using personal protective equipment, and public health measures like water treatment and soil remediation. Medical treatment focuses on supportive care and may include chelation therapy for heavy metal poisoning, which helps remove metals from the body. Monitoring and managing long-term health effects are also critical, as some damage from chronic poisoning may be irreversible.

Prevention is key to addressing chronic poisoning. This involves regulatory measures to limit the use of hazardous substances, public education to raise awareness about potential sources of exposure, and regular health screenings for at-risk populations. By identifying and mitigating the sources of chronic poisoning, significant public health benefits can be achieved, reducing the burden of disease associated with long-term toxic exposures.

Summary

- Poison management refers to the systematic approach to the prevention, diagnosis, and treatment of toxic exposures, ensuring the safety and recovery of individuals who have been poisoned.
- Antidotes are another critical aspect of poison management. For certain poisons, specific antidotes can neutralize the toxic effects or enhance the elimination of the poison from the body.
- Supportive care is essential throughout the management process. This includes monitoring and maintaining vital functions, managing symptoms, and preventing complications
- Poisoning is contact with a substance that results in toxicity. Symptoms vary, but certain common syndromes may suggest particular classes of poisons. Diagnosis is primarily clinical, but for some poisonings, blood and urine tests can help.
- Symptoms and signs of poisoning vary depending on the substance (see table Symptoms and Treatment of Specific Poisons). Also, different patients poisoned with the same substance may present with very different symptoms.
- Physical examination sometimes detects signs suggesting particular types of substances (e.g., toxidromes [see table Common Toxic Syndromes], breath odor, presence of topical drugs, needle marks or tracks suggesting injected drug use, stigmata of chronic alcohol use).
- Charcoal is usually given, particularly when multiple or unknown substances have been ingested. Use of charcoal adds little risk (unless patients are at risk of vomiting and aspiration) but has not been proved to reduce overall morbidity or mortality.
- Gastric emptying, which used to be well-accepted and seems intuitively beneficial, should not be routinely done. It does not clearly reduce overall morbidity or mortality and has risks. Gastric emptying is considered if it can be done within 1 h of a life-threatening ingestion.
- Drug-induced hypotension and arrhythmias may not respond to the usual drug treatments. For refractory hypotension, dopamine, epinephrine, other vasopressors, an intra-aortic balloon pump, or even extracorporeal circulatory support may be considered.

References

1. Anseeuw, K., Mowry, J. B., Burdmann, E. A., et al., (2016). Extracorporeal treatment in phenytoin poisoning: Systematic review and recommendations from the EXTRIP (extracorporeal treatments in poisoning) workgroup. *American Journal of Kidney Diseases, 67*(2), 187–197. https://doi.org/10.1053/j.ajkd.2015.08.031.
2. Athavale, A., Jamshidi, N., & Roberts, D. M. (2021). Kidney dysfunction has a major impact on the effect of idarucizumab for dabigatran reversal. *European Journal of Anesthesiology, 38*(9), 1005–1006. https://doi.org/10.1097/eja.0000000000001428.
3. Berling, I., King, J. D., Shepherd, G., et al.; for the EXTRIP Workgroup. (2020). Extracorporeal treatment for chloroquine, hydroxychloroquine, and quinine poisoning: Systematic review and

recommendations from the EXTRIP workgroup. *Journal of the American Society of Nephrology, 31*(10), 2475–2489. https://doi.org/10.1681/ASN.2020050564.

4. Bouchard, J., Lavergne, V., Roberts, D. M., Cormier, M., Morissette, G., & Ghannoum, M. (2017). Availability and cost of extracorporeal treatments for poisonings and other emergency indications: A worldwide survey. *Nephrology Dialysis Transplantation, 32*(4), 699–706. https://doi.org/10.1093/ndt/gfw456.

5. Bouchard, J., Roberts, D. M., Roy, L., et al., (2014). Principles and operational parameters to optimize poison removal with extracorporeal treatments. *Seminars in Dialysis, 27*(4), 371–380. https://doi.org/10.1111/sdi.12247.

6. Bouchard, J., Shepherd, G., Hoffman, R. S., et al., (2021). Extracorporeal treatment for poisoning to beta-adrenergic antagonists: Systematic review and recommendations from the EXTRIP workgroup. *Critical Care, 25*(1), 201. https://doi.org/10.1186/s13054-021-03585-7.

7. Bouchard, J., Yates, C., Calello, D. P., et al., (2022). Extracorporeal treatment for Gabapentin and Pregabalin poisoning: Systematic review and recommendations from the EXTRIP workgroup. *American Journal of Kidney Diseases, 79*(1), 88–104. https://doi.org/10.1053/j.ajkd.2021.06.027.

8. Brunet, S., Leblanc, M., Geadah, D., Parent, D., Courteau, S., & Cardinal, J. (1999). Diffusive and convective solute clearances during continuous renal replacement therapy at various dialysate and ultrafiltration flow rates. *American Journal of Kidney Diseases, 34*(3), 486–492. https://doi.org/10.1016/s0272-6386(99)70076-4.

9. Calello, D. P., Liu, K. D., Wiegand, T. J., et al., (2015). Extracorporeal treatment for metformin poisoning: Systematic review and recommendations from the Extracorporeal Treatments in Poisoning Workgroup. *Critical Care Medicine, 43*(8), 1716–1730. https://doi.org/10.1097/CCM.0000000000001002.

10. CDC. (2021). Drug Overdose Deaths in the U.S. Top 100,000 Annually. Retrieved from: https://www.cdc.gov/nchs/pressroom/nchs_press_releases/2021/20211117.htm (accessed on 3 August 2024).

11. Chan, B. S. H., & Buckley, N. A. (2014). Digoxin-specific antibody fragments in the treatment of digoxin toxicity. *Clinical Toxicology, 52*(8), 824–836. https://doi.org/10.3109/15563650.2014.943907.

12. Couriel, D., & Weinstein, R. (1994). Complications of therapeutic plasma exchange: A recent assessment. *Journal of Clinical Apheresis, 9*(1), 1–5. https://doi.org/10.1002/jca.2920090102.

13. Daly, F. F. S., Little, M., & Murray, L. (2006). A risk assessment-based approach to the management of acute poisoning. *Emergency Medicine Journal, 23*(5), 396–399. https://doi.org/10.1136/emj.2005.030312.

14. Decker, B. S., Goldfarb, D. S., Dargan, P. I., et al.; on behalf of the EXTRIP Workgroup. (2015). Extracorporeal treatment for lithium poisoning: Systematic review and recommendations from the EXTRIP workgroup. *Clinical Journal of the American Society of Nephrology, 10*(5), 875–887. https://doi.org/10.2215/CJN.10021014.

15. Decker, B. S., Kays, M. B., Chambers, M., Kraus, M. A., Moe, S. M., & Sowinski, K. M. (2010). Vancomycin pharmacokinetics and pharmacodynamics during short daily hemodialysis. *Clinical Journal of the American Society of Nephrology, 5*(11), 1981–1987. https://doi.org/10.2215/CJN.03450410.

16. Falkenhagen, D., Gottschall, S., Esther, G., Courtney, J. M., & Klinkmann, H. (1982). In vitro assessment of charcoal and resin hemoadsorbents. *Contributions to Nephrology, 29*, 23–33. https://doi.org/10.1159/000406175.

17. Ghannoum, M., & Gosselin, S. (2013). Enhanced poison elimination in critical care. *Advances in Chronic Kidney Disease, 20*(1), 94–101. https://doi.org/10.1053/j.ackd.2012.09.002.

18. Ghannoum, M., Berling, I., Lavergne, V., et al.; EXTRIP Workgroup. (2021). Recommendations from the EXTRIP workgroup on extracorporeal treatment for baclofen poisoning. *Kidney International, 100*(4), 720–736. https://doi.org/10.1016/j.kint.2021.07.014.

19. Ghannoum, M., Bouchard, J., Nolin, T. D., Ouellet, G., & Roberts, D. M. (2014). Hemoperfusion for the treatment of poisoning: Technology, determinants of poison clearance, and application in clinical practice. *Seminars in Dialysis, 27*(4), 350–361. https://doi.org/10.1111/sdi.12246.

20. Ghannoum, M., Laliberte, M., Nolin, T. D., et al.; on behalf of the EXTRIP Workgroup. (2015). Extracorporeal treatment for valproic acid poisoning: Systematic review and recommendations from the EXTRIP workgroup. *Clinical Toxicology, 53*(5), 454–465. https://doi.org/10.3109/15563650.2015.1035441.

21. Ghannoum, M., Lavergne, V., Gosselin, S., et al., (2016). Practice trends in the use of extracorporeal treatments for poisoning in four countries. *Seminars in Dialysis, 29*(1), 71–80. https://doi.org/10.1111/sdi.12448.

22. Ghannoum, M., Lavergne, V., Yue, C. S., Ayoub, P., Perreault, M. M., & Roy, L. (2010). Successful treatment of lithium toxicity with sodium polystyrene sulfonate: A retrospective cohort study. *Clinical Toxicology, 48*(1), 34–41. https://doi.org/10.3109/15563650903344785.

23. Ghannoum, M., Nolin, T. D., Goldfarb, D. S., et al., (2012). Extracorporeal treatment for thallium poisoning: Recommendations from the EXTRIP workgroup. *Clinical Journal of the American Society of Nephrology, 7*(10), 1682–1690. https://doi.org/10.2215/CJN.01940212.

24. Ghannoum, M., Roberts, D. M., Goldfarb, D. S., et al., (2022). Extracorporeal treatment for methotrexate poisoning: Systematic review and recommendations from the EXTRIP workgroup. *Clinical Journal of the American Society of Nephrology, 17*(4), 602–622. https://doi.org/10.2215/CJN.08030621.

25. Ghannoum, M., Wiegand, T. J., Liu, K. D., et al.; on behalf of the EXTRIP Workgroup. (2015). Extracorporeal treatment for theophylline poisoning: Systematic review and recommendations from the EXTRIP workgroup. *Clinical Toxicology, 53*(4), 215–229. https://doi.org/10.3109/15563650.2015.1014907.

26. Ghannoum, M., Yates, C., Galvao, T. F., et al., (2014). Extracorporeal treatment for carbamazepine poisoning: Systematic review and recommendations from the EXTRIP workgroup. *Clinical Toxicology, 52*(10), 993–1004. https://doi.org/10.3109/15563650.2014.973572.

27. Gosselin, S., Juurlink, D. N., Kielstein, J. T., et al.; on behalf of the EXTRIP Workgroup. (2014). Extracorporeal treatment for acetaminophen poisoning: Recommendations from the EXTRIP workgroup. *Clinical Toxicology, 52*(8), 856–867. https://doi.org/10.3109/15563650.2014.946994.

28. Gummin, D. D., Mowry, J. B., Beuhler, M. C., et al., (2021). 2020 Annual report of the American Association of Poison Control Centers' National Poison Data System (NPDS): 38th Annual report. *Clinical Toxicology (Phila), 59*(12), 1282–1501. https://doi.org/10.1080/15563650.2021.1989785.

29. Hoegberg, L. C. G., Shepherd, G., Wood, D. M., et al., (2021). Systematic review on the use of activated charcoal for gastrointestinal decontamination following acute oral overdose. *Clinical Toxicology (Phila), 59*(12), 1196–1227. https://doi.org/10.1080/15563650.2021.1961144.

30. Hoffman, R. S. (2003). Thallium toxicity and the role of Prussian blue in therapy. *Toxicology Reviews, 22*(1), 29–40. https://doi.org/10.2165/00139709-200322010-00004.

31. Holstege, C. P., & Borek, H. A. (2012). Toxidromes. *Critical Care Clinics, 28*(4), 479–498. https://doi.org/10.1016/j.ccc.2012.07.008.

32. Holubek, W. J., Hoffman, R. S., Goldfarb, D. S., & Nelson, L. S. (2008). Use of hemodialysis and hemoperfusion in poisoned patients. *Kidney International, 74*(10), 1327–1334. https://doi.org/10.1038/ki.2008.462.

33. Isbister, G. K., Balit, C. R., Whyte, I. M., & Dawson, A. (2003). Valproate overdose: A comparative cohort study of self-poisonings. *British Journal of Clinical Pharmacology, 55*(4), 398–404. https://doi.org/10.1046/j.1365-2125.2003.01772.x.

34. Juurlink, D. N., Gosselin, S., Kielstein, J. T., et al., (2015). Extracorporeal treatment for salicylate poisoning: Systematic review and recommendations from the EXTRIP workgroup. *Annals of Emergency Medicine, 66*(2), 165–181. https://doi.org/10.1016/j.annemergmed.2015.03.031.

35. Kielstein, J. T., Schmidt, J. J., & Ghannoum, M. (2022). Effectiveness of CytoSorb in cases of acute amitriptyline intoxication is not proven. *Journal of Clinical Pharmacy and Therapeutics, 47*(3), 420. https://doi.org/10.1111/jcpt.13483.

36. Lanese, D. M., Alfrey, P. S., & Molitoris, B. A. (1989). Markedly increased clearance of vancomycin during hemodialysis using polysulfone dialyzers. *Kidney International, 35*(6), 1409–1412. https://doi.org/10.1038/ki.1989.141.

37. Lavergne, V., Nolin, T. D., Hoffman, R. S., et al., (2012). The EXTRIP (extracorporeal treatments in poisoning) workgroup: Guideline methodology. *Clinical Toxicology, 50*(5), 403–413. https://doi.org/10.3109/15563650.2012.683436.

38. Mactier, R., Laliberte, M., Mardini, J., et al., (2011). Extracorporeal treatment for barbiturate poisoning: Recommendations from the EXTRIP workgroup. *American Journal of Kidney Diseases, 64*(3), 347–358. https://doi.org/10.1053/j.ajkd.2014.04.031

39. Maduell, F., Navarro, V., Cruz, M. C., et al., (2002). Osteocalcin and myoglobin removal in on-line hemodiafiltration versus low- and high-flux hemodialysis. *American Journal of Kidney Diseases, 40*(3), 582–589. https://doi.org/10.1053/ajkd.2002.34918.

40. Mowry, J. B., Burdmann, E. A., Anseeuw, K., et al.; on behalf of the EXTRIP Workgroup. (2016). Extracorporeal treatment for digoxin poisoning: Systematic review and recommendations from the EXTRIP workgroup. *Clinical Toxicology, 54*(2), 103–114. https://doi.org/10.3109/15563650.2015.1118488.

41. Mowry, J. B., Shepherd, G., Hoffman, R. S., et al., (2021). Extracorporeal treatments in poisoning: Extracorporeal treatments for isoniazid poisoning: Systematic review and recommendations from the EXTRIP workgroup. *Pharmacotherapy, 41*(5), 463–478. https://doi.org/10.1002/phar.2519.

42. Mydlik, M., Derzsiova, K., Bucek, J., Horky, K., Jarcuska, J., & Takac, M. (1983). Use of charcoal haemoperfusion in 55 acute poisonings. *Life Support Systems, 1*(suppl 1), 53–56.

43. Ouellet, G., Bouchard, J., Ghannoum, M., & Decker, B. S. (2014). Available extracorporeal treatments for poisoning: Overview and limitations. *Seminars in Dialysis, 27*(4), 342–349. https://doi.org/10.1111/sdi.12238.

44. Proudfoot, A. T., Krenzelok, E. P., & Vale, J. A. (2004). Position paper on urine alkalinization. *Journal of Toxicology Clinical Toxicology, 42*(1), 1–26. https://doi.org/10.1081/clt-120028740.

45. Rahman, M. H., Haqqie, S. S., & McGoldrick, M. D. (2006). Acute hemolysis with acute renal failure in a patient with valproic acid poisoning treated with charcoal hemoperfusion. *Hemodialysis International, 10*(3), 256–259. https://doi.org/10.1111/j.1542-4758.2006.00105.x.

46. Roberts, D. M., Gallapatthy, G., Dunuwille, A., & Chan, B. S. (2016). Pharmacological treatment of cardiac glycoside poisoning. *British Journal of Clinical Pharmacology, 81*(3), 488–495. https://doi.org/10.1111/bcp.12814.

47. Roberts, D. M., Yates, C., Megarbane, B., et al., (2015). Recommendations for the role of extracorporeal treatments in the management of acute methanol poisoning: A systematic review and consensus statement. *Critical Care Medicine, 43*(2), 461–472. https://doi.org/10.1097/ccm.0000000000000708.

48. Shalkham, A. S., Kirrane, B. M., Hoffman, R. S., Goldfarb, D. S., & Nelson, L. S. (2006). The availability and use of charcoal hemoperfusion in the treatment of poisoned patients. *American Journal of Kidney Diseases, 48*(2), 239–241. https://doi.org/10.1053/j.ajkd.2006.04.080.

49. Skinner, C. G., Chang, A. S., Matthews, A. S., Reedy, S. J., & Morgan, B. W. (2012). Randomized controlled study on the use of multiple-dose activated charcoal in patients with supratherapeutic phenytoin levels. *Clinical Toxicology, 50*(8), 764–769. https://doi.org/10.3109/15563650.2012.716159.

50. Vale, J., Krenzelok, E. P., & Barceloux, V. D. (1999). Position statement and practice guidelines on the use of multi-dose activated charcoal in the treatment of acute poisoning. *Journal of Toxicology Clinical Toxicology, 37*(6), 731–751. https://doi.org/10.1081/clt-100102451.

51. Wong, A., Hoffman, R. S., Walsh, S. J., et al.; for the EXTRIP Workgroup. (2021). Extracorporeal treatment for calcium channel blocker poisoning: Systematic review and recommendations from the EXTRIP workgroup. *Clinical Toxicology (Phila), 59*(5), 361–375. https://doi.org/10.1080/15563650.2020.1870123.

52. Yates, C., Galvao, T., Sowinski, K. M., et al.; the EXTRIP Workgroup. (2014). Extracorporeal treatment for tricyclic antidepressant poisoning: Recommendations from the EXTRIP workgroup. *Seminars in Dialysis, 27*(4), 381–389. https://doi.org/10.1111/sdi.12227.

TOXICOKINETICS AND TOXICODYNAMICS

4

Contents

Introduction

Two key ideas in the study of toxicology are toxicokinetics and toxicodynamics, both of which are essential to comprehending how harmful substances interact with the body and cause negative effects. The study of how toxic substances are absorbed, distributed, metabolized, and excreted (ADME) within the body is known as toxicokinetics. It includes the mechanisms through which poisons enter the body, pass through different organs and tissues, go through biotransformation, and eventually leave the body. Through ingestion, inhalation, dermal contact, or injection, toxicants can enter the bloodstream and reach their target tissues through a process known as absorption. Toxins are distributed throughout the body through the bloodstream, with the help of various elements including tissue perfusion, blood flow, and the chemical and physical characteristics of the toxin. The term "metabolism," also known as "biotransformation," describes how the body's enzymes, which primarily reside in the liver, chemically change toxins to create metabolites that can differ in toxicity from the original compound. Last but not least, excretion is the process by which poisons and their metabolites are eliminated from the body, generally by the kidneys (urine), liver (bile), lungs (breath), and skin (sweat). Determining the potential for toxicity and the proper management of exposures, as well as forecasting a substance's distribution, metabolism, and elimination, depend on understanding of its toxicokinetic properties.

The biochemical and physiological effects of toxic substances on the body's cells, tissues, and organ systems are the main focus of toxicodynamics, on the other hand. It looks at how toxicants affect physiological functions, interact with cellular components, and have negative effects. When toxicants bind to particular receptors, enzymes, proteins, or other molecular targets in the body, changes in cellular function, signaling pathways, and homeostatic mechanisms occur. This process is known as toxicodynamics. Toxicodynamics can have a wide range of effects, such as cellular damage, inflammation, oxidative stress, genotoxicity, neurotoxicity, reproductive toxicity, or carcinogenicity, depending on the type of toxicant and how it works. The amount and duration of exposure, the route of exposure, the chemical makeup, and characteristics of the toxicant, as well as individual factors like age, sex, genetics, and pre-existing medical conditions, all impact toxicodynamics. Toxicodynamics clarifies the mechanisms behind toxic effects, which aids in identifying important cellular targets, toxicity pathways, and possible exposure or effect biomarkers. This information can be used to inform risk assessment, hazard identification, and the creation of therapeutic interventions or preventive measures.

Orientation and Directional Terms:

Term	Definition	Illustration
Toxicokinetics	The description of both what rate a chemical will enter the body and what occurs to excrete and metabolize the compound once it is in the body.	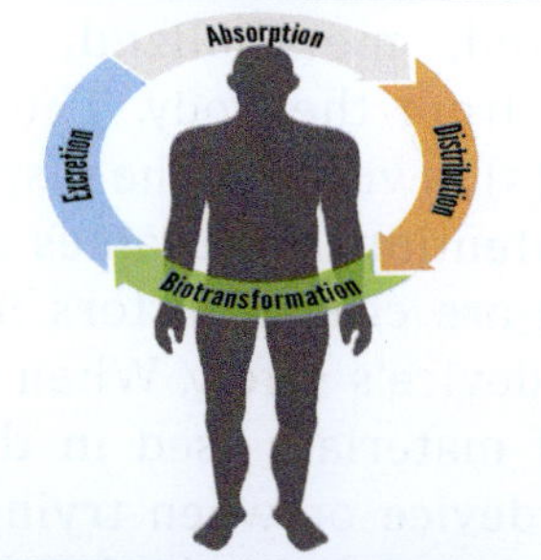
Cellular function	Cellular functions are defined by dynamic assembly, rearrangement, and disassembly of biomolecules to achieve control and specificity.	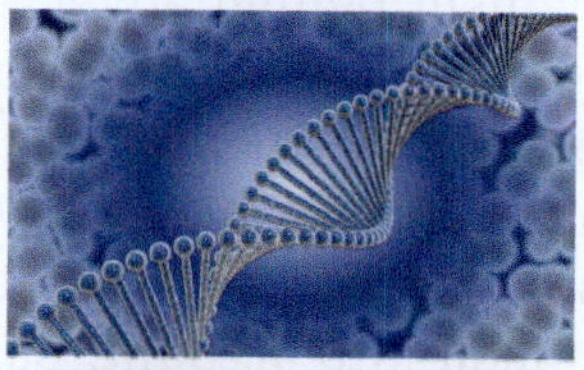
Oncology	Oncology is a branch of medicine that deals with the study, treatment, diagnosis, and prevention of cancer.	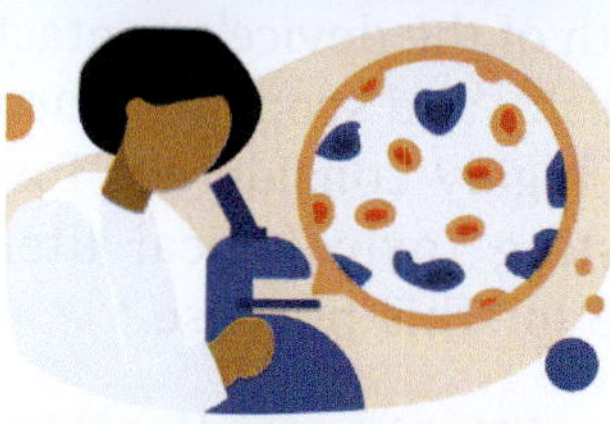
Biomonitoring	Biomonitoring refers to the measurement of chemicals in human body fluids and tissues, such as blood, urine, breast milk, saliva, and hair.	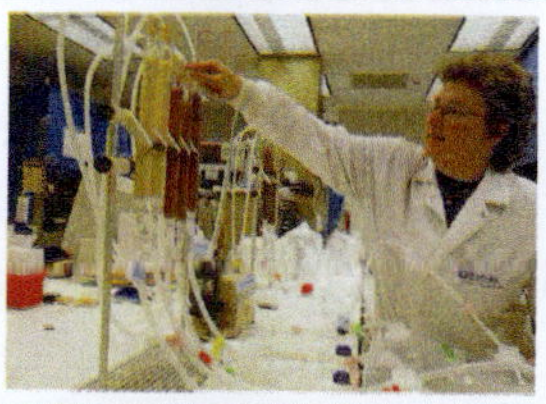
Metabolism	The whole sum of reactions that occur throughout the body within each cell and that provide the body with energy.	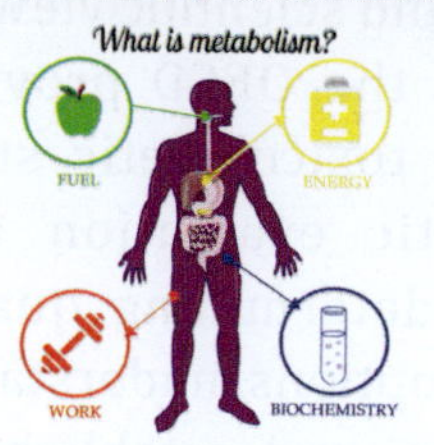

4.1. Basics of Toxicokinetics

The term "toxicokinetics" refers to the process by which foreign substances are absorbed, distributed, metabolized, and eventually excreted from the body. The stability of the material(s) in vivo and the disposal of intended and unintentional leachables and degradation products are critical factors in determining a medical device's safety. When determining the safety of materials used in the creation of a medical device or when trying to understand the mechanism behind adverse reactions that have been observed, toxicokinetic studies can be helpful. If medical devices containing active ingredients fall under the purview of toxicokinetic studies, pharmaceutical legislation must be taken into account. Based on the type and length of the device's contact with the body, the necessity and scope of toxicokinetic studies must be highly considered. Toxicokinetic data and existing toxicological literature may be adequate for this purpose.

Toxicokinetics studies involve collecting data on the kinetics of drug and device exposure in the body, as well as assessing toxicity. These studies help estimate the level of toxicity observed in exposed materials, which is crucial in the development of devices, both from regulatory and scientific viewpoints. Regulatory bodies like the OECD provide guidelines for conducting toxicokinetic studies in animals. Toxicokinetic evaluation aids in selecting materials, determining quantities, exploring alternative options, understanding toxicological mechanisms, and establishing safe exposure levels in clinical trials. These studies also contribute to reducing the number of animals used in research. The use of advanced LC/MS technology allows for precise quantitative analysis of chemicals with high sensitivity and selectivity, detecting test compound concentrations in fluids and tissues as required. Validation methods with known compounds ensure accurate extraction and detection of low-level chemical substances in test materials.

4.1.1. Relation to Pharmacokinetics

Determining the correlation between a compound's toxicity and systemic exposure is a pharmacokinetics application. It is mainly used to establish correlations between animal exposures from toxicology experiments and human exposures that correspond to those animal exposures. To ascertain the possible consequences of releasing chemicals into the environment, it can also be utilized in environmental risk assessments. Toxicokinetics and toxicodynamics can be combined to quantify toxic effects. Ecotoxicology makes use of toxicokinetic-toxicodynamic (TKTD) models. Parallel to this, physiological pharmacokinetic models are called physiological toxicokinetic models, and they are used to explain and forecast how a toxicant will behave in an animal's body. For instance, they can be used to predict which body parts (compartments) a chemical will likely enter (e.g., liver, spleen, fat, etc.), as well as whether and how quickly the chemical is anticipated to be metabolized or eliminated.

4.1.2. Processes and Goal Analysis

Toxicokinetic investigations in animals are the first step towards characterizing the PK/PD effects. Toxicokinetic analysis's main objective is to link toxicity results to the appropriate exposure level to an experimental drug compound. Toxicokinetic studies are frequently carried out using drug concentrations that are substantially higher than those that are therapeutically irrelevant and are predicted to cause toxic effects. During the later nonclinical and clinical stages of the drug development process, safer dosing strategies can be developed based on the knowledge gathered from these studies. Variations in dosages between the two types of studies also result in technological modifications to solubility, absorption, metabolism, protein binding, and pre-systemic clearance. These variations, which are impacted by the dosage, highlight important differences in the study's design and interpretation. An efficient method for translating drug discovery entails the rigorous selection and application of nonclinical models, following established protocols. Clinical trial teams, biostatisticians, and PK and PD scientists use the data from these studies to inform the design of their trials. Scientists review and assess nonclinical TK data in human trial doses to ensure they adhere to the guidelines outlined in FDA guidance M3(R2) Nonclinical Safety Studies. Accordingly, the maximum recommended starting dose for participants in human studies is based on nonclinical no observable adverse effect (NOAEL) data in pertinent animal species, which has been adjusted to the human equivalent dose.

To scale between species and simulate across various populations, dose scaling makes use of either allometric scaling or modeling/simulation with specialized software. Nonclinical data inform the selection of toxicity assessments for clinical trials, guaranteeing that shortcomings found in animal studies are successfully addressed in later human studies. Nonclinical evidence that the drug is hitting its target informs the selection of efficacy PD biomarkers in clinical trials; this is especially important in areas like neurodegenerative diseases and oncology. Various PD assessments are available to thoroughly evaluate the cognitive and behavioral effects of drugs that are active in the CNS. A chemical can interact with an animal in four possible ways: ADME. The term "absorption" refers to a chemical's entry into the body through the food, water, soil, or air. A chemical can spread to different parts of the body by diffusion or other biological processes once it has entered the body. At this stage, the substance may go through metabolism and change into different substances or metabolites. These metabolites may or may not be more or less toxic than the original substance. The metabolites may exit the body, change into new substances, or stay within the body's compartments following this possible biotransformation.

Several different approaches may be used in a well-designed toxicokinetic study, depending on the scientific question that needs to be addressed. The biological persistence, tissue and whole body half-lives, and potential for bioaccumulation of a chemical can be determined through carefully monitored acute and repeated toxicokinetic animal studies. The pharmacokinetic profiles may alter as exposure time or dosage increases. Exposure to real-world environmental factors typically takes the form of low-level mixtures from food, water, tobacco products, and the air. Due to chemical interactions, and competitive or synergistic processes, mixture effects may differ from individual chemical toxicokinetic profiles. For additional reasons, characterizing the toxicokinetics of individual chemical constituents found in mixtures is equally important because details about the behavior or fate of each individual chemical can provide insight into the results of biomonitoring studies conducted on humans, wildlife, and the environment.

4.1.3. Role of Toxicokinetics in Male and Female Reproductive Toxicity

The assessment of a compound's pharmacokinetics (PK) at dosages utilized in toxicity investigations is known as TK. A great review on toxicokinetic principles and how they apply to toxicology research, has been published. Its primary goal is to correlate the dose given with the systemic exposure and toxic effects seen in all subtypes of nonclinical toxicity studies. TK is defined as the generation of PK data to evaluate systemic exposure, either as a crucial part of carrying out nonclinical toxicity studies or in specially designed supportive studies. The interpretation of toxicological results and their applicability to clinical safety concerns may be done using these data. According to ICH guidelines, TK should increase the usefulness of the toxicological data produced, facilitating direct comparison with clinical data and aiding in the interpretation of toxicity study, ultimately evaluating risk and safety in humans. The evaluation of systemic exposure facilitates the interpretation of dose-response relationships, which may be nonlinear because of processes that are involved in the compound's absorption, distribution, metabolism, and elimination being induced, altered, or saturated. Moreover, TK data can be utilized to rule out the possibility that a lack of toxicological response results from insufficient drug exposure. In most cases, the administered dose is less relevant to the safety assessment as the systemic exposure at the NOAEL. These drug exposures can be contrasted with human exposures found in clinical trials.

The usual method for obtaining TK data is to measure the drug/metabolite concentrations in plasma, serum, blood, or urine samples obtained from test animals used for main toxicology or satellite testing. PK parameters for exposure, such as maximum plasma concentration (C_{max}), time of maximum plasma concentration (Tmax), and area under the plasma (or serum) concentration versus time curve (AUC), are typically the focus of the studies. Prior to now, the goal of TK research was straightforward, i.e., in recent years, it has developed into a potent tool that aids in the rationalization of species, dose selection, dosing vehicles, dosing frequency, and ultimately, human safety margin assessments (i.e., confirmation of the drug administration in toxicity studies). It is the proportion of an animal's AUC or C_{max} at a NOAEL dose to what humans can achieve at a therapeutic dose. This will guarantee a safe and well-tolerated initial dose of the new chemical entity (NCE) for human use. As a result, during the past 20 years, TK has grown to be a crucial component of pharmaceutical safety assessment.

TK is important for many kinds of drug toxicity studies, including those that are genetic, reproductive, subchronic, acute, dose range-finding, repeat dose, safety pharmacology, carcinogenicity, and bridging. It should be noted that not all ICH guidelines specifically identify TK as a necessary component. For this reason, ICH S3A is typically the most appropriate guideline when discussing TK's role in various study types. Reproductive toxicity studies are usually carried out subsequent to phase I safety and tolerability investigations and are not usually included in the package for an investigational new drug that is being submitted for approval in human studies. However, fast enrollment of women of childbearing potential in phase I and early phase II studies is necessary for many medications, particularly those that target diseases specific to women. Pre-first-in-human reproductive toxicity studies are carried out in these circumstances to guarantee target population safety and facilitate quick enrollment in phase II trials.

The ICH guidelines mention the following regarding the application of TK evaluations in reproductive toxicity studies, such as fertility studies, as well as studies in pregnant and lactating animals:

- Maternal toxicity is typically dose-limiting for these studies, but plasma concentrations are important for assessing the NOAEL, safety margins, and next steps forward.
- Consideration should be given to the possibility that kinetics will often differ in pregnant and nonpregnant animals and therefore must be characterized for both conditions.
- Plasma is the standard matrix. It is also appropriate to study embryo–

fetal transfer and secretion in milk not as specific study objectives related to developmental toxicology but as separate programs.

Studies on reproductive toxicity are usually carried out on rats or rabbits. It is not necessary, but "good to have," TK data from the fertility, perinatal, and postnatal studies, since they have already been generated in repeat dose rat studies. This will help to confirm whether there are any differences in exposure between pregnant and nonpregnant animals. TK is included by many sponsors in either the primary study or the dose range-finding study because of the observed PK profile differences for specific compounds in pregnant animals. To have a valid program for human safety assessment, regulations require that human metabolites be present in plasma in at least one reproductive toxicology species. The limit of exposure to reproductive toxicity is typically governed by maternal toxicity, according to the ICH Harmonized Tripartite Guideline, "Detection of toxicity to reproduction for medicinal products." Therefore, although TK monitoring in studies of reproductive toxicity might be useful in some cases—particularly when studying compounds with low toxicity—such information is not required for all compounds. The exposures obtained by dosing at various stages of the reproductive process could be usefully determined using TK principles, in cases where adequate systemic exposure may be questioned due to lack of pharmacological response or toxic effects."

The relationship between the exposure in the dam and the secondary effects in the fetus caused by the pharmacological action of the drug in the dam is the most valuable information that can be gathered from TK data as part of reproductive toxicology studies. Drug exposures in the dam may be associated with secondary effects on the fetus, even though direct extrapolation of TK data in the interpretation of primary effects on the fetus is unlikely. There is the highest chance of malformations during organogenesis, which occurs in rats between days 6 and 15 and in humans between days 18 and 60 of gestation,. Therefore, the relationship between drug exposure in the conceptus and time during the sensitive stages of gestation determines the direct developmental effect on the fetus. Measuring the drug exposure in the dam during TK during reproductive toxicity studies is important because it can be connected to therapeutic human exposure (AUC or C_{max}). Any of the TK parameters between pregnant and nonpregnant dams may vary because of pregnancy-related increases in plasma and total body water, increases in renal plasma flow and glomerular filtration, and decreases in the concentration of specific plasma proteins. Similar differences in human PK may exist based on the difference in PK of drugs between pregnant and nonpregnant animals.

However, studying particular human populations, such as patients with higher plasma volume, high renal clearance, etc., is the best way to determine whether such differences in PK actually exist. Whichever parameter primarily affects the TK will determine which TK parameters should be examined in studies of reproductive toxicity, such as embryo-fetal studies. C_{max} and valproic acid's embryo-fetal toxicity are connected. AUC influences the toxicity of cyclophosphamide and retinoids. Phenytoin is one medication whose toxicity is influenced by both C_{max} and AUC. Importantly, the test medication must be given to the animals in sufficient amounts during the dosing interval. If adequate exposures are not obtained within the dose interval, either the drug needs to be infused intravenously, or the animals need to be dosed more than once daily. It should be mentioned that the PK and the bioanalytical phase of any research on reproductive toxicity that is carried out in accordance with GLP must likewise comply with GLP.

- **Fertility and Embryo-Fetal Development Study in Rats.** A typical embryo-fetal study involves dosing male rats 4–10 weeks before mating. Blood samples for TK do not need to be obtained for a 4-week study if the findings from a previous study of the same length can be extrapolated. Samples can be taken at the conclusion of week 10 for a 10-week study, and if the PK is linear, day 1 data can be extrapolated from earlier research. Females typically receive treatment for two to four weeks before mating until the hard palate closes. Samples can only be taken at the conclusion of the study to characterize the TK, since day one data can be extrapolated from earlier research.
- **Pre- and Postnatal Development Studies in Rats.** In this study, female rats were dosed from the time of implantation until the end of lactation. There is no need to draw blood during this study to study the TK because the exposures in it can be extrapolated from other studies. On the other hand, one should try to ascertain the pups' drug exposure through breastfeeding.
- **Placental Transfer Studies.** Studies on the placental transfer of drugs evaluate the radioactivity of mother blood and fetal tissue to gather information on this topic. Rats, rabbits, and humans share many morphological similarities and differences in the yolk sac and chorioallantoic placenta. As a result, it seems doubtful that standard placental transfer research—where fetal exposure is assessed following the closure of the hard palate—would be sufficient to establish a link between embryo-fetal exposure to an NCE and a developmental consequence. Most chemicals are not significantly different in the placental transfer process despite the obvious variations between animal placentas. In addition to physicochemical characteristics, physiological parameters, and gestational age also influence the relative distribution of a drug between the embryo-fetal and maternal units. Therefore, distributional evidence can only be obtained for that specific gestational period from placental transfer studies that are limited to one accession during gestation. Since the unbound free drug is what passes through the placenta and is available for distribution, consideration should also be given to the drug's protein binding.
- **Milk Transfer Studies.** Lipophilic drugs are likely to be excreted in the milk of nursing females, meaning that while the pups are sucking, they will be exposed to the parent drug or its metabolites. As a result, the drug label ought to include a warning about the possible risks of drug ingestion through breast milk in newborn humans. Research on the amount of drug excretion in animal milk is not a reliable indicator of the amount of milk transfer in humans,

so it is debatable whether this kind of research should be routinely conducted. Research on labeled compounds in rats could yield more details. Additionally, because newborns and adults may have different metabolic profiles, blood samples from pups can be taken to measure drug levels. When determining the likelihood that the fetus will be exposed to NCE, TK may be a very useful tool. The determination of animal-to-human exposure ratios, which eventually computes the safety margins, is the primary use of TK data in reproductive toxicity studies. Disparities in the way that pregnant and nonpregnant women respond to drugs could be useful in closely observing clinical trials carried out in pregnant women or in post-marketing surveillance following the introduction of new drugs. Studies on TK should be meticulously planned and designed to yield the most information possible, ultimately ensuring human safety.

4.2. Chemistry of Toxicodynamics

In pharmacology, the term "pharmacodynamics" refers to the dynamic interactions between a toxicant and a biological target, as well as the biological effects that result. A biological target can bind proteins, ion channels, DNA, or a range of other receptors. It is also referred to as the site of action. Toxins can interact with these receptors once they enter an organism, changing it structurally or functionally. Which receptors are targeted and the overall toxic effect at the cellular and organismal levels will depend on the toxicant's mode of action, which is dictated by its chemical properties. Quantitative structure-activity relationships (QSARs) have been used to classify toxicants based on their chemical properties, making it possible to predict their toxic action from these properties alone. Carcinogens and hormone-disrupting chemicals, such as endogenous estrogen derivatives (EDCs) are two examples of toxicant classes that can function as QSARs. Natural steroid hormones normally cause transcriptional activation, which EDCs mimic or prevent. These substances can interact with thyroid hormone, estrogen, and androgen receptors. Toxins like polychlorinated biphenyls (PCBs) and dichlorodiphenyltrichloroethane (DDE) may be a part of this mechanism. Substances that cause cancer are categorized as carcinogens, which are another class of chemicals. They can be either nongenotoxic or genotoxic. Toxicants like carbon tetrachloride (CCl_4) and polycyclic aromatic hydrocarbons (PAHs) fall into these categories.

Using TKTD models, the toxicodynamics process can be applied to environmental risk assessment. Time-varying exposure, carry-over toxicity, organism recovery time, mixture effects, and extrapolation to untested chemicals and species are among the phenomena covered by TKTD models. These kinds of models have advantages over more conventional modeling techniques, which makes them potentially more useful for risk assessment.

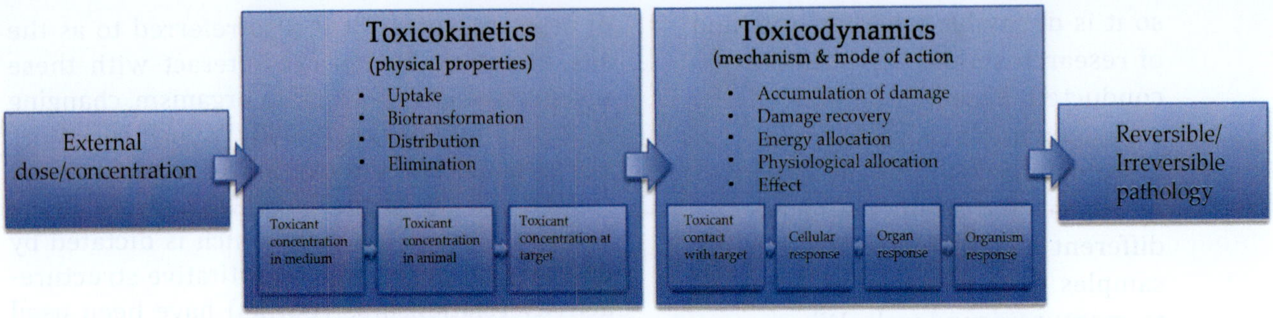

Figure 4.1. *A box model explaining the processes of toxicokinetics and toxicodynamics.*

Source: https://upload.wikimedia.org/wikipedia/en/thumb/1/18/Diagram_showing_the_conceptual_pathway_of_toxicokinetics_and_toxicodynamics.png/220px-Diagram_showing_the_conceptual_pathway_of_toxicokinetics_and_toxicodynamics.png.

Toxicodynamics deals with the interactions between a toxicant and a biological target, as well as the structural or functional changes in a cell that may eventually result in a toxic effect. Toxicokinetics describes changes in the concentrations of a toxicant over time due to the uptake, biotransformation, distribution, and elimination of toxicants. The toxicant may be able to interact with the biological target, depending on its proximity and chemical reactivity. High-affinity binding sites improve the selectivity of interactions between a toxicant and the biological target, allowing for more precise interactions. Toxicology may, therefore, primarily manifest in particular tissues or organs. Receptors in the cytoplasm, nucleus, and cell surface are frequently the targets. Toxicants can harm by either blocking a natural response or causing an unneeded reaction. Irreversible harm may start at the molecular level and spread to higher organizational levels if the biological target is important and the damage is great enough.

4.2.1. Endocrine Disruptors

EDCs are generally considered toxicants that either mimic or block the transcriptional activation normally caused by natural steroid hormones. These chemicals include those acting on androgen receptors, estrogen receptors and thyroid hormone receptors.

4.2.1.1. Effects of Endocrine Disruptors

Endocrine-disrupting substances can affect hormone synthesis, storage and release, transport and clearance, receptor recognition and binding, and postreceptor activation, among other aspects of the endocrine system. Exposure to EDCs in wildlife can lead to alterations in reproductive anatomy, decreased viability of offspring, altered hormone secretion or activity, and altered fertility. Offspring's reproductive anatomy may be especially impacted by maternal exposure. This includes the uterus, vagina, fallopian tubes, and mammary glands in females, and testes, epididymitis, prostate, and seminal vesicles in men. Fish exposed to EDCs have also been linked to thyroid abnormalities, reduced fertility, poor hatching success, de-feminization and masculinization of female fish, and immune system changes.

Theo Colborn's book Our Stolen Future made endocrine disruption known as a xenobiotic's mode of action. Endocrine disrupting substances are known to build up in bodily tissue and are incredibly enduring in the environment. Several known EDCs are toxicants, such as phthalates, phytoestrogens, pesticides, and certain commercial and industrial products. These substances can disrupt hormones in the body in a number of ways. Two other well-established mechanisms are the activation of the estrogen receptor and the inhibition of the androgen receptor, although the mechanism linked to the thyroid hormone receptor remains unclear.

4.2.1.2. Androgen-Receptor Mediated

Due to their interactions with the androgen receptor, some toxicants can disrupt hormones. Chemicals that function in this way include DDE, which is one of DDT's many environmental metabolites. DDT is still widely present in the environment, along with its metabolite DDE, even though its production is prohibited in the Western world due to its extreme persistence. DDE is mediated by the androgen receptor (AR) and functions as an antiandrogen by changing the expression of particular androgen-regulated genes. As it diffuses into the cell, the lipophilic substance DDE attaches itself to the AR. The receptor binds to the androgen response element on DNA, but this binding inactivates the receptor. It can have major repercussions for exposed wildlife as this suppresses the transcription of androgen-responsive genes. Two pesticides—dicofol and DDT—as well as their metabolites were spilled into Lake Apopka, Florida, in 1980. After a thorough investigation, researchers found that the young alligators in this lake had abnormal testicular and ovarian morphology, low clutch viability, elevated juvenile mortality, and changed plasma hormone concentrations.

4.2.1.3. Estrogen-Receptor Mediated

Interactions between toxicants and the estrogen receptor can potentially lead to endocrine disruption. The mechanism of PCBs has been thoroughly investigated. Because of their insulating qualities, these substances have been used as coolants and lubricants in transformers and other electrical equipment. PCBs are purely anthropogenic substances that are still widely present in the environment despite being produced no longer in the United States due to the harmful health effects of exposure. PCBs are xenoestrogens that act through the estrogen receptor to produce an enhancing (as opposed to an inhibiting) response. Because they mimic the effects of estrogen, these are frequently referred to as estrogen mimics. PCBs often accumulate in sediments and cause organisms to bioaccumulate them. These substances attach to the estrogen receptor after diffusing into the nucleus.

The heat shock proteins 59, 70, and 90 interact with the estrogen receptor to maintain it in an inactive conformation. The estrogen receptor is triggered upon binding of the toxicant, forming a homodimer complex that searches the DNA for estrogen response elements. A particular protein is produced when the complex binds to these elements, causing the rearrangement of the gene's chromatin and transcription. By doing this, PCBs trigger an estrogenic reaction that can impact a variety of bodily processes. These impacts are noted in a number of aquatic species. Due to bioaccumulation, marine mammals frequently have extremely high PCB levels. Research has shown that PCBs cause reproductive impairment in the *Phoca vitulina*, or harbor seal. Comparable outcomes have been observed in the California sea lion (*Zalophys californianus*), the ringed seal (*Pusa hispida*), and the grey seal (*Halichoerus grypus*). Uterine occlusions and stenosis were discovered in the grey seals and ringed seals, resulting in infertility. It has also been observed that male fish will produce vitellogenin when exposed to xenoestrogens like PCBs. Normally produced by female fish, vitellogenin is a protein found only in very small amounts in male fish eggs. This is frequently employed as an EDC biomarker.

4.2.2. Carcinogens

All substances that are known to cause cancer are considered carcinogens. Because different carcinogenic toxicants have different mechanisms of action, the toxicodynamics of carcinogens can be complicated. Carcinogens are categorized as either genotoxic or nongenotoxic due to their complex nature.

4.2.2.1. Effects of Carcinogens

Although human exposure to carcinogens is typically linked to their effects, toxicants that cause cancer can also affect species other than mammals. Numerous investigations have demonstrated that fish species can also develop cancer. Environmental toxicants have been connected to neoplasms that develop in epithelial tissue, including the liver, gastrointestinal tract, and pancreas. Fish livers are the preferred organ for carcinogens to cause hepatocellular and biliary lesions.

4.2.2.2. Genotoxic Carcinogens

Reactive metabolites of genotoxic carcinogens can interact with DNA and genetic material directly or indirectly. Aquatic organisms are susceptible to genotoxic carcinogens, such as PAHs. When coal, wood, or petroleum products do not burn completely, PAHs are released into the atmosphere and become widely distributed. Numerous studies have established that some PAH compounds, such as benzo(a)pyrene, benzo(a)anthracene, and benzofluoranthene, are bioavailable and cause liver diseases like cancer in wild fish populations, even though PAHs do not bioaccumulate in vertebrate tissue. The creation of DNA adducts is one way that genotoxic carcinogens work. The PAH compound is metabolized and ready for biotransformation as soon as it enters an organism. The PAH compound can be activated by the biotransformation process and changed into a very reactive intermediate called a diol epoxide. These diol-epoxides form stable adducts inside the DNA structure by covalently bonding with base pairs of DNA, usually guanine and adenine. DNA base pair binding with diol epoxides prevents the polymerase from carrying out replication. This blockage, by decreasing repair activity, ultimately leads to an increase in DNA damage. These mechanisms lead to the hypothesis that PAH compounds are involved in the initial stages of carcinogenesis as well as their early promotion. In fish exposed to PAHs, a variety of liver lesions develop, some of which indicate hepatocarcinogenicity.

4.2.2.3. Nongenotoxic Carcinogens

Since they are not directly carcinogenic, nongenotoxic, or epigenetic, carcinogens are distinct from genotoxic carcinogens and somewhat more ambiguous. Nongenotoxic carcinogens do not directly harm genes; instead, they operate through secondary mechanisms. This kind of carcinogenesis modifies the expression or repression of specific genes through a range of cellular processes rather than altering the DNA sequence. Since these toxicants do not act directly on DNA, the mechanism is not well understood. Oxidative stress, peroxisome proliferation, apoptosis suppression, changes in intercellular communication, and manipulation of metabolizing enzymes can all modify the expression of genes from nongenotoxic carcinogens.

For aquatic vertebrates, carbon tetrachloride is one example of a likely nongenotoxic carcinogen. Carbon tetrachloride has been utilized historically as an industrial solvent in petroleum refinement, and in the manufacture of pharmaceuticals. As a result of its extensive industrial use and environmental release, drinking water has been found to contain carbon tetrachloride, raising concerns for aquatic life. Carbon tetrachloride has a high hepatotoxic content, which may be related to liver cancer. According to research on cancer in mice, carbon tetrachloride can result in both benign and malignant liver tumors in rainbow trout. Carbon tetrachloride forms free radicals that cause oxidative stress, which is how it functions as a nongenotoxic carcinogen. It has been suggested that the CYP2E1 enzyme converts carbon tetrachloride into trichloromethyl and trichloromethyl peroxy radicals after it enters the body. Attacks on polyunsaturated fatty acids in the cellular membrane by the more reactive radical trichloromethyl peroxy can result in the formation of fatty acid free-radicals and initiate lipid peroxidation. The cellular membrane is under attack, which makes it more permeable and allows enzymes to seep out, upsetting the calcium homeostasis of the cell. Hepatic damage results from the activation of calcium-dependent degradative enzymes and cytotoxicity brought on by this loss of calcium homeostasis. The liver's regenerative and proliferative changes during this period may raise the frequency of genetic damage, which could lead to an increase in cancer cases.

4.2.3. Applications

The possible consequences of releasing a toxicant into the environment can be ascertained by combining toxicokinetics and toxicodynamics in environmental risk assessment. TKTD models are the most popular way to incorporate this.

4.2.3.1. Setup of Toxicokinetic-Toxicodynamic Models

Using the recently defined terms for TKTD, models were created that simulate exposure-related changes in internal concentration (TK) and damage (TD). To identify the characteristics of toxicants that determine TK and those that determine TD, TK and TD are divided apart in the model. TK process parameter values must be acquired prior to using this kind of model. It is necessary to estimate the TD parameters second. For parameterization, each of these procedures needs a sizable database of toxicity data. To calculate recovery times for organisms, predict toxic effects, and establish extrapolations to the toxicity of untested toxicants and species, one can use the TKTD model once all the parameter values have been established and standard scientific precautions have been followed.

4.2.3.2. History of Toxicokinetic-Toxicodynamic Models

It has been suggested that TKTD modeling can help with the problems that risk assessments are currently facing. Two factors led to the development of TKTD models. One is that toxicity and risk assessment does not take time into account. Time has been considered in some of the earliest TKTD models, including the Critical Body Residue (CBR) model and the Critical Target Occupation (CTO) model. However, these models have been criticized for being designed for extremely specific situations, such as toxicants that act irreversibly or reversibly. DEBtox, which can simulate sublethal endpoints, and hazard versions of the CTO, which consider stochastic death rather than individual tolerance, are further extrapolations of the CTO and CBR models. Adding a damage state variable to TKTD models was a crucial next step in the process. For toxicants that interact with their targets reversibly, modeling intermediate recovery rates can be achieved without making the assumptions of instant recovery (CBR model) or irreversible interactions (CTO model) by employing damage as a toxicodynamic state-variable. The Threshold Damage Model and the Damage Assessment Model (DAM) are two TKTD models that take damage into account. There are numerous distinct TKTD approaches for seemingly simple endpoints. A previous publication reviewed the underlying presumptions and theories for each to develop a general unified threshold model of survival (GUTS).

4.2.3.3. Advantages of Risk Assessment

As referenced above, TKTD models have several advantages to traditional models for risk assessments. The principal advantages to using TKTD models are:

- The consequences of time-varying or repeated exposures can be explained and simulated by the TKTD model.
- Carry-over toxicity as well as delayed effects can be simulated, whether the carry-over toxicity is due to TK or TD or both. In this way, TKTD models can quantify risks from pulsed or fluctuating exposures.
- Organism recovery time depends on the time course of TK and TD, which makes the TKTD models suitable for calculating organism recovery time.
- TKTD models have the potential to predict the effects of mixtures, including both environmental and chemical stressors and also be used as mechanism-based extrapolation to untested toxicants or untested species.
- Linking TKTD models with Individual Based Models (IBM) may improve risk assessment of toxicants by simulating temporal aspects as well as ecological aspects.

The incorporation of chemical concentrations and temporal dimensions in TKTD models makes them potentially more powerful than traditional dose-response models, adding to their advantages. There is growing potential to apply these findings in risk assessment to enable a more scientifically based risk assessment that is less dependent on animal testing. Toxicodynamic modeling, such as TKTD models, has been demonstrated to be a valuable tool for toxicological research. All in all, these kinds of models are helpful instruments for risk assessment because they can formalize information about the toxicity of toxicants and organism sensitivity, generate new theories, and simulate temporal aspects of toxicity.

4.3. Chemistry, Exposure of Toxicokinetics, and Toxicodynamics

4.3.1. Physical and Chemical Properties

Mercury has several chemical species that are important to toxicology. These include the organic forms methyl- and ethylmercury, as well as the inorganic forms elemental or metallic Hg (Hg^0), mercurous Hg (Hg^{1+}), and mercuric Hg (Hg^{2+}). While there are numerous organic Hg compounds, MeHg is the focus of this chapter. Table 4.1 displays the composition, molecular formula, and physical and chemical characteristics of a few compounds containing mercury. The Agency for Toxic Substances and Disease Registry (ATSDR) Toxicological Profile for Mercury (Update) contains a more comprehensive table of physical and chemical characteristics of some mercury compounds. Information on a few toxicologically significant mercury compounds is summarized in Table 4.2.

Table 4.1. *Physical and Chemical Properties of Some Toxicologically Relevant Mercury Compounds*

Chemical Name	Elemental Mercury [a]	Mercuric Chloride	Mercurous Chloride [b]	Methylmercuric Chloride [c]	Dimethylmercury
Molecular formula	Hg^0	$HgCl_2$	Hg_2Cl_2	CH_3HgCl	C_2H_6Hg
Molecular structure		Cl-Hg-Cl	Cl-Hg-Hg-Cl	CH_3-Hg-Cl	CH_3-Hg-CH_3
Molecular weight	200.59	271.52	472.09	251.1	230.66
Solubility	5.6×10^{-5} g/L at 25°C	69 g/L at 20°C	2.0×10^{-3} g/L at 25°C	0.100 g/L at 21°C	1 g/L at 21°C
Density	13.534 g/cm³ at 25°C	5.4 g/cm³ at 25°C	7.15 g/cm³ at 19°C	4.06 g/cm³ at 20°C	3.1874 g/cm³ at 20°C
Oxidation state	+1, +2	+2	+1	+2	+2

[a]*Also known as metallic mercury.*

[b]*Also known as calomel.*

[c]*Methylmercuric chloride is used experimentally to investigate the effects of methylmercury.*

Source: *https://nap.nationalacademies.org/read/9899/chapter/4.*

Table 4.2. *Summary Table Comparing Toxicologically Relevant Mercury Species*

Methylmercury (CH_3Hg^+)	Elemental Mercury (Hg^0)	Mercuric Mercury (Hg^{2+})
Sources of Exposure		
Fish, marine mammals, crustaceans, animals, and poultry fed fish meal	Dental amalgams, occupational exposure, Caribbean religious ceremonies, fossil fuels, incinerators	Oxidation of elemental mercury or demethylation of MeHg; deliberate or accidental poisoning with $HgCl_2$
Biological Monitoring		
Hair, blood, cord blood	**Urine, blood**	**Urine, blood**
Toxicokinetics		
Absorption		
Inhalation: Vapors of MeHg absorbed	Inhalation: Approximately 80% of inhaled dose of Hg^0 readily absorbed	Inhalation: Aerosols of $HgCl_2$ absorbed
Oral: Approximately 95% of MeHg in fish readily absorbed from GI tract	Oral: GI absorption of metallic Hg is poor; any released vapor in GI tract converted to mercuric sulfide and excreted	Oral; 7–15% of ingested dose of $HgCl_2$ absorbed from the GI tract; absorption proportional to water solubility of mercuric salt; uptake by neonates greater than adults

Dermal: In guinea pigs, 3–5% of applied dose absorbed in 5 hrs	Dermal: Average rate of absorption of Hg^0 through human skin, 0.024 ng/cm^2 for every 1 mg/m^3 in air	Dermal: In guinea pigs, 2–3% of applied dose of $HgCl_2$ absorbed
Distribution		
Distributed throughout body since lipophilic; approximately 1–10% of absorbed oral dose of MeHg distributed to blood; 90% of blood MeHg in RBCs	Rapidly distributed throughout the body since it is lipophilic	Highest accumulation in kidney; fraction of dose retained in kidney dose dependent
MeHg-cysteine complex involved in transport of MeHg into cells		
Half-life in blood, 50 d; 50% of dose found in the liver; 10% in the head.	Half-life in blood, 45 d (slow phase); half-life appears to increase with increasing dose	Half-life in blood, 19.7–65.6 d; 1st phase, 24 d, 2nd phase, 15–30 d
Readily crosses blood-brain and placental barriers	Readily crosses blood-brain and placental barriers	Does not readily penetrate blood-brain or placental barriers
		In neonate, mercuric Hg not concentrated in kidneys; therefore, more widely distributed to other tissues
		In fetus and neonate, blood-brain barrier incompletely formed, so mercuric Hg brain concentrations higher than those in adults
Biotransformation		
MeHg slowly demethylated to mercuric Hg (Hg^{2+})	Hg^0 in tissue and blood oxidized to Hg^{2+} by catalase and hydrogen peroxide (H_2O_2); H_2O_2 production the rate-limiting step	Hg^0 vapor exhaled by rodents following oral administration of mercuric Hg
Tissue macrophages, intestinal flora, and fetal liver are sites of tissue demethylation		Mercuric Hg not methylated in body tissues but GI microorganisms can form MeHg
Mechanisms of demethylation unknown; free radicals demethylate MeHg in vitro; bacterial demethylation enzymes studied extensively, none has been characterized or identified in mammalian cells		
Does not bind or induce metallothionein		Binds and induces metallothionein
Excretion		
Daily excretion, 1% of body burden; the major excretory route is bile and feces; 90% excreted in feces as Hg^{2+}; 10% excreted in urine as H^{g2}+	Excreted as Hg^0 in exhaled air, sweat, and saliva, and as mercuric Hg in feces and urine	Excreted in urine and feces; also excreted in saliva, bile, sweat, exhaled air, and breast milk

Lactation increases clearance from blood; 16% of Hg in breast milk is MeHg		
Half-Life elimination		
(Whole body) 70–80 d; dependent on species, dose, sex, and animal strain	58 d	1–2 mo
Toxicodynamics		
Critical target organ		
Brain, adult and fetal	Brain and kidney	Kidney
Causes of Toxicity		
Demethylation of MeHg to Hg^{2+} and the intrinsic toxicity of MeHg	Oxidation of Hg^0 to Hg^{2+}	Hg^{2+} binding to thiols in critical enzyme (e.g., cysteine) and structural proteins
Latency period		
In Iraq, from weeks to month; in Japan, more than a year; differences suggested to be caused by Se in fish; no toxic signs during latency period		
Mobilization		
DMPS, DMSA	After oxidation to Hg^{2+}: DMPS, DMSA	DMPS, DMSA
Possible Antagonists		
Selenium, garlic, zinc		

Source: https://nap.nationalacademies.org/read/9899/chapter/4. DMPS, 2,3-dimercapto-1-propane sulfonate; DMSA, meso 2,3-dimercaptosuccinic acid; GI, gastrointestinal tract; RBC, red blood cells are some examples of abbreviations. (Aschner, M., N.B. Eberle, and H.K. Kimelberg. 1991).

The solubility of elemental mercury in water is 5.6×10^{-5} g/L at 25°C. At 20°C, mercuric chloride has a solubility of 69 g/L, which is significantly higher. By contrast, an organic mercury compound with a solubility of 0–100 g/L at 21°C, such as methylmercury chloride, is much less soluble in water. A highly hazardous byproduct of the chemical synthesis of mercury is dimethylmercury (Nierenberg et al., 1998); it also has a water solubility of only 1.0 g/L at 21°C. MeHg chloride is relatively lipid soluble due to its low water solubility. As will be covered later in this chapter, the varying degrees of toxicity caused by the various forms of mercury may be related to their solubility.

4.3.2. Methods of Chemical Analysis

Atomic absorption spectrometry (AAS), atomic fluorescence spectrometry (AFS), gas chromatography (GC)-electron capture, X-ray fluorescence (XRF), and neutron activation analysis (NAA) are among the techniques used to analyze mercury (Hg) in biological samples. Additionally, anodic stripping voltammetry (ASV) has been employed. Only cold vapor (CV)-AAS can detect mercury at parts per billion among those methods; GC-electron capture can distinguish MeHg from other species. Hair mercury content has been analyzed using CV-AAS, AFS, XRF, and NAA. Prior to being measured, mercury must be reduced to its elemental form in biological samples. The most common applications for CV-AAS are blood and urine Hg measurements. For instance, the most widely used technique for analyzing mercury in biological samples, CV-AAS, entails reducing the mercury in the sample to elemental mercury by reducing it with stannous chloride. Without chemically reducing the sample, the analysis is performed to quantify inorganic mercury. The amount of organic mercury that was present in the sample is indicated by the difference between the total mercury concentration and the inorganic mercury concentration.

The strain FB1 of *Pseudomonas putida* can also be used to analyze biological materials containing mercury. Methane gas and elemental mercury are produced by these bacteria from MeHg. Due to the minimal amount of chemical interference, this method is among the most precise and dependable for measuring mercury levels. With a coefficient of variation of 1.9%, it can identify 15 ng of mercury in 1 g of biological tissue. Novel techniques, like inductively coupled plasma-mass spectrometry (ICPMS), have been developed to analyze mercury levels in biological samples. The majority of the new techniques are pricey and out of the reach of most labs. The instrument costs between $150,000 and $250,000, and the annual cost of gases and maintenance is more than $35,000. During sample preparation and analysis, care must be taken to eliminate or prevent contamination by mercury ions (Hg) regardless of the analytical method employed. It is necessary to acid wash all glass and plasticware used in the specimen collection and analysis. Furthermore, precautions must be taken to prevent losses from elemental mercury and mercury ion volatilization, particularly when concentrating or preserving the samples. For many processes, the sample must be broken down before being reduced. Data are required to validate the methods and their application in a particular laboratory when trying to quantify the amount of mercury present, particularly in biological samples. Every analysis method is subject to significant variances. Measuring the concentration of mercury in blood, urine, or both is necessary for the biological monitoring of inorganic mercury, which includes elemental mercury. Biological MeHg monitoring typically entails determining the amount of Hg present in blood, scalp hair, or both. Because the mercury included in hair is stable, hair segments can be analyzed to determine the historical record of exposure to mercury through a process known as longitudinal timing. The presence of Hg on the hair surface because of external deposition is one factor that can cause errors in hair Hg analysis. This error is reduced when the hair sample is thoroughly cleaned before analysis.

An excellent summary of the analytical methods for determining various species of Hg in biological specimens, including blood, urine, hair, breath, and tissues, as well as in environmental samples.

4.3.3. Exposures to MeHg in the Population of USA

Fish, marine mammals, and crustaceans are the main sources of mercury exposure in humans. Variations in MeHg exposure in the U.S. are caused by fish consumption, which accounts for nearly all of the exposure and varies depending on the type of fish consumed, which is population are determined by the unique traits of fish consumption. Additionally, exposure differs based on the typical kinds and quantities of fish eaten in various US regions. In the US, the amounts of mercury found in commercial fish and seafood vary by roughly two orders of magnitude. For instance, the Hg content of shark exceeds 1 ppm, whereas that of herring is roughly 0:01 ppm. There is little evidence to support the theory that fish consumption is higher overall in coastal areas. Furthermore, recreational fishermen as well as particular ethnic and cultural subgroups, may be more exposed. Fish consumption by species and portion size has been accounted for in dietary assessment studies, which have served as the foundation for population-based estimates of MeHg exposure in the US. An estimation of the average mass of fish consumed (in grams per day) can be obtained by combining the intake frequency by species with the portion size by species for each individual consumer.

The EPA's report to Congress includes summaries of these studies that provide data at the national level. The gram-per-day amount of each species consumed by each individual is multiplied by the characteristic MeHg concentration of each species (microgram per gram), and the summation across species yields the average intake of MeHg by each individual (microgram/day) in order to estimate population-based MeHg exposure from such studies. An estimate of the intake of MeHg in the underlying population can then be obtained from the distribution of individual intakes for the study sample. The recall and recording of intake frequency and portion size, incorrect species identification, extrapolation of short-term dietary studies to long-term average exposure, and the out-of-date and incomplete national database on average MeHg concentrations of various fish species are among the uncertainties in such assessments. Additionally, estimates usually differ based on how long the fish-intake data was collected over (e.g., 1-day memory compared to 1-week memory). The EPA analysis of MeHg intake based on fish consumption data for a month is shown in Table 4.3 for both the general population and the population of women of childbearing age. In general, estimates based on intake from these data are less than those based on dietary data collected over one day. Additionally, data from New Jersey derived from a 7-day recall survey are shown in Table 4.3. These figures imply that the population in that American region has greater intakes than the U.S. A. populace as a whole. Therefore, the population may underestimate their exposure to large subpopulations. Data from the National Health and Nutrition Examination Survey (NHANES IV) and the Continuing Survey of Food Intakes by Individuals (CFSII) may eventually provide information on fish consumption in the area. Additionally intended to provide data on MeHg exposure in the U.S. is NHANES IV. S. numbers.

Table 4.3. *Estimated Average MeHg Intake for the U.S. Population and for New Jersey Fish Consumers*

Average Daly Intake of MeHg (μg/day) [a]				
Percentiles of the Population	General Population		Women of Childbearing Age	
	U.S. [b,c]	New Jersey [d]	U.S. [b,e]	New Jersey [c,f]
50th	1.4	3.1	0.6	3.2
75th	3.5	5.8	1.8	5.4
90th	9.1	13.1	4.8	10.8
95th	15.6	21.1	7.8	15.7
99th		49.9	22.2	26.5

[a]Assuming body weight of 70 kg for the general population and 60 kg for women of childbearing age.
[b]Data from EPA 1997a.
[c]Unweighted average across ethnic groups.
[d]Data from Stern et al., 1996.
[e]Women 15–45 years old.
[f]Women 18–40 years old.
Source: https://www.ncbi.nlm.nih.gov/books/NBK225779/table/ttt00004/?report=objectonly.

There is insufficient data to determine whether eating fish meal-fed animals or poultry would increase one's exposure to mercury. Since young children may be more susceptible to those mercurials than adults, the use of organic mercury compounds as preservatives in vaccinations and medical preparations is also a source of exposure. There are up to 219 of these items in use. At concentrations of 0.01% and 0.00002%, respectively, phenolmercuric acetate (PMA) and sodium ethylmercurithiosalicylate (TM) are the most commonly used compounds. According to FDA estimates, those vaccine and medical preparation manufacturers use between 75 and 80 kg of Hg compounds annually. Clinicians have received an interim report that addresses the risks related to the use of thimerosal in vaccines, the main way that Americans are exposed to elemental mercury. Mercury vapor emitted from dental amalgams is the cause of the population. Every year, dentists use about 300 metric tons of mercury to make amalgams. Roughly half of the amalgams used in the US are made of mercury. According to a study on college students with dental amalgams, the amalgams' Hg vapor was responsible for two-thirds of the mercury excreted in the urine. There's evidence that mercury vapor from dental amalgams seeps into bodily tissues, including the brain, where it oxidizes to form inorganic mercury. After receiving amalgam fillings labeled with radioactive mercury, pregnant sheep quickly developed radioactivity in both the mother's and the fetus' tissues. The amount of amalgams in the mouth and the amount of mercury in human tissues—including the brain—have been shown to significantly positively correlate. If no fish with high MeHg concentrations is consumed, the mean total mercury concentration in whole blood is most likely between 5 and 10 μg/L. Since the retention of inorganic mercury is much lower than that of organic and elemental mercury, exposure to mercury vapors from amalgams is most likely the cause of this concentration. Additionally, the amount of MeHg exposure from non-fish sources is extremely low.

Accidents in chloralkali plants have resulted in occupational exposure to elemental mercury. There are additional possible occupational exposures to elemental mercury, though. Additionally, elemental mercury is used in religious rites by certain Caribbean faiths. Due to elemental mercury's intriguing physical characteristics, children have been known to play with it that could seriously contaminate areas used for play and living. Dental offices, hospitals, and laboratories are the primary sources of elemental mercury in wastewaters. Humans have been exposed to mercury through intentional or unintentional means (e.g., occupational exposures) and mercuric chloride poisonings.

4.3.4. Toxicokinetics

4.3.4.1. Absorption and Distribution

- Methylmercury

MeHg is found in most fish. In the US, the mercury content of many freshwater fish is more than 2–3 parts per million. People who regularly consume fish across the globe may have levels in their hair of more than 10 parts per million. It has been discovered that the gastrointestinal (GI) tract absorbs approximately 95% of the mercury (Hg) in fish consumed by humans and 95% of the methylmercuric nitrate administered orally to volunteers. While the main focus of this report is on MeHg toxicity after ingestion, it should be remembered that MeHg is also easily absorbed through the skin and lungs. It is thought that after inhalation exposure, there is a high degree of absorption. MeHg enters red blood cells after being absorbed into the bloodstream. Red blood cells' hemoglobin binds more than 90% of the mercury (MeHg) present in blood. The distribution of mercury compounds in three male volunteers in good health who were given oral [^{203}Hg]-methylmercuric nitrate (Cappon, C.J., and J.C. Smith, 1978). Within 15 minutes of administration, 203Hg was detected in the blood, and it peaked in 3–6 h. Red blood cells had a concentration ten times higher than plasma. MeHg binds to hemoglobin's β chain's cysteine residues 93 and 112 as well as α chain's residue number 104. Cysteine residues with numbers 104 and 112 can be found in the hemoglobin molecule's contact junction. Since number 93 is on the outside of the hemoglobin molecule, it is out of the junction and readily binds to MeHg. Animal species vary in the quantity and location of their hemoglobin's junctional and external cysteine residues. A comprehensive table containing information on the hemoglobin of eight different animal species. Additionally, some MeHg is bonded to plasma proteins. The percentage of total mercury found as inorganic mercury in whole blood, plasma, breast milk, liver, urine, and other tissues in humans exposed to high daily oral doses of mercury was 7%, 22%, 39%, 16%–40%, and 73%, respectively. Total mercury concentrations in the cerebrum, cerebellum, heart, and spleen were on the order of tens of ng/g. MeHg accounted for about 80% of the total mercury content in those organs. Methylmercurmade up 33%, 15%, and 1% of the mercury in the kidney cortex, liver, and kidney medulla, respectively. Only roughly 5% of total blood and 20% of scalp hair contain inorganic mercury when fish that have high MeHg concentrations are consumed. It is important to note that the precise form(s) in which mercury exists in the body is still a mystery. MeHg ions in aqueous solutions are hydrated. Hg-substituted oxonium ions are produced by pH-dependent processes (Figure 4.2). For instance, the cysteinate has a linear C—Hg—S composition. MeHg transport may be impacted by the chemistry and formation of Hg-substituted oxonium ion complexes, although researchers who focus on this kind of transport generally overlook them (Ballatori and Clarkson, 1983, 1982).

$$CH_3Hg(OH_2)^+ + OH^- \rightleftharpoons CH_3HgOH + H_2O$$

$$CH_3Hg(OH_2)^+ + CH_3HgOH \rightleftharpoons (CH_3Hg)_2OH^+ + H_2O$$

$$CH_3HgOH + (CH_3Hg)_2OH^+ \rightleftharpoons (CH_3Hg)_2O^+ + H_2O$$

Figure 4.2. *Hg-substituted oxonium ions formed in aqueous solution.*

Source: https://www.ncbi.nlm.nih.gov/books/NBK225779/bin/200032fc004401.jpg.

In the brain, where it is gradually demethylated to inorganic mercuric mercury, about 10% of the body's MeHg load is located (refer to Figure 4.3). Additionally, MeHg is easily transferred to the developing brain of the fetus. MeHg is thought to cross the blood-brain barrier through the MeHg-l-cysteine complex, which is carried by the leucine-preferring l-system amino acid carrier. This theory is supported by data from rat experiments. MeHg-cysteine is liberated in vitro from a MeHg-glutathione complex through the involvement of dipeptidases and γ-glutamyltransferase. This suggests that the transport of MeHg into endothelial cells may indirectly involve glutathione. It would be anticipated that the MeHg-cysteine or MeHg-glutathione complex would dissolve in water. That would refute the theory that lipid solubility in bodily fluids and tissues is the reason for the brain's quick uptake of mercury.

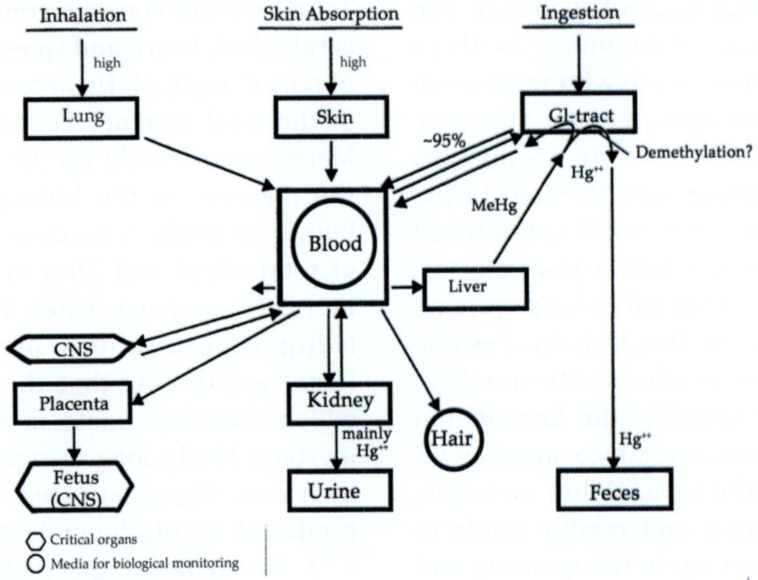

Figure 4.3. *Methylmercury kinetics.*

Source: https://www.ncbi.nlm.nih.gov/books/NBK225779/bin/200032fc004402.jpg.

MeHg sensitivity is highest in the cerebrum and cerebellum, according to a case study of family members who consumed tainted pork and experienced classic symptoms of the illness. Upon autopsy of one female member, several years later, analyses of different brain regions showed a correlation between regional brain mercury concentrations and the degree of brain damage. Between 82 and 100% of the total Hg was inorganic, indicating that most of the MeHg had been transformed into inorganic Hg during that time. The cerebellum and cerebrum had the highest concentrations of mercury. Studies using Magnetic Resonance Imaging (MRI) revealed brain damage in other family members' cerebellum, parietal cortices, and calcarine cortices. Since those brain regions are in charge of sensations, balance, and coordination, it is thought that damage to those regions is the root cause of many of their enduring clinical symptoms.

- Dimethylmercury

Accidental exposure to dimethylmercury, a highly toxic form of mercury, has resulted in fatalities. A chemistry professor at Dartmouth College passed away 298 days after multiple drops of dimethylmercury landed on her latex gloves. The substance was quickly absorbed through her skin, and the gloves did not seem to serve as a barrier. After being exposed, her blood mercury level was 1,000 µg/L six to seven months later. The usual range of mercury concentrations in blood is 1 to 8 µg/L. According to studies on mice, dimethlymercury, which is incredibly toxic, needs to be converted to MeHg to enter the brain.

- Elemental Mercury

Elemental mercury vapor enters the lungs quickly and is absorbed. 75–85% of a dose inhaled by a human is absorbed. Less than 0.01% of liquid or vaporized elemental mercury is absorbed from the GI tract (Bornmann et al., 1970). Less than 3% of the total amount absorbed by the skin in humans exposed to elemental mercury vapor came from the skin; 97% came from the lungs. Elemental mercury diffuses quickly through the lungs and dissolves quickly in blood lipids due to its high lipid solubility. Its uncharged state with an intermediate molecular weight and size could also contribute to its easy translocation from air to blood. It is found all over the body and can easily pass through the blood-brain barrier and the placenta (see Figure 4.4). Mercury is oxidized to produce mercuric mercury. The red blood cell to plasma Hg ratio eventually reaches 1:1.

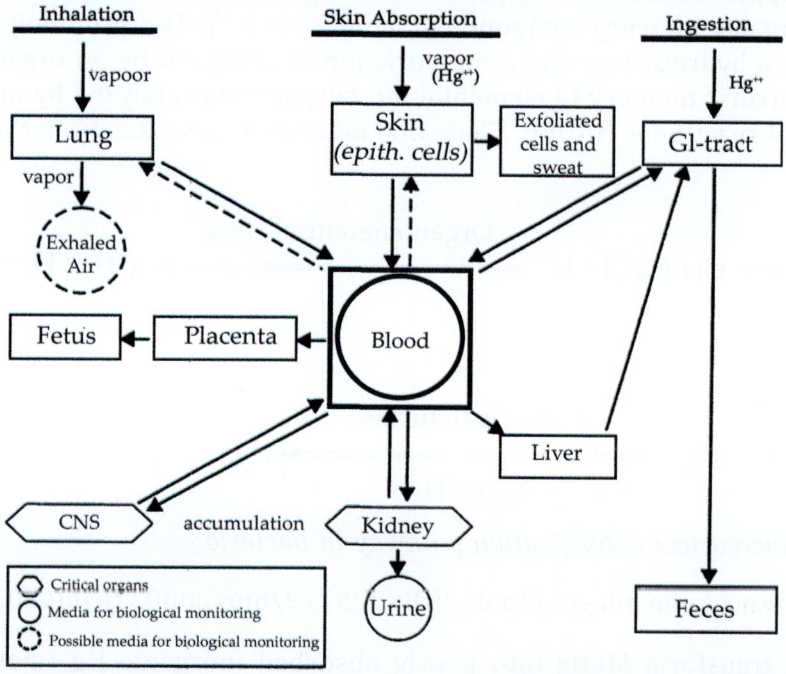

Figure 4.4. *Inorganic mercury kinetics. This diagram is complicated by the fact that inhaled vapor is oxidized to Hg++ so that both species are present. The inhaled vapor is highly mobile, readily crosses cell membranes, the blood-brain barrier, and the placenta.*

Source: https://www.ncbi.nlm.nih.gov/books/NBK225779/figure/mmm00004/?report=objectonly.

- Inorganic Mercury

The GI tract absorbs between 7 and 15% of the mercuric chloride that is consumed. The mercuric salt's water solubility determines how much of it is absorbed. Mercuric mercury has a strong affinity for sulfhydryl groups found in plasma and red blood cells. According to reports, the blood's half-life is between 19 and 65 points per day. The kidneys have the largest concentration of mercuric mercury buildup. In the kidneys of rats, metallothionein binds to a significant portion of the inorganic mercury. MeHg, on the other hand, has little affinity for metallothionein. Mercuric mercury does not easily pass through the placenta or the blood-brain barrier due to its ionic charge (Fritzinger, 1983)

4.3.4.2. Biotransformation

Tissues transform MeHg into mercuric Hg. Rats and the majority of other species have very slow rates of demethylation. There is debate over the processes by which mercury is changed from mercury ions to mercury ions. The enzymes in-charge of the biotransformation in mammalian tissues have never been found. There has been an increased focus on looking into the potential function of a free radical mechanism. Furthermore, it has been demonstrated that glutathione can further enhance the similar degradation activity of γ-globulin and serum albumin. Tissue demethylation occurs in fetal liver, tissue macrophages, and intestinal flora. Numerous methods for detoxifying heavy metals (Aposhian, et al., 1983) are demonstrated by experiments conducted on bacteria. As an illustration, certain metals are actively moved outside of the cell (e.g., arsenite), and other metals are trapped within cells by protein binding. A microbial organomercurial resistance system detoxifies organic mercury compounds (see Figure 4.5). The protonolysis of the carbon-Hg bond to produce a hydrocarbon and a mercuric ion is catalyzed by an organomercurial lyase. The reduction of mercuric mercury to elemental mercury is then catalyzed by mercuric reductase. The coenzyme in that reaction is NADPH. Elemental mercury evaporates from the bacterial culture due to its volatility.

$$\text{Equation 1: } CH_3HgCl + H^4 \xrightarrow{\text{Organomercurial lyase}} CH_4 + Hg^{2+} + Cl^-$$

$$\text{Equation 2: } Hg^{2+} \xrightarrow[\text{NADPH}]{\text{mercuric reductase}} Hg^0$$

Figure 4.5. *Organomercurical detoxification pathway in bacteria.*

Source: https://www.ncbi.nlm.nih.gov/books/NBK225779/bin/200032fc004801.jpg.

Intestinal flora transform MeHg into poorly absorbed inorganic Hg (mercuric ion), which reduces MeHg's GI absorption. Escherichia coli has been used to purify organomercurial lyase. The plasmid R831 contains the enzyme's encoding. Enzyme activity does not require cofactors, and there are no metals in the structure of the enzyme. In primary, secondary, and tertiary alkyl, vinyl, allyl, and aryl organomercurial salts, the enzyme can catalyze the protonolysis of the C-Hg bond to the hydrocarbon and mercuric ion. Cysteine is the most active thiol compound and is required for the demethylation of organic mercurials to occur. Mammals do not contain enzymes that are comparable to those found in bacteria. It is believed that the mammalian brain uses a free-radical mechanism to demethylate mercury, which could do away with the requirement for those enzymes. Another possibility is that the enzymes are still unidentified.

The liver homogenates from rats, mice, and guinea pigs for the presence of enzymes that could break down organic mercury compounds. MeHg was not broken down, but phenylmercuric acetate and methoxyethylmercury chloride were, despite the presence of a minimum level of activity. Rat kidney and liver to cleave phenylmercuric acetate (PMA) and ethylmercury chloride, but no action against mercury was observed. Catalase and hydrogen peroxide (H2O2) in blood and tissues oxidize elemental mercury vapor to mercuric mercury (Berlin 1986). Production of H2O2 is the step that limits the rate. Elemental mercury vapor has been found in the expired air following the oral administration of mercury to rodents, suggesting that some elemental mercury metabolism must have taken place. Mammals do not methylate mercuric mercury; nevertheless, intestinal flora has a limited capacity to methylate Hg2+.

- Excretion

MeHg is excreted from the human body mainly through the bile and feces, with approximately 1% being eliminated daily. About 90% of a dose of MeHg is excreted in the feces, while 10% is excreted via urine. Some biliary MeHg is reabsorbed, but MeHg complexed with glutathione is eliminated through the bile. In one study, only 33% of an orally administered dose of MeHg was excreted in feces over 49 days, with a small amount excreted in urine. The half-life of MeHg in the body was found to be around 70–80 days in humans. Elimination rates of MeHg vary depending on species, dose, sex, and animal strain.

It is important to remember that newborn rats and monkeys have restricted bile excretion of mercury. As a result, they excrete MeHg more slowly than mature animals. Furthermore, during this nursing phase, their intestinal flora may also be less capable of demethylating MeHg. In the event that both of those human phenomena hold true, newborns may be especially vulnerable to MeHg exposure. The main cellular defense against MeHg toxicity might be GSH. One important mechanism for MeHg excretion from the cell and defense against MeHg toxicity is GSH complexation with MeHg. MeHg levels in guinea pig, human, and rat breast milk have all been measured. As a result, breast milk is regarded as a route of excretion, but it also serves as a vital conduit for exposure for newborns who are nursing. MeHg has been found to make up 16% of the Hg in human breast milk. That percentage is significantly less than the percentage of mercury in whole blood found as MeHg. It was discovered that in animals, the total mercury content of the plasma was proportionate to the total mercury content of the breast milk.

Sweat, saliva, feces, urine, and exhaled air all contain trace amounts of elemental mercury vapor. Elemental mercury levels in the urine and exhaled air are very low. Saliva and sweat usually excrete very little. In humans, the hair-life for total body mercury excretion was 58 days. Additionally, the body oxidizes elemental mercury to mercuric mercury, which is expelled in the urine and feces. This is supported by the finding that the Hg content in feces increases and is four times higher than that in urine following exposure to Hg vapor. Within a few days of mercuric Hg being administered orally to humans, 85% of it was eliminated through the feces. The epithelium of the small intestine, the colon, and bile secretion all contribute to the excretion of mercury in feces. In addition, breast milk, sweat, urine, and lungs all expel mercury. When tracking inorganic mercury biologically, urinary excretion is helpful. The half-life of absorbed inorganic mercury is thought to be 40 or 67 days. A 35-day half-life was reported by WHO. When exposed to inorganic mercury at work, humans excrete three different forms of the element in their urine: a metallic form, an Hg-cysteine complex, and a large unidentified complex.

4.3.5. Mobilization of Body Hg

Inorganic and organic mercury are excreted in the urine, and the body burden is decreased by synthetic chelating or complexing agents that compete with endogenous ligands for mercuric or organic mercury. Two compounds that have been used therapeutically are meso 2,3-dimercaptosuccinic acid (DMSA, succimer) and 2,3-dimercapto-1-propane sulfonate (DMPS, Dimaval, and Unithiol). The less-toxic, water-soluble chemical analogs of 2,3-dimercapto-1-propanol (British Anti-Lewisite BAL dimercaprol) are DMPS and DMSA. Because BAL is lipid soluble, it needs to be injected deeply into the muscle. DMPS and DMSA can be taken orally. A DMPS injectable preparation is available. Approximately 55% of patients who receive BAL experience one or more side effects, the majority of which are not life-threatening. Whether BAL will remain useful as a therapeutic is debatable because it redistributes mercury, raising brain mercury concentrations in animals exposed to mercury. In 1958, DMPS was added to the official Soviet drug arsenal. It was later made available to the West in 1978. Over the past eighteen years, several reviews of DMPS and other chelating agents have been published. The German and Chinese equivalents of the U.S. have authorized its use. S. FDA stands for Food and Drug Administration. Alternative medicine doctors have used DMPS elsewhere, including the United States, because they are worried about the toxicity of dental amalgams. It was recently used to raise the amount of Hg excreted in the urine of eight people who had been exposed to mercurous Hg. Rats' brain Hg concentration is not increased by DMPS, in contrast to BAL. Hg intoxication has been treated with DMSA, despite its unapproved use for this purpose. In 1990, the FDA approved its use for treating children whose blood lead concentration was 45 μg/dL or higher.

4.3.6. Chemical forms of Hg in Toxicity

MeHg is slowly biotransformed to inorganic Hg in the brain, as demonstrated by numerous human and animal model experimental studies. The brain's biotransformation mechanism for mercury from mercury ions to inorganic mercury is still poorly understood, despite the fact that the rate of demethylation of mercury in the brain seems to be dose-related. Total Hg concentrations were significantly elevated (71–300 times greater than controls) in several brain regions of a patient who passed away about 21 years after consuming MeHg-contaminated pork. Inorganic mercury made up at least 82% of the mercury in the patient's brain. In most areas of her brain, 100% of the mercury was in the inorganic form. A Minamata patient who passed away eighteen years after the exposure had similar outcomes.

Additionally, after administering MeHg and assessing the brain for total and inorganic Hg from days to years after exposure, experimental studies have documented a gradual increase in the concentration of inorganic Hg in the brain in a number of species. The brains of monkeys given high doses of mercury every day for extended periods of time showed notable levels of inorganic mercury. Of the brain Hg, 10 to 33% was inorganic by 69–166 weeks. MeHg was given to female *Macaca fascicularis* monkeys on a daily basis for a maximum of eighteen months. After six to twelve months of exposure, and then eighteen months later, when the brains were analyzed for mercury species, inorganic mercury accounted for approximately 9% of the total mercury. It was 74% six months after a 12-month exposure concluded. The authors claimed that they thought the demethylation of mercury in the brain produced inorganic mercury. ".

Questions concerning the species responsible for the poisonings in Iraq have also been raised, in addition to the question of whether organic or inorganic Hg mediates MeHg toxicity at the cellular level. Certain grain seeds in the Iraqi poisoning incident seemed to contain phenyl Hg rather than MeHg. Without a doubt, however, gas chromatography detected MeHg in the blood of the majority of the exposed population, and the blood's phenyl Hg would have swiftly transformed into inorganic Hg. Furthermore, barley seeds contained phenyl mercury, even though no barley was used to make bread.

4.3.7. Toxic Effects and Target Organs

It is currently widely accepted that the brain is the key organ for MeHg toxicity. Although the developing nervous system seems to be more sensitive, both the adult and fetal brains are vulnerable to MeHg toxicity (see Figure 4.3). Prenatal exposure damages the fetal brain throughout, and at high doses, it results in effects in the offspring that are almost identical to cerebral palsy caused by other factors, according to studies on the Minamata disaster in Japan. Adults exposed to mercury had focal lesions. It takes time to notice the neurotoxicity of chronic low-level mercury exposure. Usually, a latent period of at least one month takes place. Other negative consequences (e.g., MeHg) levels that cause negative effects in the nervous system are higher than those that have been shown to cause effects in the cardiovascular and immune systems. But those effects haven't been investigated as thoroughly as the neurotoxic effects. The kidney and brain are the target organs of elemental mercury. It is thought that the mercuric form is the cause of elemental mercury toxicity. The blood-brain barrier is easily crossed by elemental mercury vapor inhaled, which oxidizes to mercuric mercury. The latter solidifies into a bond with brain macromolecules. Mercuric mercury from such sites does not appear to be removed quickly by any endogenous mechanism. Tremors, psychological issues, gingivitis, and behavioral changes are indicators of severe exposure in people who work with elemental mercury vapor.

Mercuric Hg toxicity primarily targets the kidneys, where Hg accumulates. The early indicators of renal damage from Hg compounds include elevated levels of N-acetyl-β-glucoseaminidase, β2-microglobulin, and retinol-binding protein in the urine. The exact mechanism of this toxicity is not fully understood, but it is known that mercuric Hg has a strong attraction to sulfhydryl groups. The formation of Hg sulfhydryl complexes has a high affinity, with formation constants reaching approximately 1030. Mercuric Hg forms stronger bonds with sulfhydryl groups compared to carboxyl or amino groups, making it more likely to bind to critical enzymes and proteins with active sulfhydryl centers throughout the body.

4.3.8. Biochemical Mechanisms of Toxicity

A thorough review has been conducted on experimental investigations into potential biochemical mechanisms of mercury toxicity. Possible mechanisms have included disruption of microtubules, induction of lipid peroxidation, disruption of mitochondria, and disrupted protein synthesis. Another theory for the mechanism of developmental toxicity is the disruption of cell-surface recognition. When it comes to the neurotoxic symptoms linked to adult exposure to mercury, there are currently no conclusive data that identify a single mechanism as the primary cause. Although biochemical and ultrastructural alterations in the mitochondria have long been reported following MeHg exposure in rats, the evidence does not support the theory that these alterations serve as the main cause of MeHg toxicity. The cellular damage caused by mercury exposure may involve free-radical-induced lipid peroxidation because antioxidants, like vitamin E and selenium, provide some protection in vivo against MeHg neurotoxicity. Yet, for a variety of reasons, lipid peroxidation does not seem to be the essential process that results in cell death.

MeHg has been shown to cause disruption in protein synthesis, which is thought to be the main cause of MeHg neurotoxicity. On the other hand, inorganic Hg was ten times more effective than MeHg as an inhibitor of cell-free protein synthesis in rats. MeHg-stimulated protein synthesis has also been documented. Mitotic arrest is one of the most accurate markers of mercury exposure in mice. On postnatal day 2, a single 4-mg/kg dose of mercury led to a brain Hg concentration of only 1.8 μg/g of tissue. In the cerebellum of exposed mice, the ratio of late mitotic figures to total mitotic figures was markedly decreased, suggesting mitotic arrest. MeHg toxicity may also be caused by oxidative stress. The main antioxidant in the cell is glutathione. Glutathione concentrations decrease and then rise following exposure to mercury. MeHg-resistant cells exhibited a four-fold increase in glutathione concentrations and a faster rate of MeHg efflux than normal cells.

A different theory that explains MeHg toxicity is the disruption of microtubules within the cytoskeleton of neurons. Tubulin, the protein monomers that make up microtubules, contain thiols to which mercury binds. This prevents the microtubules from depolymerizing and repolymerizing. Disruption of microtubule assembly could cause cellular processes to malfunction since many cell functions, such as cell division and migration, depend on the disintegration and assembly of microtubules. MeHg has been demonstrated to impede the progression of the cell cycle in primary rat brain cells in vitro. Because the developing nervous system undergoes a great deal of cell migration and division, it would be especially vulnerable to those effects. The foundation of therapeutic approaches after exposure to MeHg and Hg vapor is the ability to exchange thiols. The neurotoxic effects of combined exposure to mercury and mercury vapor are similar, but they are more severe than those that result from exposure to each element separately. The biochemistry of the inorganic Hg cation (Hg^{2+}), which causes toxicity after exposure to Hg vapor, and MeHg+ share many similarities. Both cations have a strong affinity for SH groups, and they react quickly to associate and dissociate. Both are present in tissues attached to proteins, cysteine, and glutathione, which are small and large molecular weight thiol-containing molecules. The mobility and toxicity of mercury in the body are thought to be caused by the creation of Hg thiol bonds.

In vivo conversion of organic and elemental mercury to inorganic mercury occurs eventually, even though the exposure patterns, TK, and TD of the various mercury species are typically investigated independently. Table 4.4 lists the approximate daily intake and retention of each type of mercury. The body retains between 3 and 17 μg of mercury per day, according to estimates for dental amalgams. The range of estimated daily MeHg retention is 1 to 6 μg. Individuals with higher fish consumption will have a different ratio of MeHg to total Hg. According to Table 4.4's data, the average exposure to mercury from dental amalgams may be significantly higher than the average exposure to mercury from mercury amalgams. But there aren't enough data available to make a conclusive comparison.

Table 4.4. *Estimated Daily Intake and Retention (micrograms per day) of Total Hg and Hg Compounds in the General Population Not Occupationally Exposed to Hg*

Exposure	Elemental Hg Vapor	Inorganic Hg Compounds [b]	MeHg
Air	0.030 (0.024) [b,c]	0.002 (0.001) [b,c]	0.008 (0.0064) [b,c]
Food Sources			
Fish	0 [b,c]	0.600 (0.042) [b,c]	1 [d,e,f], 3 [e,g,h], 6 [c,g,h]
Non-Fish	0 [b,c]	3.6 (0.25) [b,c]	0 [b,c]

Drinking water	0 [b, c]	0.050 (0.0035) [b, c]	0 [b, c]
Dental amalgams	3.8–21 (3–17) [b, c]	0 [b, c]	0 [b, c]
Total	3.9–21 (3.1–17)	4.3 (0.3)	1–6 (1–6)

[a]Retention is assumed to be 95% of intake for MeHg, 80% for elemental Hg vapor, and 7% for inorganic Hg compounds.

[b]Data from IPCS 1991.

[c]Mean value.

[d]Data are for United States nationwide (per capita), calculated assuming a body weight of 70 kg (EPA 1997).

[e]Median value.

[f]Equivalent data for women of childbearing age: median = 1, assuming a body weight of 60 kg.

[g]Data are for the general population of reproductive age in New Jersey fish consumers, calculated assuming a body weight of 70 kg (Stern et al., 1996).

[h]Equivalent data for women of childbearing age: mean = 5, median = 3, assuming a body weight of 60 kg.

Source: https://www.ncbi.nlm.nih.gov/books/NBK225779/table/ttt00005/?report=objectonly.

MeHg is converted to inorganic Hg in situ in the brain, albeit very slowly. In the brain, elemental mercury is oxidized to inorganic mercury as well. Uncertainty surrounds the source of MeHg toxicity at the cellular level: the parent compound itself, the inorganic Hg that is its metabolite, or free radicals produced during MeHg metabolism to inorganic Hg. If MeHg's inorganic metabolite is the most toxic form of the metal, then exposure to elemental Hg (especially from dental amalgams) and MeHg may result in cumulative doses of inorganic Hg to the brain. This remains true even when considering the oxidation of elemental mercury in the blood prior to its absorption into the brain. For this reason, dental amalgams and other additional chronic sources of Hg exposure should be taken into account in risk-assessment models for MeHg. Uncertainty regarding the precise mechanisms through which mercury specifically causes neurodevelopmental toxicity complicates these considerations. These mechanisms may differ from those causing neurotoxicity in adults. However, understanding the mechanisms of mercury toxicity in the brain is vital research priority because of the possible consequences of additive toxicity from dental amalgams and fish consumption.

A Closer Look

Nanotoxicokinetics

A specialized branch of toxicokinetics that studies the absorption, distribution, metabolism, and excretion (ADME) of nanomaterials, including nanoparticles (NPs), within biological systems. With the rapid advancement of nanotechnology, engineered nanomaterials are increasingly utilized in various industries, including medicine, cosmetics, electronics, and environmental applications. This widespread use raises concerns about their potential health impacts, necessitating a thorough understanding of how these materials interact with biological systems at the nano scale.

One of the defining characteristics of nanoparticles is their small size, typically less than 100 nanometers in diameter, which confers unique physical and chemical properties compared to their bulk counterparts. These properties, such as high surface area to volume ratio, can enhance their reactivity and biological interactions, potentially leading to unforeseen toxicological effects. The study of nanotoxicokinetics is crucial for predicting these effects and ensuring safe design and use of nanomaterials.

Absorption of nanoparticles can occur through various routes, including inhalation, ingestion, dermal contact, and intravenous injection, particularly in medical applications like drug delivery systems. Due to their small size, nanoparticles can penetrate biological barriers more easily than larger particles. For instance, they can cross the epithelial layers of the respiratory and gastrointestinal tracts, enter the bloodstream, and even penetrate the blood-brain barrier, raising concerns about their potential to reach and accumulate in sensitive organs.

Once absorbed, the distribution of nanoparticles within the body depends on their size, shape, surface charge, and coating materials. Nanoparticles can travel through the circulatory system and accumulate in organs like the liver, spleen, kidneys, and lungs. The high surface reactivity of nanoparticles can also lead to interactions with cellular components, potentially causing oxidative stress, inflammation, and other cellular responses. Understanding these distribution patterns is essential for assessing the risk of chronic exposure and potential long-term health effects.

Metabolism of nanoparticles involves biotransformation by biological systems, which can alter their physicochemical properties and toxicity. Enzymatic processes, similar to those that metabolize conventional drugs and chemicals, can modify the surface characteristics of nanoparticles, potentially influencing their reactivity and interactions with biological molecules. However, the metabolism of nanoparticles is not fully understood and can vary significantly depending on the material and its surface modifications. This area of study is critical for determining how long nanoparticles persist in the body and their potential to cause harm over time.

Excretion of nanoparticles from the body occurs primarily through renal and biliary pathways, but their small size can also facilitate removal via the respiratory tract or skin. The efficiency of excretion processes can be influenced by the nanoparticle's properties, such as size, surface charge, and hydrophilicity. Inefficient excretion can lead to bioaccumulation, where nanoparticles persist in the body, potentially leading to adverse effects.

Nanotoxicokinetics is a rapidly evolving field that integrates principles from pharmacokinetics, toxicology, and nanotechnology to understand the complex behaviors of nanoparticles in biological systems. Research in this area aims to elucidate the mechanisms underlying the ADME processes of nanoparticles, develop predictive models for their biological interactions, and establish safety guidelines for their use. This knowledge is essential for ensuring that the benefits of nanotechnology are realized while minimizing potential risks to human health and the environment.

Summary

- TK and TD are two fundamental concepts in the field of toxicology, each playing a crucial role in understanding how toxic substances interact with the body and produce adverse effects.
- TD, on the other hand, focuses on the biochemical and physiological effects of toxic substances on the body's cells, tissues, and organ systems. It examines how toxicants interact with cellular components, disrupt normal physiological processes, and produce adverse effects.
- TK describes the ADME, with time, of foreign compounds in the body. Essential to the evaluation of the safety of a medical device is consideration of the stability of the material(s) in vivo and the disposition of intended and unintended leachables and degradation products.
- The characterization of PK/PD effects starts with toxicokinetic studies in animals. The primary goal of toxicokinetic analysis is to correlate toxicity findings with the corresponding level of exposure to an experimental drug compound.
- The most useful piece of information that can be collected from TK data, as a part of reproductive toxicology studies, is the relationship between the exposure in the dam and the secondary effects caused in the fetus by the pharmacological action of the drug in the dam.
- Placental transfer studies provide information on the placental transfer of drugs by assessing the radioactivity in fetal tissue and maternal blood. There are many morphological differences and similarities in yolk sac and chorioallantoic placenta between rats, rabbits, and humans.
- Drugs that are lipophilic are likely to be excreted in milk of lactating females, and hence the pups will be exposed to the parent drug or its metabolites during suckling. The drug label should accordingly mention the warning of potential risks from drug consumption via breast milk in human infants.
- TS, termed pharmacodynamics in pharmacology, describes the dynamic interactions of a toxicant with a biological target and its biological effects. A biological target, also known as the site of action, can be binding proteins, ion channels, DNA, or a variety of other receptors.
- Endocrine disrupting chemicals can interfere with the endocrine system in a number of ways including hormone synthesis, storage/release, transport and clearance, receptor recognition and binding, and postreceptor activation.
- Toxicants may also cause endocrine disruption through interacting with the estrogen receptor. This mechanism has been well-studied with PCBs. These chemicals have been used as coolants and lubricants in transformers and other electrical equipment due to their insulating properties.

References

1. Aaseth, J., Jacobsen, D., Andersen, O., & Wickstrom, E. (1995). Treatment of mercury and lead poisoning with dimercaptosuccinic acid and sodium dimercaptopropane-sulfonate: A review. *Analyst, 120*(3), 853–854. https://doi.org/10.1039/AN9952000853.
2. Aberg, B., Ekman, L., Falk, R., Greitz, U., Persson, G., & Snihs, J. O. (1969). Metabolism of methyl mercury (203Hg) compounds in man. *Archives of Environmental Health, 19*(4), 478–484. https://doi.org/10.1080/00039896.1969.10665285.
3. American Academy of Pediatrics. (1999). Thimerosal in vaccines—An interim report to clinicians. Committee on Infectious Diseases and Committee on Environmental Health. *Pediatrics, 104*(3), 570–574. https://doi.org/10.1542/peds.104.3.570.
4. Aposhian, H. V. (1983). DMSA and DMPS: Water-soluble antidotes for heavy metal poisoning. *Annual Review of Pharmacology and Toxicology, 23*, 193–215. https://doi.org/10.1146/annurev.pa.23.040183.001205.
5. Aposhian, H. V., & Aposhian, M. M. (1990). Meso-2,3-dimercaptosuccinic acid: Chemical, pharmacological and toxicological properties of an orally effective metal chelating agent. *Annual Review of Toxicology, 30*, 279–306. https://doi.org/10.1146/annurev.tox.30.022190.152233.
6. Aposhian, H. V., Bruce, D. C., Alter, W., Dart, R. C., Hurlbut, K. M., & Aposhian, M. M. (1992a). Urinary mercury after administration of 2,3-dimercaptopropane-1-sulfonic acid: Correlation with dental amalgam score. *FASEB Journal, 6*(7), 2472–2476. https://doi.org/10.1096/fasebj.6.7.1518341.
7. Aposhian, H. V., Maiorino, R. M., Gonzalez-Ramirez, D., Zuniga-Charles, M., Xu, Z., Hurlbut, K. M., Junco-Munoz, P., Dart, R. C., & Aposhian, M. M. (1995). Mobilization of heavy metals by newer, therapeutically useful chelating agents. *Toxicology, 97*(1–3), 23–28. https://doi.org/10.1016/0300-483X(95)03106-9.
8. Aposhian, H. V., Maiorino, R. M., Rivera, M., Bruce, D. C., Dart, R. C., Hurlbut, K. M., Levine, D. J., Zheng, W., Fernando, Q., Carter, D., & Aposhian, M. M. (1992b). Human studies with the chelating agents DMPS and DMSA. *Clinical Toxicology, 30*(4), 505–528. https://doi.org/10.3109/15563659209019153.
9. Aposhian, M. M., Maiorino, R. M., Xu, Z., & Aposhian, H. V. (1996). Sodium 2,3-dimercapto-1-propanesulfonate (DMPS) treatment does not redistribute lead or mercury to the brain of rats. *Toxicology, 109*(1), 49–55. https://doi.org/10.1016/0300-483X(96)03568-4.
10. Arenholt-Bindslev, D., & Larsen, A. H. (1996). Mercury levels and discharge in waste water from dental clinics. *Water, Air, & Soil Pollution, 86*(1–4), 93–99. https://doi.org/10.1007/BF00345271.
11. Aschner, M., Eberle, N. B., & Kimelberg, H. K. (1991). Interactions of methylmercury with rat primary astrocyte cultures: Methylmercury efflux. *Brain Research, 554*(1–2), 10–14. https://doi.org/10.1016/0006-8993(91)90617-R.
12. Atchison, W. D., & Hare, M. F. (1994). Mechanisms of methylmercury-induced neurotoxicity. *FASEB Journal, 8*(9), 622–629. https://doi.org/10.1096/fasebj.8.9.8089735.
13. ATSDR (Agency for Toxic Substances and Disease Registry). (1999). *Toxicological Profile for Mercury* (Update). U.S. Department of Health & Human Services, Agency for Toxic Substances

and Disease Registry. Retrieved from: https://www.atsdr.cdc.gov/toxprofiles/tp46.html (accessed on 3 August 2024).

14. Bakir, F., Damluji, S. F., Amin-Zaki, L., Murthadha, M., Khalidi, A., Al-Rawi, N. Y., Tikriti, S., Dhahir, H. I., Clarkson, T. W., Smith, J. C., & Doherty, R. A. (1973). Methylmercury poisoning in Iraq. *Science, 181*, 230–241. https://doi.org/10.1126/science.181.4096.230.

15. Baldi, F., & Filippelli, M. (1991). New method for detecting methylmercury by its enzymic conversion to methane. *Environmental Science & Technology, 25*(2), 302–305. https://doi.org/10.1021/es00013a015.

16. Ballatori, N. (1991). Mechanisms of metal transport across liver cell plasma membranes. *Drug Metabolism Reviews, 23*(1–2), 83–132. https://doi.org/10.3109/03602539109007008.

17. Ballatori, N., & Clarkson, T. W. (1982). Developmental changes in the biliary excretion of methylmercury and glutathione. *Science, 216*(4541), 61–63. https://doi.org/10.1126/science.7085238.

18. Baron Jr., S., Haykal-Coates, N., & Tilson, H. A. (1998). Gestational exposure to methylmercury alters the developmental pattern of trk-like immuno-reactivity in the rat brain and results in cortical dysmorphology. *Developmental Brain Research, 109*(1), 13–31. https://doi.org/10.1016/S0165-3806(98)00043-0.

19. Begley, T. P., Walts, A. E., & Walsh, C. T. (1986). Bacterial organomercurial lyase: Overproduction, isolation, and characterization. *Biochemistry, 25*(22), 7186–7192. https://doi.org/10.1021/bi00377a006.

20. Berlin, M. (1986). Mercury. In L. Friberg, G. F. Nordberg, & V. B. Vouk (Eds.), *Handbook on the Toxicology of Metals* (2nd ed., pp. 387–445). Elsevier.

21. Bernard, S., & Purdue, P. (1984). Metabolic models for methyl and inorganic mercury. *Health Physics, 46*(3), 695–699. https://doi.org/10.1097/00004032-198403000-00014.

22. Bluhm, R. E., Bobbitt, R. G., Welch, L. W., Wood, A. J. J., Bonfiglio, J. F., Sarzen, C., Heath, A. J., & Branch, R. A. (1992). Elemental mercury vapor toxicity, treatment, and prognosis after acute, intensive exposure in chloralkali plant workers: Part I: History, neuropsychological findings and chelator effects. *Human & Experimental Toxicology, 11*(3), 201–210. https://doi.org/10.1177/096032719201100305.

23. Bornmann, G., Henke, G., Alfes, H., & Mollmann, H. (1970). Intestinal absorption of metallic mercury. [in German]. *Archives of Toxicology, 26*(3), 203–209. https://doi.org/10.1007/BF00317186.

24. Brown, N. L., Ford, S. J., Pridmore, R. D., & Fritzinger, D. C. (1983). Nucleotide sequence of a gene from the Pseudomonas transposon Tn501 encoding mercuric reductase. *Biochemistry, 22*(17), 4089–4095. https://doi.org/10.1021/bi00285a013.

25. Burbaker, P. E., Klein, R., Herman, S. P., Lucier, G. W., Alexander, L. T., & Long, M. D. (1973). DNA, RNA and protein synthesis in brain, liver and kidneys of symptomatic methylmercury treated rats. *Experimental & Molecular Pathology, 18*(3), 263–280. https://doi.org/10.1016/0014-4800(73)90017-3.

26. Cappon, C. J., & Smith, J. C. (1978). A simple and rapid procedure for the gas-chromatographic determination of methylmercury in biological samples. *Bulletin of Environmental Contamination and Toxicology, 19*(5), 600–607. https://doi.org/10.1007/BF01685596.

Chapter

5

CLASSES OF TOXICANTS

Contents

Introduction

There are numerous classification schemes for toxic substances, primarily driven by the requirements and preferences of the classifier. Since there isn't a single classification scheme that works for the entire spectrum of hazardous chemicals, the best classification scheme may combine several schemes based on different attributes. Both the biological and chemical characteristics of the toxin may be included in toxicity classifications; nevertheless, visibility factors also play a significant role in toxicity. The sources of toxins include minerals, animals, plants, and artificial substances; the physiological state includes solid, liquid, gaseous, and dust toxicants; the focus organ or system includes hepatotoxicants, hematotoxicants, pulmotoxicants, nephrotoxicants, and so on, in terms of their chemical nature and structure (metals, nonmetals, acids, and alkalis), as well as their analytical behavior (metals, volatile toxicants, cyanides, and metallic carbides), and the types of toxic effects they can cause (chronic, acute, sub-acute, etc.). Use (insecticides, rodenticides, herbicides, fungicides, food additives, etc.) and toxic effects (teratogens, carcinogens, mutagens, and clastogens) depend on factors such as mechanism of action, health, and environmental effects.

Orientation and Directional Terms:

Term	Definition	Illustration
Biochemical conversion	It is the process where microorganisms break down the biomass to produce useful end products.	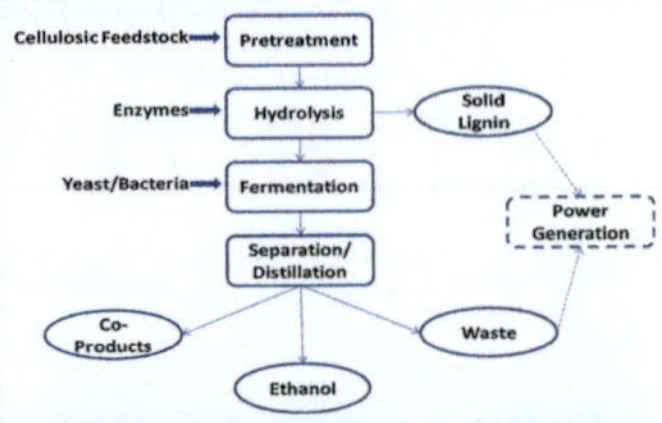
Enzymatic systems	There are several enzyme systems that catalyze reactions to neutralize free radicals and reactive oxygen species. These enzymes include: superoxide dismutase. glutathione peroxidise.	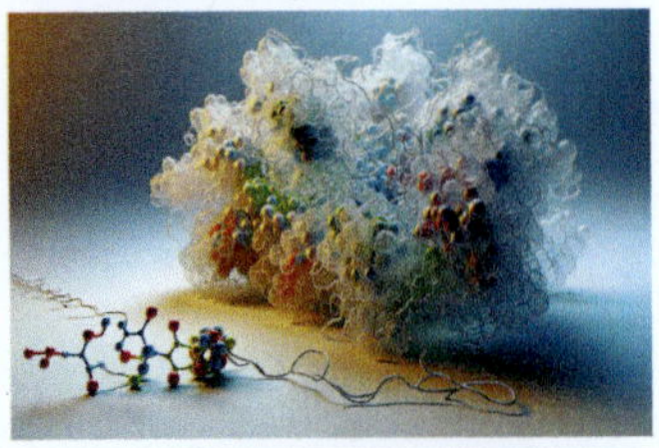
Cytochrome	Cytochrome contains a heme prosthetic group embedded within a porphyrin ring. Porphyrin rings are comprised of four pyrrole structures.	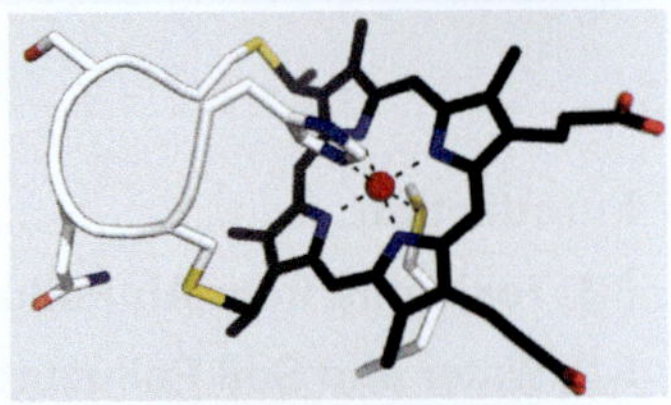
Biotransformation	A metabolic process that takes place mainly in the liver and helps to facilitate the excretion of both exogenous and endogenous substances.	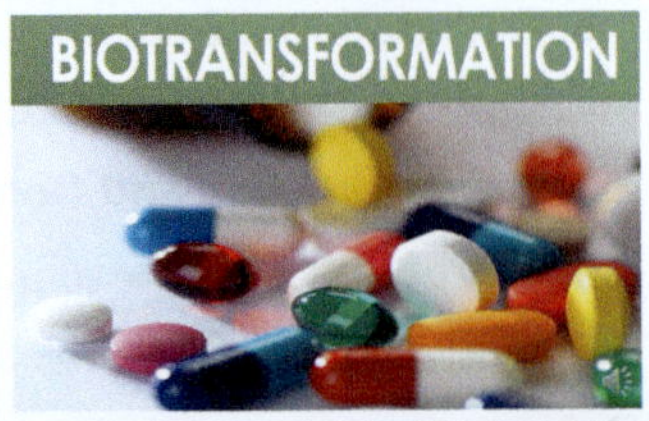
Bioinorganic chemistry	Bioinorganic chemistry is an important field that helps scientists to analyze the relationship between different metals, inorganic substances, and organisms.	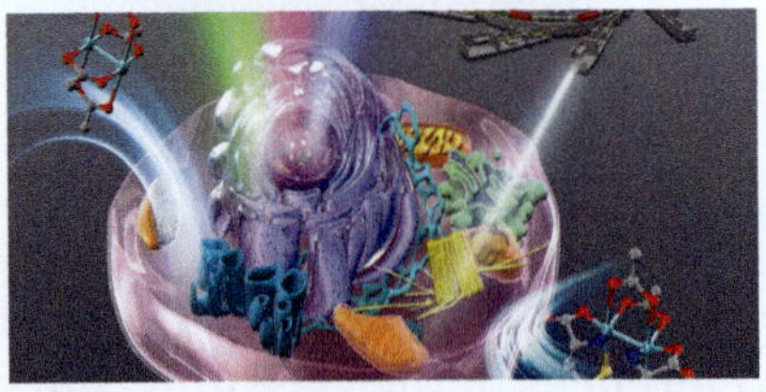

5.1. Toxicants from Air Pollution

The use of burning wood for cooking and heating by humans is most likely what started the air pollution problem. For millennia, people used fireplaces in such a way that smoke-filled living rooms. The construction of chimneys allowed for the separation of combustion products and cooking odors from living areas and their outdoor venting. With the discovery of soft coals and their use as fuel, carbon smoke started to cause problems in urban areas. Fuel smoke had become an issue in London by the thirteenth century. In 1273, Edward I enacted the first air pollution control law, which forbade burning coal during meetings of the National Assembly, saying that "everyone understands within the tone of my voice that coal-burning is forbidden, and anyone found guilty of it will lose his head". London's smoking pollution problem persists in spite of these and later royal decrees, as shown in Figure 5.1.

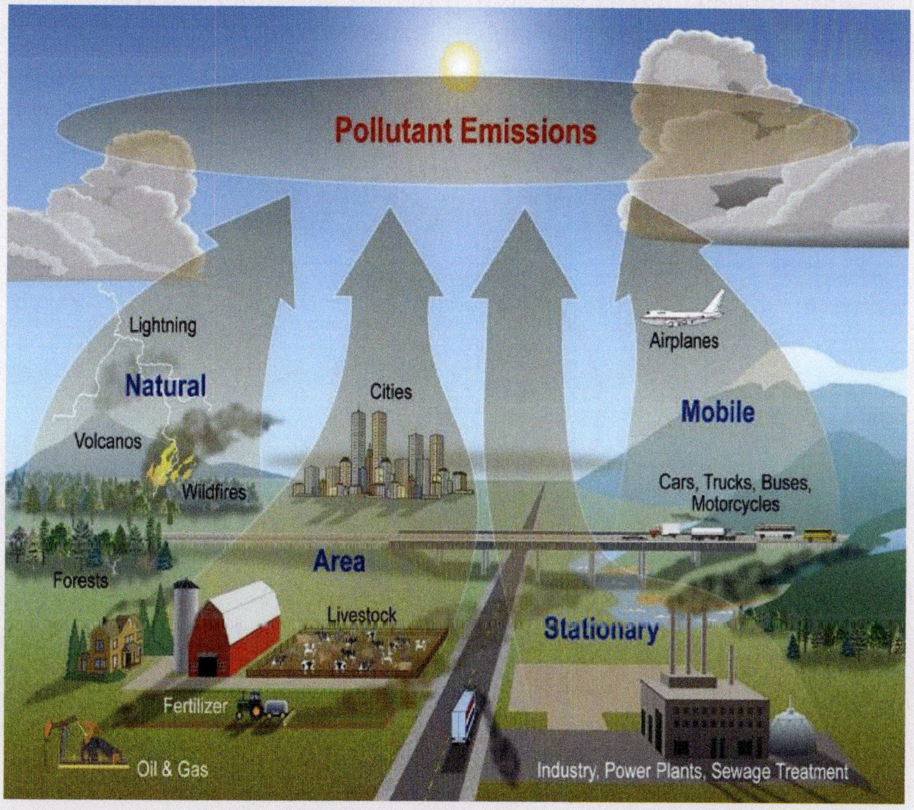

Figure 5.1. *Illustration of pollution sources in the air.*

Source: https://media.licdn.com/dms/image/D4D22AQHGiC8Pdnid-w/feedshare-shrink_800/0/1698149806886?e=2147483647&v=beta&t=W3TtZxq3AdlUpbD8QKgvjZw9P8zm0A_ZKlVQZHLrDtw.

With rising domestic and industrial coal consumption, particularly in large cities, air pollution has only gotten worsened. According to Pinkerton and Joad (2006), the most significant change that occurred there in the 20th century was the massive increase in the number of vehicles, which went from almost nonexistent at the beginning of the century to a million in a matter of years. In certain industrialized countries, not much had been done to control air quality until long after

World War II. Two serious pollution incidents that resulted in the death of humans due to high levels of pollutants spurred action. In the small western Pennsylvanian steel plant community of Donora, something happened in 1948. Late October saw the formation of severe smog in the area, and a weather inversion made it impossible for pollutants to escape. The pollution's effects were directly to blame for twenty-one deaths. The story "Donora" brought attention to the issue of air pollution in the US.

5.1.1. Types of Air Pollutants

What does it mean to have clean air? Pollution-free air is the air that would have existed if humans and their activities had not existed on Earth, meaning that natural point sources such as volcanoes and forest fires would not have contaminated the air. The true makeup of "non-polluted" air is unknown because humans have been contaminating the atmosphere for centuries. Organic pollutants include gases and smoke from volcanoes, terpenes from trees, and smoke from wildfires. (Figure 5.2).

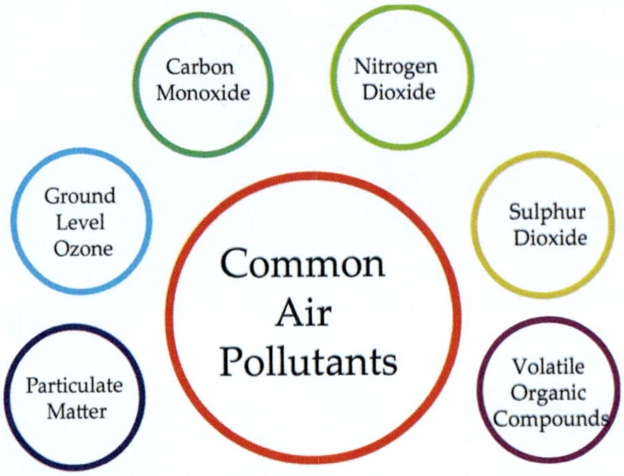

Figure 5.2. *Schematic of pollutant types in the air.*

Source: https://www.researchgate.net/publication/347081919/figure/fig1/AS:1022724583485446@1620847950827/common-air-pollutants.jpg.

Gaseous Pollutants. Such substances include gases at room temperature and atmospheric pressure, along with vapors evaporating from solid or liquid. Hydrocarbons, Carbon monoxide (CO), hydrogen sulfide (H_2S), oxides of nitrogen (NxOy), ozone (O_3) and other oxidizing agents, sulfur oxides (SxOy), and CO_2 are some of the most dangerous pollutants.

Pollution concentrations are often measured in micrograms per cubic meter (g/m^3) and parts per million (ppm) per volume for toxic gases, with 1 ppm equaling one part pollutant per million parts (10^6) of air.

- **Particulate Pollutants:** Air may sustain fine particles or liquid. The following are some examples of various sorts of particulates :
- **Dust:** Particles with a diameter of roughly 100 m originate straight from the chemicals being employed (e.g., sawdust, coal dust, cement dust, ash, grain dust).

- **Fumes:** Suspended particles with a diameter of 1 m are generally released during mechanical or chemical operations (e.g., lead and zinc oxides).
- **Mist:** Droplets of liquid floating in the air have a radius of less than 2.0 m (e.g., sulfuric acid mist).
- **Smoke:** Improper fossil fuel combustion produces solid particles (size range 0.05–1.0 m).
- **Aerosol:** Solids (diameter range 0.05–1.0 m) are produced by incorrect fossil fuel burning.

5.1.2. Examples of Air Pollutants

Acute pollution events, such as those in London and Donora provide the majority of data on the impacts of air pollution on people. Chemical irritation of the pulmonary system may cause illness, with particular sensitive groups of people being much more affected:

- Extremely young toddlers with underdeveloped circulatory and respiratory systems.
- The old, whose cardiovascular and pulmonary systems are in bad condition; and
- Those suffering from cardio-respiratory disorders, including asthmatic, emphysema, or cardiovascular disease, and smoking are also more vulnerable to air pollution.

The combined action of particles and sulfur dioxides (SO_2) seems to be responsible in the majority of instances; no single pollutant seems to be to blame. (Figure 5.3).

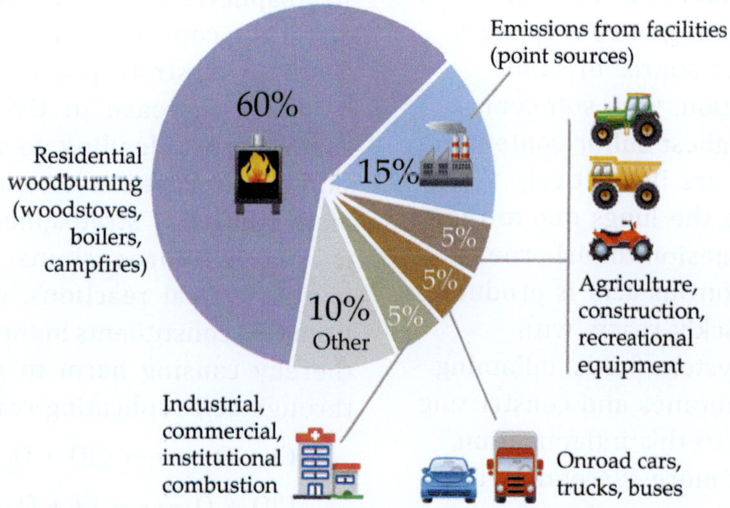

Figure 5.3. *Illustration of different sources of emission percentages.*

Source: https://image.slidesharecdn.com/presentation1-211208140839/75/Pollution-control-35-2048.jpg.

- **Carbon Monoxide:** Hemoglobin (Hb) and carbon monoxide combine fast to form carboxyhemoglobin (COHb), which blocks the flow of oxygen to tissues. The sensitivity of hemoglobin to CO is approximately 210 times higher than its oxygen requirement. Five percent COHb blood content, or equilibrium at about 45 parts per million CO, has been associated with cardiovascular effects. At 100 parts per million CO, headaches, nausea, dizziness, and breathing difficulties can happen. An acute level of 1000 ppm is always fatal. Severe traffic congestion has been known to cause carbon monoxide concentrations to reach 400 parts per million (ppm); additionally, smokers have a higher body weight of CO overall than non-smokers. Low CO concentrations may have unknown long-term effects, but they are likely to exacerbate respiratory and cardiac conditions. One type of sulfur compound is sulfur oxide. The industrial burning of coal appears to be the main source of sulfur dioxide pollution, with soft coal having the highest sulfur content. Sulfur oxides are ineffectively expelled from the lungs due to their continued adhesion to airborne particles. Sulfurous acid is produced when SO_2 quickly reacts with respiratory system fluids, inflaming mucous membranes and constricting bronchi. Due to this inflammation, the airway is more susceptible to additional airborne toxins.

- **Nitrogen Oxides:** Nitrogen dioxide (NO_2) is one lung irritant that is common in photochemical smog, which has been related to both bleeding and pulmonary edema. Nitrogen oxides are a significant cause of photochemical smog and ozone depletion, despite the fact that they can also contribute to acid deposition.
- **Ozone:** When nitrogen dioxide is exposed to ultraviolet (UV) light during smog, a very disagreeable and oxidizing gas is produced. Lung congestion, edema, and bleeding may result from the ozone created as a result (Shen, 2015; Castell et al., 2005).

NO_2 + UV light ----→ NO + Ož

Ož + O_2 ----→ O_3

At this point, it's critical to distinguish between "good" and "poor" ozone. Toxic tropospheric ozone is found between zero and ten miles above the surface of the Earth. To block out incoming UV light, stratospheric ozone—found at a height of about 30 miles above the Earth's crust—is crucial. The thinning stratospheric ozone layer has been the subject of recent concern. It is estimated that a 1% decrease in stratospheric ozone would result in a 2% increase in UV rays reaching the earth's crust, leading to a 10% increase in skin cancer cases. It is believed that one of the main causes of stratospheric ozone depletion is chlorofluorocarbons (CFCs). Through photochemical reactions, chlorine is released from CFC constituents in the earth's atmosphere, thereby causing harm to stratospheric ozone through self-replicating reactive species.

$Cl + O_3$ ----→ $ClO + O_2$

$ClO + O$ ----→ $Cl + O_2$

Every chlorine atom may damage up to 10,000 layers of ozone before even being inactivated by methane and nitrogen dioxide. International agreements are progressively phasing out the use of CFC chemicals (Nazaroff & Weschler, 2004).

5.2. Water and Soil Pollutants

Given that soil covers a large portion of the planet's surface and water covers three-quarters of it should come as no surprise that the final drains with the highest levels of anthropogenic pollutants are both soil and water. In most developing countries, the primary concern regarding water contamination was the potential health effects caused by pathogens until recently. However, the focus has shifted to chemical pollutants as treatment techniques in the US and other developed countries have all but eliminated bacterial disease-causing microorganisms from the water system (Figure 5.4).

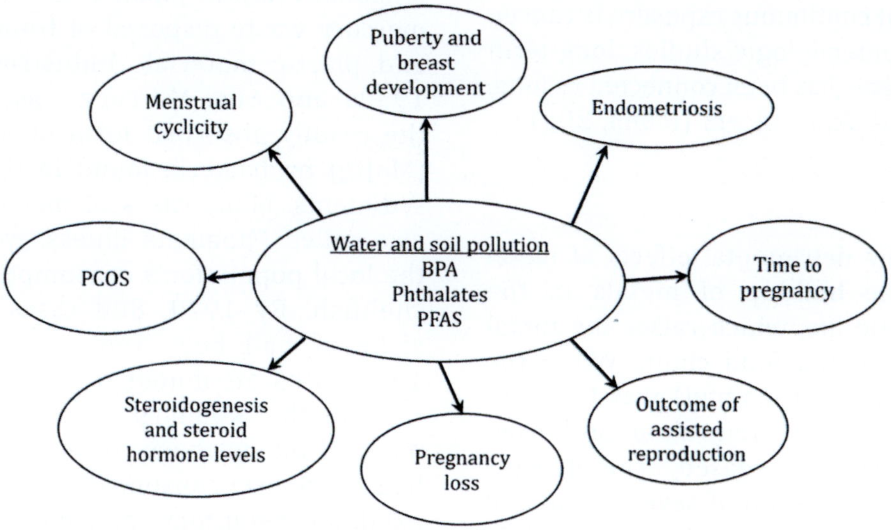

Figure 5.4. *Potential reproductive hazards of BPA, phthalates, and PFAS.*

Source: https://www.researchgate.net/publication/330352148/figure/fig2/AS:963513874915328@1606731017045/Potential-reproductive-hazards-of-BPA-phthalates-and-PFAS.png.

5.2.1. Examples of Water and Soil Pollutants

There are three types of metals that are environmentally hazardous:

- metals that have been linked to cancer;
- metals that transfer willingly in soil; and
- Metals that are passed down the food chain.

5.2.2. Lead

The two heavy metals that present the greatest health risk when ingested through groundwater are lead (Pb) and arsenic. Lead soldering and lead pipes are the main sources of lead in drinking water. Concerns should also be raised about lead leaks from hazardous locations and soil contaminated by leaded gasoline fallout. Children frequently suffer from lead poisoning, especially in inner-city and elderly residential complexes where children may swallow paint colors contaminated with lead.

5.2.3. Arsenic

Drinking water tainted with arsenic is at risk from the dissolution of inorganic toxic elements used in pesticide spray, burning of coal and oil containing arsenic, and smelting runoff from mining waste. Long-term high exposure levels may cause symptoms such as stomach discomfort, nasal congestion, hyperkeratosis, and irregular skin pigmentation. The main risk at lower levels of continuous exposure is cancer. According to epidemiologic studies, long-term exposure to arsenic has been connected to lung, lymph node, and skin cancers (Monn, 2001).

5.2.4. Cadmium

One of the many detrimental effects of metal pollution is the buildup of metals in the tissues of aquatic life, which raises the metal concentrations in the food chain. When the illness Itai-Itai (painful-painful) was found in some regions of Japan, worries about prolonged cadmium exposure increased. The disease presents as a combination of severe bone and joint disease and severe renal impairment in areas where rice is heavily contaminated with cadmium. The land being irrigated with water containing cadmium emissions from industrial sources is what caused this pollution. Fish consumed after being caught in rivers close to smelting facilities in Japan has also been connected to cadmium poisoning (Manning and Keane, 1988).

5.2.5. Mercury

Minamata Bay in Japan was contaminated by mercury waste disposed of from the chemical and plastic materials industries during the 1950s and 60s. Mercury was changed into the readily absorbed form of methylmercury (MeHg) by bacteria found in the underwater sediments. Many cases of mercury poisoning, also called Minamata illness, were caused by the local population's consumption of fish and shellfish. By 1970, 800 cases of Minamata sickness had been reported, with at least 107 deaths attributed to mercury poisoning. Despite the women's apparent good health, many of the newborns of these mothers—who had previously consumed contaminated fish—exhibited symptoms and mental deficiencies similar to those of cerebral palsy (Scow and Johnson, 1996) (Figure 5.5).

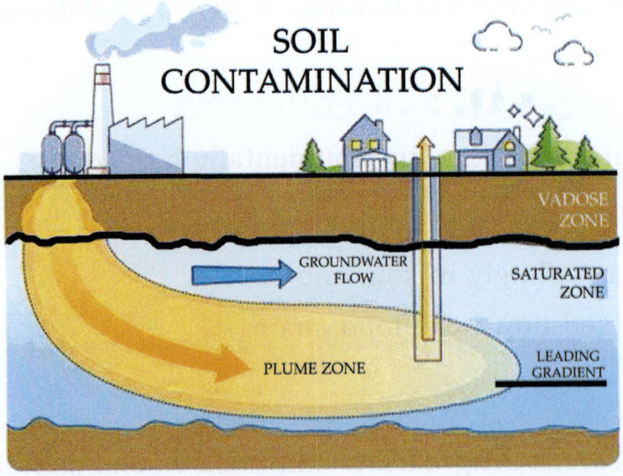

Figure 5.5. *Diagram of the issue of soil contamination and subterranean water pollution.*

Source: https://www.shutterstock.com/shutterstock/photos/2069527187/display_1500/stock-vector-soil-contamination-and-underground-water-pollution-problem-outline-diagram-labeled-educational-2069527187.jpg.

Two important nutrients, phosphates, and nitrates, have been steadily increasing in natural streams since the mid-1960s. Nitrate pollution is caused by fertilizers, wastewater treatment plant output, sewage systems, and dung leachate. Fertilizer nitrates seep out of soils rapidly, and drainage and leachate are thought to allow up to 40% of applied nitrates to enter water sources. Only 20 to 25% of applied nitrates leach into the water because fertilizer phosphates, on the other hand, prefer to be absorbed or bonded to sand grains. Phosphate detergents are an additional source of phosphate that have received a lot of media attention lately (Mostert et al., 2010). Overnutrition can cause "algal blooms" or eutrophication in ponds, lakes, estuaries, and very slow-moving rivers; therefore, the environment may be concerned about the rise in these nutrients, particularly phosphates. The algal bloom stops the atmosphere from reoxygenating the water and reduces light penetration. Microbial degradation happens when a thick algal bloom dies, creating anaerobic conditions and the death of a variety of aquatic life. High phosphate levels and algal blooms are rarely a problem because running streams are continuously washed away, and algae do not concentrate (Havlikova and Kroeze, 2006).

Petroleum and/or oils are common environmental contaminants in today's world, whether they come from oil truck leaks or spent oil from individual cars. Daths of many birds at sea can also be attributed to oil spills. that only a tiny portion of seriously polluted birds recover after de-oiling or hand feeding. Additionally, oil builds up on rocks and sand, making it impossible to enjoy the location until a costly cleanup is finished. Among the animals affected are shrimp, barnacles, mussels, and crabs. These animals also ingest toxic hydrocarbons. It is unclear how long-term effects will affect aquatic species, and they might be worse than previously believed (Hirano and Tamae, 2011). Volatile organic compounds are among the other common contaminants found in groundwater (VOCs). Among them are petroleum products and volatile organic compounds, or VOCs. Both types of chemicals are used extensively in many industries, such as paints, laundry services, rust remover, and the military. Subterranean tanks used to hold hydrocarbons eventually eroded or flowed onto the surface. The 11 volatile organic compounds (VOCs) on the EPA's National Priority List are trichloroethylene, vinyl chloride, toluene, xylene, benzene, chloroform, ethylbenzene, tetrachloroethylene, 1,1,1-trichloroethane, trans-1,2dichloroethane, and dichloromethane (Loureiro et al., 2018).

In certain parts of the world, natural radiation levels such as radon contribute to radioactive fallout; however, the contamination of surface and groundwater by radiation compounds produced during the fabrication of nuclear weapons and nuclear fuel is a particular cause for concern. Most of these locations have remained undiscovered due to government surveillance (Copaciu et al., 2016). Acids from mine runoff and rainfall have severely contaminated the majority of freshwater lakes and rivers. Because acids have the ability to release hazardous metals into solutions and lower water's pH to lethal levels, they are particularly dangerous (Havugimana et al., 2017). The amount of organic PCB chemicals found in water and soil increases yearly. Among them are phenols, solvents, cyanides, plasticizers, PCBs, and a host of other industrial compounds. Traditionally used as coolants in power transformers, PCBs are recognized byproducts of the manufacturing of plastics, lubricants, rubber, and paper. They are stable, lipid-soluble, and degrade gradually in tissues. Due to these characteristics, the aggregate can be found in large quantities in fish and waterfowl; in 1969, PCBs were linked to the deaths of thousands of seabirds in the Irish Sea (Crouau et al., 1999). Due to industrial accidents and widespread use of herbicides 2,4,5-T, dioxin has contaminated large areas of soil and water, resulting in the extremely hazardous compound TCDD (2,3,7,8-tetrachlorodibenzo-p-dioxin). Tiny amounts of TCDD were discovered to be a pollutant during the manufacturing of herbicides. In Vietnam, the US Army used the herbicide Agent Orange extensively as a dispersant (Zhang and Zhang, 2022). With LD50 values of 0.022 mg/kg for male mice, 0.045 mg/kg for female rats, and 0.0006 mg/kg for female guinea pigs (the most susceptible species examined), TCDD is one of the most toxic synthetic chemicals for laboratory animals. In addition, it has been demonstrated to cause birth defects at concentrations as low as 1 to 3 ng/kg and to be fetotoxic to pregnant rats at doses as low as 1/400 of the LD50. TCDD causes cancer in mice and rats, with the liver being the main organ impacted. Although chronically low exposure to TCDD is thought to contribute to carcinogenic effects and sexual abnormalities, it does not appear to be particularly acutely harmful to humans (Cakmak et al., 2018).

5.3. Occupational Toxicants

Professional toxicology has a long history that stretches back to ancient nations and is concerned with evaluating workplace hazards. In the first century AD, Greek historian Strabo wrote of the arsenic mines in Pants: "The air in mine would be both dangerous and difficult to tolerate on the reason of the awful scent of the metal, so the employees are condemned to a premature death" (Cope, 2004). The 19th century saw the rise of industrialization, which led to the development of modern models of industrial disorders. One such model is chronic mercurialism, brought on by exposure to mercuric nitrate, which is used to "felt" animal furs. The phrase "mad as a hatter" was coined to characterize the tremors known as "hatters' shakes," specifically felt by hat manufacturers, who were particularly vulnerable. The risk of various occupational chemicals causing cancer has come under increased scrutiny recently (Sharma et al., 2020) (Figure 5.6).

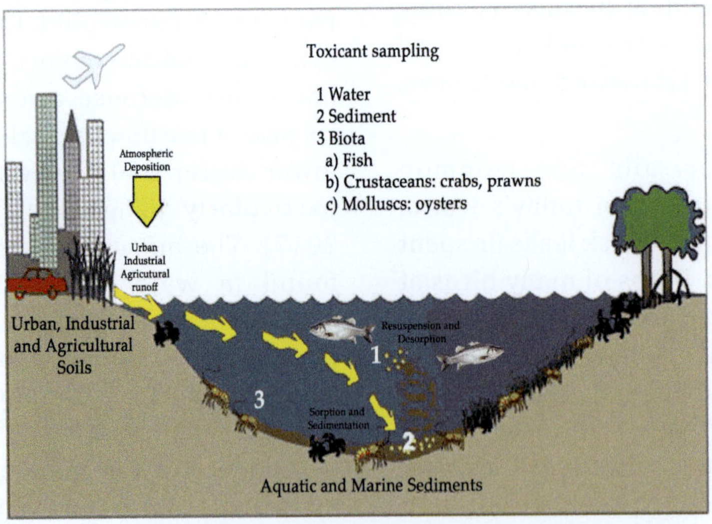

Figure 5.6. *Illustration of toxicants' passage through Moreton Bay is shown as a conceptual model.*

Source: https://ozcoasts.org.au/wp-content/uploads/2016/09/toxicants.gif.

- **Examples of Industrial Toxicants:** Carcinogen exposure is mostly due to life factors like tobacco smoking, although the profession is also a major source of carcinogen exposure (Costa et al., 2017).

With a biological half-life of up to thirty years, cadmium is a cumulative toxicant for humans. More than 70% of the cadmium in blood is bound to red blood cells; cadmium mainly builds up in the kidney and liver, where it binds to metallothionein. After chronic cadmium poisoning, the kidneys are the crucial organ to target in humans, and the first telltale sign of kidney damage is elevated protein urine (Zawadzki et al., 2016,). Hexavalent chromium is the source of chromium toxicity; it is absorbed more quickly through the GI tract and lungs than through the skin. All of the following are signs of professional chromium (Cr6+) exposure: dermatitis, nasal septum, ulcers on the arms and hands, perforation of the (possibly caused by chromic acid), infections of the throat and liver, and bronchitis. Employees of chromate plants are 20 times more likely to develop lung cancer than the general population due to chromate, a carcinogen that causes bronchogenic carcinoma. Compounds containing trivalent chromium have poor absorption. According to Zhang et al., chromium is a non-accumulative substance that is rapidly removed from the body through urine. (2021). Due to its widespread toxicity in the environment, exposure conditions have an impact on the amount of lead that is considered healthy in the body. Ten percent or less of the lead that is consumed enters the bloodstream, whereas only about half of the lead produced in the lungs is absorbed. Lead exposure is no longer a major occupational hazard, but environmental contamination is still widespread (Ng and Amini, 2021). Because lead inhibits the formation of porphyrins and heme, lead toxicity screening procedures look for suppression of the enzyme Aminolevulinic Acid Dehydratase (AAD) or the presence of coproporphyrin and aminolevulinic acid (ALA) in urine (UCP). The metabolism of inorganic lead and calcium are closely related, and too much lead can be stored in the bones for a long time. Inorganic lead poisoning manifests as fatigue, dysphagia, anemia, colic, and neuritis. Children who suffer from severe lead poisoning may experience encephalopathy, mental retardation, and in rare instances, poor vision (Lichtfouse, 2009) (Figure 5.7).

Benzene was widely used in the rubber industry as a rubber latex agent in the latter half of the 1800s. High concentrations of solvent were released into the atmosphere as a result of benzene's volatile nature, which also made it so desirable to industry. Rubber cement based on benzene is employed in the shoe manufacturing, processing, and packaging industries. Despite the fact that benzene poisoning cases had been reported as early as 1897 and that additional research and warnings were published in the 1920s, benzene's exceptional solvent properties allowed for its continued widespread use. There were cases of benzene toxicity during the 1930s printing industry's use of benzene as a toner solvent. Today, the annual consumption of benzoene exceeds 11 billion liters of water (Preuss et al., (2003)). Benzene is an inhaled steroid that impacts the bone marrow's hematopoietic cells. Over time, there may be a decrease in the quantity of platelets, white blood cells, and red blood cells, or any combination of these. Long-term exposure to benzene can cause aplastic anemia and grave bone marrow damage. Exposure to benzene has been connected to leukemia (Frigerio et al., 2019).

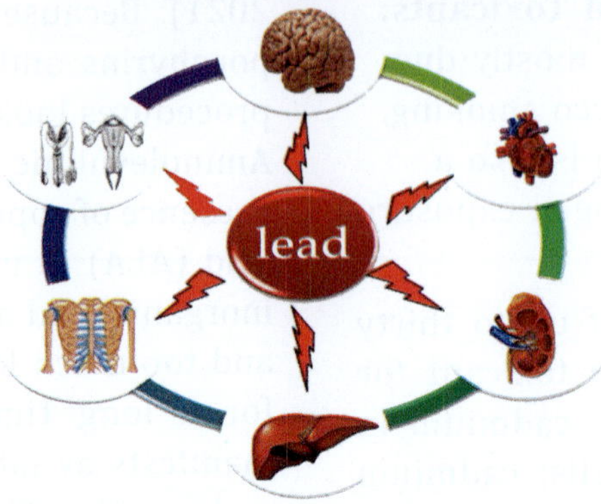

Figure 5.7. *Systems affected by lead toxicity.*

Source: https://www.researchgate.net/profile/Manodeep-Chakraborty/publication/326565451/figure/fig1/AS:651726969393153@1532395226965/Systems-affected-by-lead-toxicity.png.

5.3.1. Metal Toxicants

The majority of metals are typically found in low and distributed concentrations because they are found naturally in rocks, soil, ores, air, and water. Because they increase metal concentrations where human activities occur, human impacts represent the most significant human exposures and have toxicological significance (Levander, 1977).

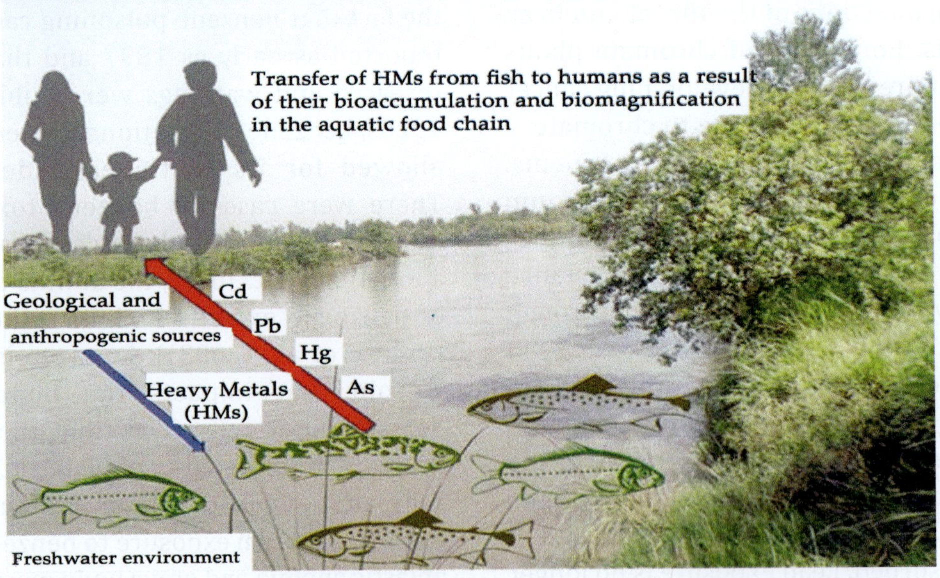

Figure 5.8. *Image of heavy metals transferred trophically from freshwater fish to people in the human food chain.*

Source: https://media.springernature.com/m312/springer-static/image/art%3A10.1007%2Fs10311-018-0734-7/MediaObjects/10311_2018_734_Fig1_HTML.jpg?.

For the majority of human history, metals have been used to make tools, machinery, and other objects. Smiling and mining produced the metals needed for these uses. These actions led to an increase in the concentration of metals in the surrounding environment. Recently, metals have been found to have many uses in industry, health, and agriculture. These procedures have increased exposure for end users of various products as well as for professionals working with metal (Khan et al., 2011). Many metals have a wide range of toxicological properties despite the great diversity of toxic metals and poisonous qualities. A brief description of some of the most pertinent subjects is provided in the section that follows. A metal needs to pass through the cell surface and enter the cell in order to manifest its toxicity. Any metal that is always in a lipid-soluble form, such as mercury, can pass through membranes with ease; other metals, such as cadmium-metallothionein, can be absorbed into cells through endocytosis (e.g., lead) are taken up through passive diffusion. In most cases, interactions between the free metal and the cellular targets lead to metal toxicity. Targets include different cellular membranes and/or particular metabolic processes (Sharma et al., 2019) (Figure 5.8).

5.3.2. Lead

Lead has been used for so long, and is one of the most common hazardous metals. Air, water, and food can all expose someone. Other industrial uses, such as batteries, have remained mostly unaffected, but major ones, like paint pigments and fuel additives, were removed from the country. Two additional sources of lead are ceramic tiles found in food containers and pipes (Klaine et al.). (2008). The skin, GI tract, and respiratory system are the three entry points for inorganic lead (Pb) into the body. In children, inorganic lead crosses the placenta with ease and enters the brain stem more efficiently than it does in adults. Although lead is typically distributed throughout the blood, kidneys, and liver, prolonged exposure can detect up to 95% of the body's lead load in bone cells (Flora et al., 2006). The main organs affected by lead poisoning are the neurological and hematologic systems. Heme synthetase (HS) and ALAD are the two most vulnerable enzymes among the many that are involved in heme synthesis susceptible to lead reduction. Biochemical effects may manifest at lower levels, even though clinical anemia is only identified with significant lead exposure. As a result, lead poisoning may be diagnosed by ALAD restriction or the presence of ALA in the urine (Ju-Nam and Lead, 2008). Since the neural systems of newborns and young children are still developing, lead poisoning may also have an impact on them. Even at moderate levels of exposure, children may show signs of hyperactivity, poor attention span, mental impairments, and vision impairment. Children and adults may be more severely affected by encephalopathy. Due to arterioles and capillaries being damaged, lead results in cerebral edema and neuronal degeneration. According to Flora et al., ataxia, coma, convulsions, and stupor are clinical indicators of this injury. 06). Another mechanism that is damaged by lead is the reproductive organs. In addition to miscarriages and abnormal offspring, lead poisoning can cause reproductive toxicity in both men and women (Fabrega et al., 2011 and Handy et al., 2008).

5.3.3. Mercury

Elements of mercury (Hg^0), organic methylmercury (CH_3Hg), inorganic mercurous (Hg^+), mercuric (Hg^{2+}) salts, and dimethylmercury (CH_3HgCH_3) and organic methylmercury (CH_3Hg) molecules are all found in nature. The process of breathing nearly entirely absorbs pollutants in the type of mercury vapor, while swallowed elemental mercury also isn't quickly absorbed and therefore is generally innocuous. Elemental mercury may pass the BBS and enter the neurological system once ingested. Most people who are exposed to elemental mercury do so at work (Schroeder & Munthe, 1998).

The increased concern over exposure to organic mercury compounds stems from environmental contamination. MeHg, an extremely poisonous form that can easily cross membranes, is the result of the conversion of inorganic mercury to organic mercury by sulfate-reducing microbes. The consumption of seafood contaminated with mercury or seeds treated with mercury fungicides has been linked to numerous significant outbreaks of mercury poisoning (Harris et al., 2003). Minamata Bay was contaminated by mercury waste that was disposed of in the 1950s and 1960s from a chemical and plastics plant in Japan. Mercury was converted into absorbable MeHg by bacteria found in the aquaculture sediments. Numerous cases of Minamata disease, or mercury poisoning, were caused by the local population's consumption of fish and seafood. By 1970, there had been 800 confirmed cases of Minamata sickness, and at least 107 deaths linked to mercury poisoning. Even though their moms appeared to be in good health, many newborns whose mothers had eaten tainted fish displayed symptoms resembling neurological palsy and mental deficiencies. The nervous system is primarily impacted by organic mercury, and the developing brain is more susceptible to mercury poisoning than the adult brain (Clarkson, 1997). Inorganic mercury salts, which are primarily nephrotoxicants, are primarily found in the renal tubule cells. Mercury interacts with the amino groups of membrane proteins, compromising the stability of the membrane and leading to oliguria, uremia, and anuria (Langford and Ferner, 1999).

5.3.4. Cadmium

The majority of cadmium is naturally occurring in zinc and lead ores, and it is released into the air by miners and smelters who process these ores. In industry, cadmium is utilized as a pigment in paints and plastics, as well as in alloys, alkali battery packs, electroplating, and other processes. g. nickel-cadmium batteries) (Bidari et al., 2013). The primary sources of indoor cadmium exposure are industrial and smelting-related groundwater pollution, as well as the use of wastewater as a fertilizer for food crops. Leafy green vegetables, grains, and cereal products are the main food sources of cadmium. There has been mention of the Itai-Itai condition, which is brought on by consuming rice contaminated with cadmium in Japan) (Telisman et al., 1986). Most of the acute effects of exposure to cadmium are due to localized inflammation. Following ingestion, nausea, abdominal pain, and vomiting are the most typical symptoms. Inhalation can result in respiratory edema and pneumonia. Chronic effects are especially concerning because cadmium has a half-life of about thirty years and is progressively eliminated from the body. Therefore, even low exposure levels have the potential to cause a large buildup of cadmium (Cambar et al., 1983). Long-term exposure would primarily affect the kidneys, with the distal tubules serving as the main site of exposure. The liver and the circulatory system produce the metal-binding protein metallothionein, which is strongly linked to cadmium. Following glomerular filtration within the kidney, CMT is efficiently taken up by the tubular cells and accumulated within the lysosomes. Following this, the CMT complex breaks down, releasing Cd+2, which inhibits lysosomal activity and damages cells (Piotrowski et al., 1974).

5.3.5. Chromium

Since chromium is naturally found in ores, the environmental risks associated with chromium increase with mining, industrial use, and smelting. Chromium is present in various alloys, colors, and stainless steel. As this metal is typically found in very small amounts in food, water, and the air, worker exposure is the most common way that people are exposed to it. There are several oxidation states of chromium, from Cr^{+2} to $Cr^{+6,}$ but only the trivalent (Cr^{+3}) and hexavalent (Cr^{+6}) forms are significant for biological processes (Rai et al., 1989). In the industry, the hexavalent form is more significant even though the trivalent molecule is more common. Despite not being soluble in water, hexavalent chromium is also absorbed through cellular membranes more quickly than trivalent chromium. In actuality, the hexavalent form is changed into the trivalent form, which has the potential to bind to internal macromolecules and become toxic. Exposure to chromium has been shown to cause lung cancer in humans. This includes employees. It is believed that chromium (C^{r+6}) carcinogenicity in the lung results from the reduction of chromium (Cr^{+6}) to C^{r+3} and the synthesis of intermediates, which causes bronchogenic carcinoma (Kimbrough et al., 1999).

5.3.6. Arsenic

The main way that humans are exposed to arsenic is through their diets, as air and water contain relatively little of the material. Nonetheless, considerable concentrations of this metalloid have been found in the water in some regions of Taiwan and South America, where inhabitants experience hyperpigmentation and hyperkeratosis of the skin. Increased exposure led to a more serious condition called "Blackfoot disease," or lower extremity gangrene. These locations may also see cases of skin cancer (Oremland and Stolz, 2003). Approximately 80% of compounds containing arsenic come from pesticides. Paints, glassware, and pigments are a few more uses. The electronics industry uses arsine gas.

There are three types of arsenic compounds:

- Pentavalent, As^{+5}, organic or arsenate compounds (e.g., alkyl arsenates);
- Trivalent, As^{+3}, inorganic or arsenate compounds (e.g., sodium arsenate, arsenic trioxide); and
- Arsine gas, ash3, a colorless gas resulting from the action of acids on arsenic.

With a TLV-TWA of 0.05 ppm, arsine gas is the most toxic type (Braman and Foreback, 1973). Microbes that metabolize arsenic to dimethyl arsenate can accumulate in fish and seafood, putting people at risk. Pollutants, including arsenic compounds, can also be discovered in well water. Because arsenite (As^{+3}) molecules are lipophilic, they can be absorbed through the skin, food, or inhalation. Within 24 h after absorption, arsenic travels throughout the body and binds to the SH groups involved in protein metabolism. A very small proportion of people pass the BBS. Arsenic can also be stored for a long period and used to replenish phosphorus in bone tissue. After acute poisoning, acute GI symptoms can appear 30 min to 2 h later. Among the symptoms are vomiting, diarrhea that is both bloody and watery, stomach pain, and burning pain in the esophagus. Possible side effects include cerebral edema, proximal neuropathic pain, vasodilation, and cardiovascular depression. Advanced poisoning manifests as nephrotoxicity failure and jaundice. Death typically results from blood flow failure in 24 to 4 days (Nordstrom, 2002). Hyperkeratosis, diarrhea, abdominal pain, and hyperpigmentation are typical signs of prolonged exposure. Pain with spherical sensory neuropathic pain is often the outcome. According to Meharg and Hartley-Whitaker (2002), delayed changes include lung cancer, anemia, skin, nasal tissue, and gangrene of the limbs.

5.4. Agricultural Chemicals

Pesticides have been used for millennia to control or eradicate pests. The ancient Romans used regular salt to suppress weeds, and the Chinese used sulfur to manage pests. The Chinese also used arsenic to manage insects. Insecticidal properties of pyrethrin, a compound present in the blooms of *Pyrethrum cineraefolium*, a chrysanthemum, were discovered in the 1800s (Hallberg, 1987). The roots of certain plant species called Derris were used by the Chinese and native Americans in South America. Its active ingredient, rotenone, was first identified in 1895 and was initially applied to insect control. Paris Green, another chemical created for pest control in the 1800s, was a mixture of copper and arsenic salts. Fungi were repelled by the Bordeaux Mixture, a mixture of lime and copper sulfate (Mann et al., 2009).

5.4.1. Pesticides

However, the development of modern pesticidal substances did not occur until the 19th century. Insect scales and red creepy crawlies were first treated with petroleum oils, which are made from raw crude oil, in the 1920s. Chlorinated hydrocarbon insecticides, such as DDT, and phenoxy acid herbicides, such as 2,4-D, were first introduced in the 1940s. Red Squill, a naturally occurring substance derived from Urginea (Scilla) Maritima bulbs, has been demonstrated to be effective in controlling rodents (Hallberg, 1987). Triazine herbicides, such as atrazine, which was introduced in the late 1950s, dominated the global herbicide market for a long time. Synthetic pyrethrins, also known as pyrethroid insecticides, are preferred due to their low toxicity, enhanced persistence compared to pyrethrins, and ease of application (e.g., insects—such as resmethrin—were and are still widely used). Families of fungicides, herbicides, and insecticides continue to be introduced into international markets when older chemicals become less popular due to pest resistance or unfavorable health effects (Gupta and Crissman, 2013) (Figure 5.9).

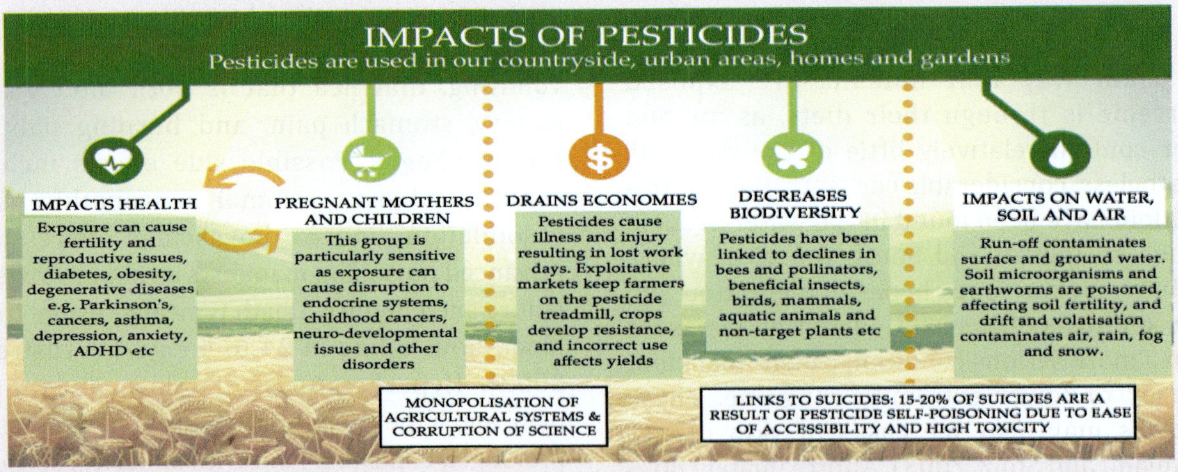

Figure 5.9. *Illustration of pesticides' effects.*

Source: https://www.kingsbridgeclimateaction.co.uk/post/pesticides-and-their-ripple-effect-on-water.

Among environmental contaminants, pesticides are special since their purpose is to kill living organisms. Ideally, pesticides should be highly selective, eradicating target species with minimal harm to non-target organisms. Conversely, the majority of insecticides lack significant selectivity (Nielsen, 1987). The benefits of applying pesticides must be weighed against the risks to human health and the environment. Pesticides have the benefit of preventing vector-borne diseases, increasing agricultural productivity, and decreasing urban pests. One major risk of pesticides getting into the food supply and environmental water systems is environmental contamination, especially when it comes to pesticide movement in the surrounding environment. Two things to consider are the ecosystem's durability and the potential for biomagnification (Grant, 1982).

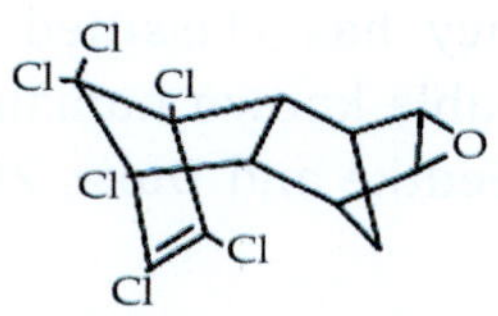

Dieldrin

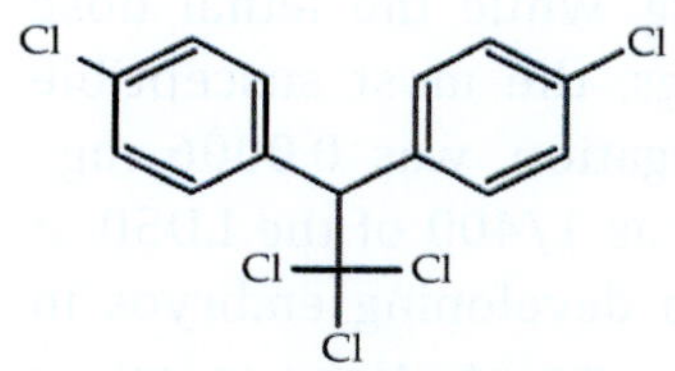

DDT

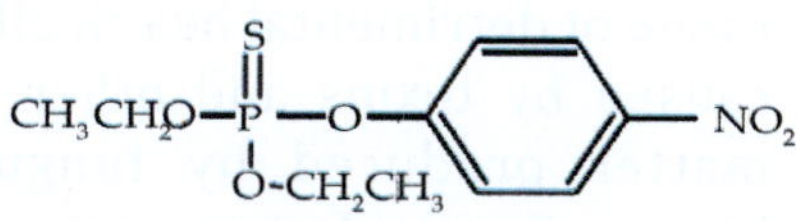

Parathion

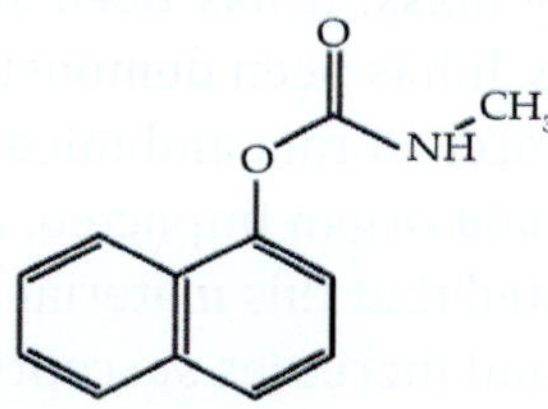

Carbaryl

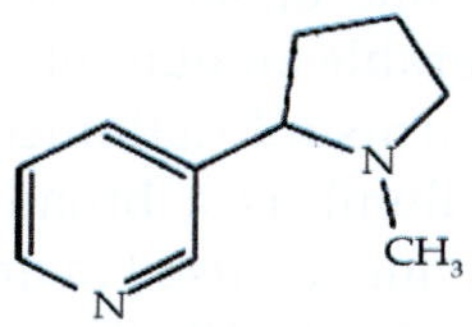

Nicotine

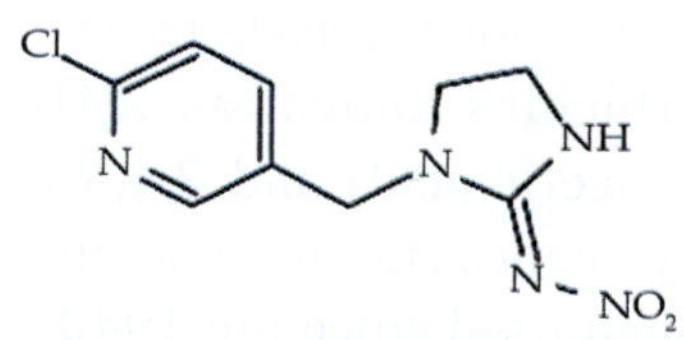

Imidacloprid

5.4.2. Herbicides

The most widely used insecticides to control weeds are herbicides. Herbicides accounted for 578 million pounds of pesticides used in the US in 1997, or roughly 47% of all pesticides applied, according to the most recent US EPA statistics. This type of herbicide can be applied to crops in a number of ways to eradicate or reduce the weed population. Examples include pre-intervention, post-emergent, and preplant integration treatments. Low-level herbicides are mainly not phytotoxic to beneficial plants, making them environmentally safe and still under development. A few of the new families, such as imidazolinones, inhibit the synthesis of branched-chain amino acids in crops by blocking the enzyme acetohydroxy acid synthesis. Since this enzyme is only present in plants, these herbicides are safe for use around fish, birds, insects, and other animals (Moreland, 1980). Long-term use of herbicides can have a negative impact on the environment. Chlorophenoxy herbicides have been used as systemic herbicides to suppress leafy plants since the 1940s. Examples of these herbicides are 2,4,5-T (2,4,5-trichlorophenoxy acetic acid) and 2,4D (2,4-dichloro phenoxy acetic acid). When ingested, these substances are not very harmful (Kudsk and Streibig, 2003).

Agent Orange, a mixture of 2,4,5-T and 2,4-D used as a defoliant by the US military during the Vietnam War, has generated much discussion due to claims made by service members regarding long-term health effects. In terms of toxicological significance, TCDD (2,3,7,8-tetrachlorodibenzodioxin) was identified as the contaminant produced during production (Morrison et al., 1992). Among all synthetic chemicals, TCDD is one of the most toxic to animals used in experiments. The lethal dose (LD) for male rats was 0.022 mg/kg, while the lethal dose for female guinea pigs, the most susceptible species under investigation, was 0.0006 mg/kg. At dosages as low as 1/400 of the LD50, it is also detrimental to developing embryos in pregnant mice, and at concentrations as low as 1 to 3 ng/kg of body mass, it has been shown to cause birth defects. It has been demonstrated that TCDD causes cancer in rats and mice, with the liver being the main organ impacted. It has also been demonstrated that this material alters the immune system and increases susceptibility in exposed animals (Ashton and Crafts, 1973). Herbicide families that have been in use for a long time continue to pose a risk to the environment. The herbicides known as 2,4D (2,4-dichloro phenoxy acetic acid) and 2,4,5-T (2,4,5-trichlorophenoxy-acetic acid) are systemic herbicides that have been used since the 1940s to control broadleaf plants. These substances don't pose much of an oral toxic threat.

Triazines, a herbicide class, continue to worry environmental and toxicologists due to pollution of surface and groundwater supplies that become publicly drinking water. Atrazine [6-chloro-N-ethyl-N'-(1-methylethyl)-1,3,5-triazine-2,4-diamine is a maize herbicide with an MCL of 3.0 g/L, and it is used largely on maize. This pesticide has been discovered in surfaces and groundwater resources all over the globe, with quantities ranging from 1 to >130 g/L (Gianessi, 2013). It has an MCL of 4.0 g/L, together with cyanazine [2–4-chloro-6-(methylamino)-1,3,5-triazin-2ylamino-2-methylpropanenitrile] and simazine (6-chloro-N,Ndiethyl-1,3,5-triazine2,4-diamine). The usage of cyanazine was phased down in 2001, with no further use allowed after 2002. Although generally harmless (e.g., atrazine has an oral LD50 of 3,100 mg/kg in rats), the main worry with these chemicals is their carcinogenic potential, and the US Environmental Protection Agency has classified all three triazines as probable known human carcinogens (category C) (Fedtke and Duke, 2005).

5.4.3. Fungicides

Fungi cause millions of dollars worth of agricultural losses in the United States each year. Moreover, new studies have shown that a range of detrimental health effects are probably caused by toxins and other airborne organic matter produced by fungus that inhabits homes. Fungicides are compounds developed to mitigate such loss and adverse health effects; some of these groups have existed for a considerable amount of time (Qu et al., 2021). Tetrachloroisophthalonitrile, also known as chlorothalonil, is a broad-spectrum fungicide that is frequently used in urban environments. It regulates about 140 different kinds of organisms and is fairly cheap. This chemical is frequently found in surface waters that enter public water supply systems due to its extensive use. Within the formulation accessible to the general public, it is essentially innocuous (Audus, 1964; Walker, 2002). One class of fungicides that ought to be avoided are the dithiocarbamates, which are sulfur compounds of dithiocarbamic acid that include the metallic diethyldithiocarbamate. The latter category (zinc ethylenebisdithiocarbamate) includes mancozeb (a coordination product of manganese ethylene bisdithiocarbamate and zinc ion), maneb (manganese ethylene bisdithiocarbamate), and zineb (manganese ethylene bisdithiocarbamate). These are all very effective fungicides that are used on ornamentals, grapes, and sugar beets, among other crops. Although generally safe (ETU), they hydrolyze to produce known carcinogens like ethylthiourea (Gianessi and Reigner, 2007).

5.4.4. Rodenticides

Rodents cause losses of 20 to 30% a year in grain and other food warehouses; this chemical family is used to keep them out. Furthermore, to carrying other organisms, fleas are a pest that spread disease (Knight et al., 1997). Among the anticoagulants that have been around for a long time is warfarin [3-(-acetonylbenzyl)-4-hydroxycoumarin]. This is a potent toxin (rat) with an oral LD50 of only 3.0 mg/kg. They sustain minor wounds from the rats' damage as they squeeze through small tunnels. Anticoagulants stop blood clots from forming, so within a week the animals die in excruciating pain. Blood donations and vitamin K are used to treat humans who are sensitized to this family of chemicals, if the poisoning is severe (Bartett et al., 2001). Certain rodenticides are harmful to the animals and are frequently used in combination with only an attractant, such as peanut butter, to help overcome the aversion to bait. With an ingested LD50 of 15 mg/kg in rats, fluoroacetamide is a potent toxin that acts rapidly. This material comes in grain or pellet form for baiting. ANTU ('-naphthylthiourea), strychnine, and thallium salts—which were marketed for years—are a few examples of fast-acting poisons. Most rodenticides have restricted uses and should only be applied by licensed pest control experts. Human rodenticide poisonings are primarily brought on by accidental or self-destructive ingestion of the chemicals (Bartlett et al., 2002) (Figure 5.10).

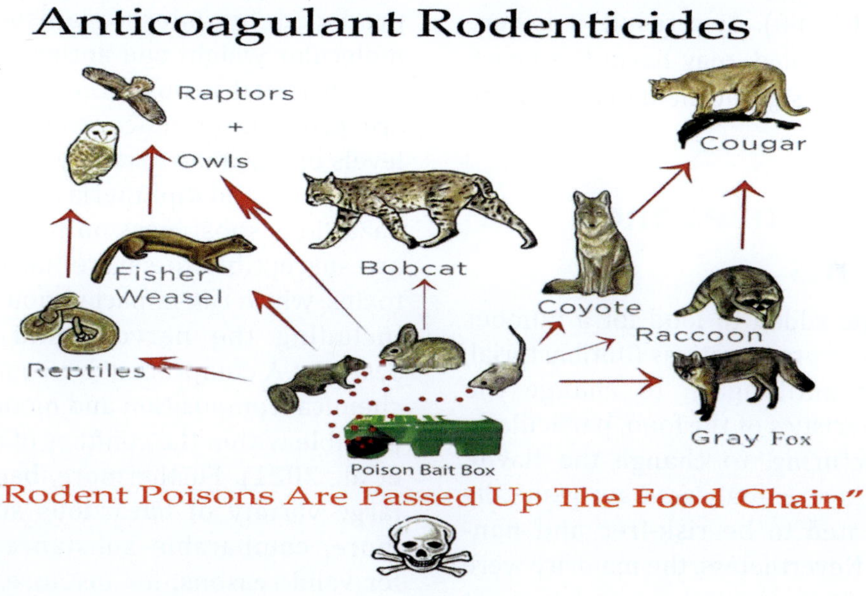

Figure 5.10. *Image of rodenticides with anticoagulants.*

Source: https://image.slidesharecdn.com/anticoagulantrodenticides-181113060609/75/Anticoagulant-rodenticides-1–2048.jpg.

5.4.5. Fumigants

Fumigants are extremely toxic gases used to get rid of soil worms and protect stored goods, especially grains. These compounds are used to treat storage facilities, freight vehicles, and homes infested with parasites such as powdered post beetles. When handling and applying this family of pesticides, extra caution is required due to the risk of inhalation and the pesticides' rapid diffusion into the respiratory system. According to Murphy (2002), fumigants are all classified as restricted-use materials that need to be handled by authorized applicators. Of all the fumigants, methyl bromide is one of the strongest. Because it kills worms, insects, and weed seeds, it is used to sterilize soil when placed beneath a soil covering and to disinfect warehouses. Large inhalations of this molecule can result in CNS effects, heart attacks, and breathing difficulties. The LC50 for inhaling air in rats is 0.06 mg/L (15 min), and for humans, it is 7900 ppm (1.5h). Methyl bromide has already been classified as an ozone depleter under the Environmental Quality Act, and its use would end by 2005 (Watt et al., 2005).

Another soil/space fumigant that has been used for a long time is chloropicrin (trichloronitromethane). This has a 150 ppm inhaling LC50 (15 min). As a result, it is very poisonous when inhaled, may harm the heart, and also can cause significant damage to the eyes (Murphy, 2018).

5.5. Food Additives and Contaminants

Chemicals can be added to food for a number of reasons, such as preservatives (antibacterial, antioxidant, or antifungal); to change the physical characteristics of the food, particularly during manufacturing, to change the flavor, color, or odor. Flavor enhancers have generally been demonstrated to be risk-free and non-toxic over time. Nevertheless, the majority were introduced when toxicological research was not as developed, and some have since been shown to be detrimental. The various types of natural food additives (Ibekwe et al., 2001; Joint et al., 2007). Next, we will discuss inorganics, nitrate and nitrite being the most important ones. Thousands, if not hundreds, of food ingredients are used worldwide, and many of them have not received enough testing. There hasn't been enough research to date on the potential for these drugs to work in concert. Not all toxins found in food are created by humans; several naturally occurring toxicants, including genetic and carcinogenic mutations, found in human nutrition are well known (Price, 1985).

5.5.1. Microbial Toxins

In contrast, pollutants produced by microorganisms that do not meet these criteria have been loosely referred to as poisons. Microbiologists typically refer to toxic chemicals produced by microorganisms that have a molecular weight and antigenic characteristics as "microbial toxins.". The majority of the first are proteins or mucoproteins with different levels of enzymatic activity. Toxins like tetanus, botulinum, and diphtheria are some of the most hazardous substances on the planet. Mammals are susceptible to severe harm from bacterial toxins, which can impact various bodily systems, including the nervous and cardiovascular systems. A comprehensive explanation of their chemical composition and mode of action is not possible within the confines of this book (Gupta et al., 2021). Furthermore, bacteria produce a large variety of hazardous substances. Once more, comparable substances may be used for valid reasons; for instance, the insecticidal properties of *Bacillus thuringiensis*, which are associated with the toxin, have long been used in agriculture (Rajkovic, 2014) (Figure 5.11).

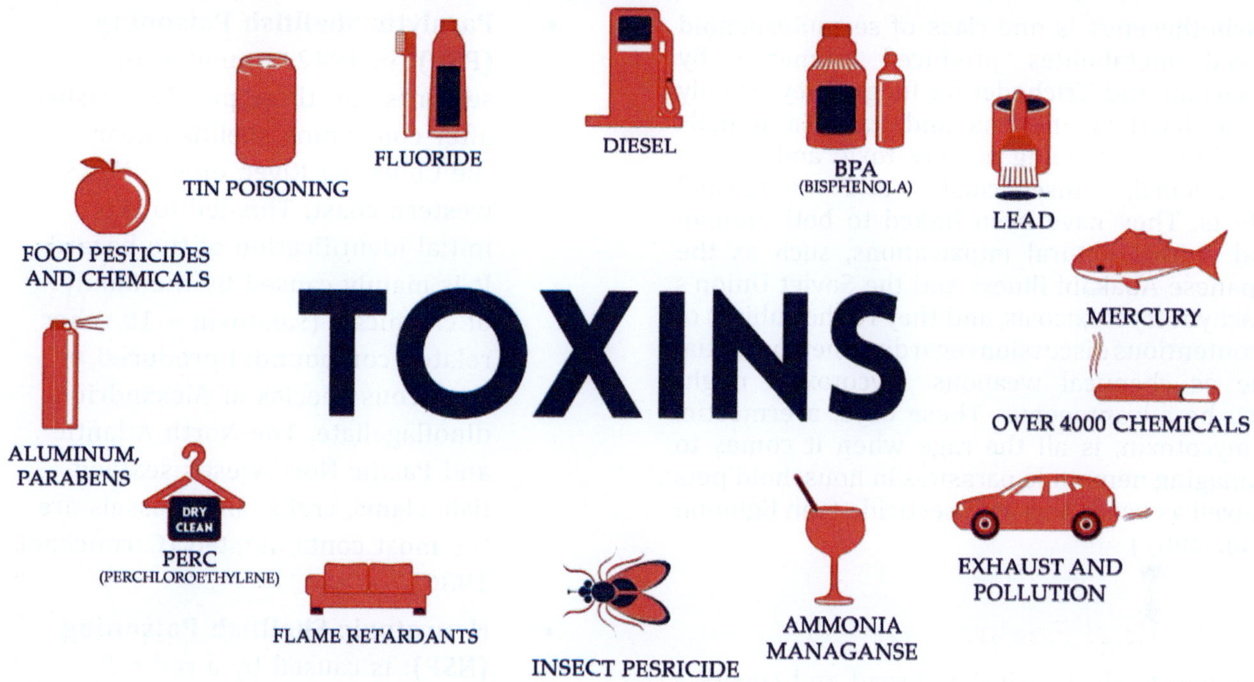

Figure 5.11. *Illustration of toxins come in a variety of forms.*

Source: https://media.licdn.com/dms/image/C5612AQGsD14Qpq9WCw/article-cover_image-shrink_720_1280/0/1623760785061?e=2147483647&v=beta&t=stdaCmvOH2Bfl_bgL3iyzrB6F2SmQAdeCZYruNI5U2g.

5.5.2. Mycotoxins

It is impossible to cover the vast range of chemical compositions and biological activities found in fungal species in a short period. Since mycotoxins lack any shared molecular properties, they cannot be classified as a separate chemical group (Richard, 2007). Particularly of interest are mycotoxins found in household pet food or even in the diet of humans. The *Claviceps* sp. generates Aspergillus sp. and ergot alkaloids. produces a variety of imperfect fungal species, primarily Fusarium sp., as well as substances similar to aflatoxins. Induced Trichothecenese production (Coulombe Jr, 1993): it is well known that ergot alkaloids are vasoconstrictors and affect the CNS. They have been connected to convulsive, severely infected ergotism (St. Anthony's fire) illnesses in the past, but because of a better knowledge of the causes and more varied modern diets, such outbreaks do not occur in humans today. As a result, animal ergotism infections are still prevalent. These substances were also used to make abortifacients. The most potent ergot alkaloids are amides of lysergic acid, which are found in the ergot alkaloids (Pitt, 2000; Schatzmayr et al., 2006). Aspergillus species, most famously A flavus, a common fungus found in grains, corn, nuts, and other foods, produce aflatoxins. Initially connected to poultry diseases such as Turkey-X, they were later shown to raise the risk of cancer in animal trials and in humans, as per epidemiological studies. Aflatoxin B1, the most potent of the aflatoxins, needs to be enzymatically activated to exert its carcinogenic effects (Speijers and Speijers, 2004).

Trichothecenes is one class of sesquiterpenoid fungal metabolites produced primarily by Fusarium and Trichoderma fungi. They usually cause diarrhea, anorexia, and ataxia in animals in addition to being acutely toxic and having bactericidal, insecticidal, and fungicidal effects. They have been linked to both human and animal natural intoxications, such as the Japanese Abakabi illness and the Soviet Union's Stachybotryotoxicosis, and they're the subject of a contentious discussion regarding their potential use as chemical weapons. Mycotoxins might also be advantageous. These days, avermectin, a mycotoxin, is all the rage when it comes to managing nematode parasites in household pets as well as using it as an insecticide (van Egmond et al., 2007).

5.5.3. Algal Toxins

The word "algal toxins" is broad and covers a range of substances made by dinoflagellates, cyanobacteria (blue-green bacteria), and diatoms. Such freshwater and marine microorganisms produce toxins that frequently accumulate in surrounding shellfish and fish, causing illness in humans and animals as well as obvious fish deaths. Algal toxins have a higher potential for human exposure and harm because, in contrast to many microbiological toxins, they are frequently heat resistant and unaffected by cooking processes. This list includes many of the most common algae toxins that poison people worldwide (Van Dolah, 2000).

- **Amnesic Shellfish Poisoning (ASP):** The first evidence of it was discovered in 1987 on Prince Edward Island, Canada, when four people perished after consuming contaminated mussels. It is brought on by the production of domoic acid by a variety of Pseudo-nitzschia diatom species. The primary contaminants are clams, crabs, and mussels from the American Pacific Coast (Collins, 1978).
- **Paralytic Shellfish Poisoning (PSP):** In 1942, a number of seabirds and three people perished after consuming shellfish near the Columbia River, on the USA's western coast. This led to the initial identification of the hazard. It is mainly caused by the family of chemicals (saxitoxin + 18 other related compounds) produced by numerous species of Alexandrium dinoflagellate. The North Atlantic and Pacific Northwest's seafood, fish, clams, crabs, and mussels are the most contaminated (Carmichael, 1986).
- **Neurotoxic Shellfish Poisoning (NSP):** is caused by a red tide generator that was first found in Florida in 1880, though there are references to earlier historical periods. People become sick from it for several days. NSP has no effect on humans, but it has been shown to harm fish, marine life, invertebrates, and seabirds. The dinoflagellate Karenia Brevis produces the brevetoxin group, which consists of brevetoxin plus ten related chemicals. k. a. The disease's cause is Gymnodinium breve. The main contaminants are clams and other filter feeders from the Southeast Atlantic and Gulf Coast, particularly North Carolina (Falconer, 1998).
- **Diarrheic Shellfish Poisoning (DSP):** In the 1960s, the first types of toxicity to humans were identified. It is not fatal, but it makes people sick for several days at a time. It is caused by substances from the okadaic acid

group (okadaic acid + 4 related medications), which are produced by various Dinophysis dinoflagellate species. The main contaminants are mussels, clams, and other shellfish from the temperate regions of the Pacific and Atlantic oceans, mostly in Japan and Europe. There were only two recorded cases of DSP in North America (Shilo, 1967).

- **Ciguatera Fish Poisoning (CFP):** CFP is a highly toxic tropical subtropical seafood that affects up to 50,000 people annually and is the most commonly reported food-borne illness disease linked to a chemical source in the United States. Although it was initially identified in 1511, S. is the most commonly reported food-borne illness disease linked to a chemical source in the United States. S. A. When people eat reef fish, they become sick (e.g., grouper, snapper), and while it is uncommon, it lasts for several days or even weeks. It is caused by the ciguatoxin group (ciguatoxin + 3 or even more similar chemicals) produced by different dinoflagellate taxa, such as Ostreopsis, Prorocentrum, and Gambierdiscus. Tropical reef fish that consume plants are some of the most susceptible to pollution (Rositano et al., 2001).
- **Cyanobacteria (Blue-Green Bacteria) Toxins:** The first reports of cyanobacteria-related poisonings date back to the late 1800s. Although poisoning humans is rare, it frequently results in the deaths of fish, cattle, other animals, birds, and aquatic invertebrates. Many biotoxins affect it, including cytotoxins produced by cyanobacteria like Microcystis, Aphanizomenon, Nodularia, Oscillatoria, and Anabaena, which include nodularin, microcystin, and anatoxin. Pollution poses a threat to all eutrophic freshwater rivers, ponds, and flows (McNabb et al., 2005).
- **Ambush Predator (Pfiesteria piscicida and Toxic Pfiesteria Complex) Toxins:** In 1991, the first members of this genus of animals were found in the estuaries of North Carolina. These were believed to produce a poison that may be harmful to humans and has been connected to multiple large fish deaths. However, the poison or poisons are still unknown, and toxicity studies are not always conclusive. In addition to Pfiesteria piscicida and Pfiesteria shumway, there could be many other unidentified, undiscovered dinoflagellate taxa connected to the potentially hazardous Pfiesteria complex that produces this toxin. The main problems are massive fish deaths in Maryland and North Carolina and possible health risks to humans. According to Lawton and Codd (1991), the range may extend from the Gulf of Mexico to Atlantic estuary waters, which include Florida, Maryland, Delaware, and North Carolina, as well as possibly to Europe.

5.5.4. Solvents

Although they are sometimes more prevalent in the workplace, solvents can also be found in homes. Many have dermatological effects like defatting or localized irritation, in addition to systemically harmful effects like effects on the CNS or, as with benzene, impacts on plasma constituents. Business solvents are typically complex mixtures of organic materials containing sulfur and nitrogen, such as petroleum and other hydrocarbon chemicals (Zuccato et al., 2000).

The following are some of the most prevalent solvents:

- Aliphatic Hydrocarbons, like hexane. These chemicals may have a linear or branched chain and are often seen in mixes.
- Halogenated Aliphatic Hydrocarbons. Methylene dichloride, Carbon tetrachloride and chloroform, and are very well examples, however chlorinated ethylenes are also commonly employed (Di Carlo et al., 1999).
- Aliphatic Alcohols. Ethanol and methanol are typical examples.
- Glycols and Glycol Ethers. Antifreeze containing propylene glycols and ethylene, for example, exposes the general population to significant levels of propylene glycols and ethylene. Glycol ethers also are commonly utilized, like methyl cellosolve.
- Aromatic Hydrocarbons. Benzene has to be the most dangerous, although other chemicals, like toluene, are sometimes utilized (Gabathuler, 2010).

5.6. Therapeutic Drugs

Almost all therapeutic medications have the potential to be toxic, leading to negative effects at certain dosages, despite the fact that pharmacology studies the therapeutic qualities of substances. An individual's risk is influenced by the type of toxic reaction, the dosage needed to cause the reaction, and the relationship between the recommended dose and the poisonous dose. The same factors that affect the toxicity of numerous other xenobiotics also affect the toxicity of drugs: individual (genetic) variation, food, age, and the availability of numerous other exogenous chemicals (Khan et al., 2021). A drug's potential risks to health must be weighed against its expected benefits, even after the risks have been evaluated. In cases where there is no other viable treatment option, it may be appropriate to utilize a highly hazardous medication with a narrow tolerance between safe and toxic dosages. However, a reasonably safe medication might not be appropriate if safer alternatives are available or if the condition being treated is not serious (Robinson and Kolb, 2004). Among the cytotoxic medications used in cancer therapy that contain carcinogens are melphalan, nitrogen mustard, methotrexate, adriamycin, an antitumor antibiotic, and an antimetabolite. Children of women exposed to diethylstilbestrol (DES), a once-common medication, have been linked to vaginal and cervical cancer (Finney, 1971). Almost every organ system may be connected to additional pharmacological adverse effects. In the 1960s, subacute myeloid-optic neuropathy (SMON) was common in Japan and was believed to be a side effect of the anti-diarrhea medication chloroquine (Enterovioform). Moreover, drugs can cause teratogenesis; the most alarming example of this is thalidomide. One common side effect of medications is skin reactions, or dermatitis; topically applied corticosteroids are one example (Piomelli et al., 2000). Blood toxicity can manifest as hemolytic anemia from methyldopa, methotrexate-induced megaloblastic anemia, and agranulocytosis induced by chlorpromazine, to name a few. There have been reports of eye toxicity, including retinotoxicity caused by thioridazine and glaucoma caused by systemic corticosteroids (Schooltink & Rose-John, 2002).

5.6.1. Drugs of Abuse

Every medication has some poison in it. Contrarily, illegal drugs are either used at doses higher than those required for treatment or don't have a therapeutic purpose. While mood, reaction time, and coordination are the main areas affected by some illegal substances, many others lead to physical dependency and have disastrous physiological effects, including fatal overdoses (Leshner and Koob, 1999). opioids like meperidine (Demerol) and heroin; central nervous stimulants like narcotics, caffeine, methamphetamine (Speed), and nicotine; central nervous depressants like ethanol, secobarbital, and methaqualone (Quaalude); and hallucinogens like lysergic acid diethylamide (LSD), tetrahydrocannabinol (THC), and phencyclidine (PCP). An additional issue of toxicology relevance is that the majority of drugs used for abuse are produced in unlicensed, shoddy facilities with no quality control. Consequently, a large number of the finished products are contaminated with chemicals whose toxicity is unknown but may be fatal. A few of these compounds' structures are shown in Figure 5.12 (Stein and Tallman, 2016).

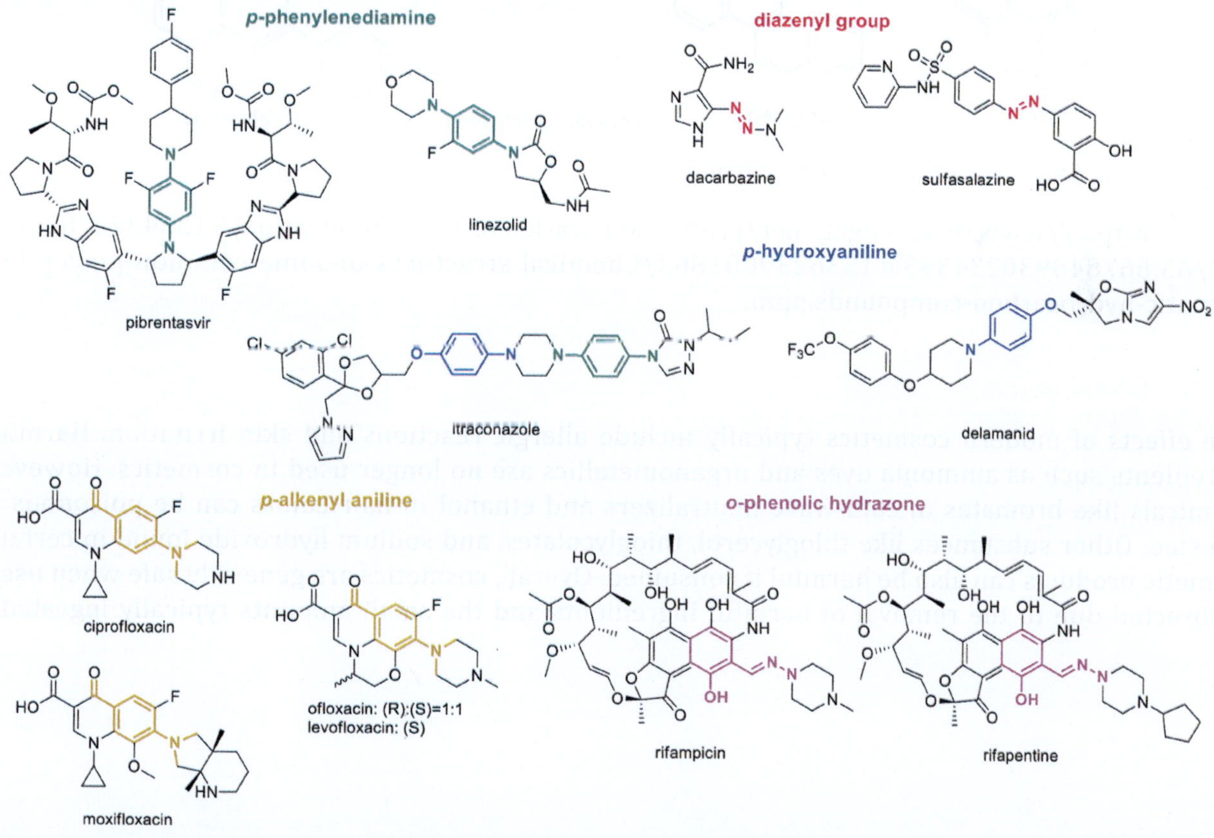

Figure 5.12. *Chemical structures of some of the essential medicines.*

Source: https://www.researchgate.net/publication/341068029/figure/fig5/AS:1008219765878785@1617389732686/Structures-of-EMs-displaying-PAINS.png.

5.6.2. Combustion Products

The most dangerous air pollutants for public health are polycyclic aromatic hydrocarbons, even though many other air pollutants are also produced by human or natural combustion. They are derived from natural product lines like crude oil and coal and are found in smokes, wood, coal, petroleum, and food products that have been broiled (Baumgartner et al., 1989). These are usually found in smoke from cigarettes, coal, oil, and wood smoke, and are linked to incomplete combustion of fossil fuel components. The metabolization, DNA connections, and other aspects of chemical carcinogenesis of the compounds have been extensively studied because some of them are carcinogenic. Some are heterocyclic, meaning they have an additional nitrogen-containing ring. Some example structures of the most studied polycyclic aromatic hydrocarbons are shown in Figure 5.13 (Rech et al., 2015).

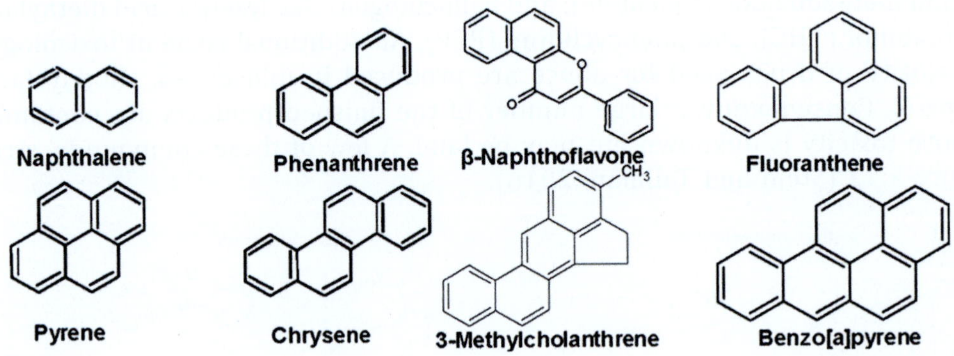

Figure 5.13. *Structure of a few hydrocarbons*

Source: https://www.researchgate.net/profile/Marwa-Elsherbiny/publication/51554320/figure/fig2/AS:667848930234393@1536239001863/Chemical-structures-of-some-common-polycyclic-aromatic-hydrocarbon-compounds.ppm.

5.6.3. Cosmetics

Side effects of modern cosmetics typically include allergic reactions and skin irritation. Harmful ingredients such as ammonia dyes and organometallics are no longer used in cosmetics. However, chemicals like bromates in cold-wave neutralizers and ethanol in hair colors can be poisonous if ingested. Other substances like thioglycerol, thioglycolates, and sodium hydroxide found in certain cosmetic products can also be harmful if consumed. Overall, cosmetics are generally safe when used as directed due to the removal of harmful ingredients and the small amounts typically ingested.

A Closer Look

Therapeutic Drug Monitoring (TDM)

A clinical practice that involves measuring specific drug concentrations in a patient's bloodstream at designated intervals to ensure optimal therapeutic levels are achieved without causing toxicity. TDM is particularly important for medications with narrow therapeutic indices, where the difference between therapeutic and toxic doses is small. The primary goals of TDM are to personalize drug dosing, maximize therapeutic efficacy, minimize adverse effects, and improve patient outcomes.

TDM is typically used for drugs that exhibit significant interindividual variability in their pharmacokinetics. This variability can arise from differences in absorption, distribution, metabolism, and excretion (ADME) among patients due to factors such as age, weight, genetics, organ function, concurrent medications, and overall health status. By monitoring drug levels, healthcare providers can adjust dosages to account for these individual differences, ensuring that drug concentrations remain within the therapeutic range.

The process of TDM involves several key steps. Initially, a baseline measurement is taken to determine the drug concentration in the patient's blood. Subsequent measurements are then performed at specified intervals, depending on the drug's half-life, to monitor its levels over time. Blood samples are the most commonly used, but other biological fluids like saliva or plasma can also be utilized. The timing of these measurements is crucial and is often aligned with the drug's pharmacokinetic profile to capture peak or trough levels, providing insights into the drug's absorption and clearance rates.

For TDM to be effective, a thorough understanding of the drug's pharmacokinetics and pharmacodynamics is essential. Pharmacokinetics involves studying how the body affects a drug, encompassing the ADME processes. Pharmacodynamics, on the other hand, examines how the drug affects the body, including its mechanism of action, therapeutic effects, and side effects. Integrating these two fields helps in interpreting TDM results accurately and making informed dosage adjustments.

Several drugs are commonly monitored using TDM due to their narrow therapeutic windows and significant variability in pharmacokinetics. These include anticonvulsants (e.g., phenytoin, valproic acid), antibiotics (e.g., vancomycin, aminoglycosides), immunosuppressants (e.g., cyclosporine, tacrolimus), and certain cardiovascular drugs (e.g., digoxin). For instance, in the case of anticonvulsants, maintaining therapeutic levels is critical to prevent seizures while avoiding toxicity that can lead to severe side effects.

TDM also plays a vital role in managing drug interactions. When patients are on multiple medications, the risk of drug interactions increases, which can alter the pharmacokinetics of the involved drugs. TDM can help detect such interactions early, allowing for timely adjustments in dosing to maintain therapeutic efficacy and prevent adverse effects.

The benefits of TDM extend beyond individual patient care to broader healthcare outcomes. By optimizing drug dosages, TDM can reduce hospitalizations due to adverse drug reactions, enhance patient compliance by minimizing side effects, and contribute to the overall effectiveness of treatment regimens. In the context of personalized medicine, TDM represents a practical approach to tailoring therapy based on the unique pharmacokinetic profile of each patient.

Summary

- Toxic substances are categorized in several different ways, based mostly on the classifier's preferences and requirements.
- Air pollution most likely began when people began to utilize burning wood for heating and cooking. The fireplace was utilized in such a manner for millennia that dwelling rooms were full of smoke.
- Polluted air has continuously worsened as domestic and industrial coal consumption has increased, especially in major cities.
- Acute pollution events, such as those in London and Donora provide the majority of data on the impacts of air pollution on people.
- Carbon monoxide quickly interacts with hemoglobin (Hb) to generate carboxyhemoglobin (COHb), obstructing oxygen delivery to tissues. The sensitivity of hemoglobin to CO is around 210 times greater than its oxygen demand.
- With water covering three-quarters of the surface of the planet and soil covering many of the rest, it is no surprise both soil and water are the final drains with the most anthropogenic pollutants. Until lately, the primary worry with water contamination was pathogen-related health impacts, and that's still the situation in most poor nations.
- Lead (Pb) and Arsenic are the two heavy metals that pose the biggest health risk when consumed via groundwater. The major sources of lead in drinking water include lead pipes and lead soldering.
- The dissolving of inorganic toxic elements once employed in pesticide spray, the burning of arsenic-containing oil and coal, and the dissolving of mining waste and smelting runoff all provide a danger to arsenic-contaminated drinking water.

References

1. Ajwa, H. A., Trout, T., Mueller, J., Wilhelm, S., Nelson, S. D., Soppc, R., & Shatley, D. (2002). Application of alternative fumigants through drip irrigation systems. *Phytopathology, 92*(12), 1349–1355. https://doi.org/10.1094/PHYTO.2002.92.12.1349.
2. Ashton, F. M., & Crafts, A. S. (1973). *Mode of Action of Herbicides* (Vol. 1, pp. 2–8).
3. Audus, L. J. (1964). *The Physiology and Biochemistry of Herbicides* (Vol. 1, pp. 4–8).
4. Bartlett, D. W., Clough, J. M., Godfrey, C. R., Godwin, J. R., Hall, A. A., Heaney, S. P., & Maund, S. J. (2001). Understanding the strobilurin fungicides. *Pesticide Outlook, 12*(4), 143–148. https://doi.org/10.1039/B101516H.
5. Bartlett, D. W., Clough, J. M., Godwin, J. R., Hall, A. A., Hamer, M., & Parr-Dobrzanski, B. (2002). The strobilurin fungicides. *Pest Management Science, 58*(7), 649–662. https://doi.org/10.1002/ps.490.
6. Baumgartner, W. A., Hill, V. A., & Blahd, W. H. (1989). Hair analysis for drugs of abuse. *Journal of Forensic Sciences, 34*(6), 1433–1453. https://doi.org/10.1520/JFS11423J.

7. Belkin, S., Smulski, D. R., Dadon, S., Vollmer, A. C., Van Dyk, T. K., & Larossa, R. A. (1997). A panel of stress-responsive luminous bacteria for the detection of selected classes of toxicants. *Water Research, 31*(12), 3009–3016. https://doi.org/10.1016/S0043-1354(97)00150-5.

8. Bidari, E., Irannejad, M., & Gharabaghi, M. (2013). Solvent extraction recovery and separation of cadmium and copper from sulphate solution. *Journal of Environmental Chemical Engineering, 1*(4), 1269–1274. https://doi.org/10.1016/j.jece.2013.09.016.

9. Braman, R. S., & Foreback, C. C. (1973). Methylated forms of arsenic in the environment. *Science, 182*(4118), 1247–1249. https://doi.org/10.1126/science.182.4118.1247.

10. Cakmak, D., Perovic, V., Kresovic, M., Jaramaz, D., Mrvic, V., Simic, S. B., & Trivan, G. (2018). Spatial distribution of soil pollutants in urban green areas (a case study in Belgrade). *Journal of Geochemical Exploration, 188*, 308–317. https://doi.org/10.1016/j.gexplo.2018.02.007.

11. Cambar, J., Cal, J. C., Desmouliere, A., & Guillemain, J. (1983). Circadian variations of the mortality of mice due to cadmium sulfate. *Comptes Rendus des Seances de l'Academie des Sciences; Serie III, Sciences de la Vie, 296*(20), 949–952.

12. Carmichael, W. W. (1986). Algal toxins. In *Advances in Botanical Research* (Vol. 12, pp. 47–101). Academic Press.

13. Castell, J. V., Donato, M. T., & Gómez-Lechón, M. J. (2005). Metabolism and bioactivation of toxicants in the lung. The in vitro cellular approach. *Experimental and Toxicologic Pathology, 57*, 189–204. https://doi.org/10.1016/j.etp.2005.06.002.

14. Clarkson, T. W. (1997). The toxicology of mercury. *Critical Reviews in Clinical Laboratory Sciences, 34*(4), 369–403. https://doi.org/10.1080/10408369708566693.

15. Collins, M. (1978). Algal toxins. *Microbiological Reviews, 42*(4), 725–746.

16. Colombo, M. (2020). EASL clinical practice guidelines for the management of occupational liver diseases. *Liver International, 40*(1), 136–141. https://doi.org/10.1111/liv.14241.

17. Copaciu, F., Opriş, O., Niinemets, Ü., & Copolovici, L. (2016). Toxic influence of key organic soil pollutants on the total flavonoid content in wheat leaves. *Water, Air, & Soil Pollution, 227*(6), 1–10. https://doi.org/10.1007/s11270-016-2934-3.

18. Cope, W. G. (2004). Exposure classes, toxicants in air, water, soil, domestic and occupational settings. In *A Textbook of Modern Toxicology* (pp. *33*, 4–7).

19. Cope, W. G., Leidy, R. B., & Hodgson, E. (2004). Classes of toxicants: Use classes. In *A Textbook of Modern Toxicology* (pp. *49*(1), 2–9).

20. Costa, C., Miozzi, E., Teodoro, M., Briguglio, G., Rapisarda, V., & Fenga, C. (2017). New insights on 'old' toxicants in occupational toxicology. *Molecular Medicine Reports, 15*(5), 3317–3322. https://doi.org/10.3892/mmr.2017.6520.

21. Coulombe, R. A., Jr. (1993). Biological action of mycotoxins. *Journal of Dairy Science, 76*(3), 880–891. https://doi.org/10.3168/jds.S0022-0302(93)77368-7.

22. Crouau, Y., Chenon, P., & Gisclard, C. (1999). The use of *Folsomia candida* (Collembola, Isotomidae) for the bioassay of xenobiotic substances and soil pollutants. *Applied Soil Ecology, 12*(2), 103–111. https://doi.org/10.1016/S0929-1393(99)00024-6.

23. Curtis, L., Rea, W., Smith-Willis, P., Fenyves, E., & Pan, Y. (2006). Adverse health effects of outdoor air pollutants. *Environment International, 32*(6), 815–830. https://doi.org/10.1016/j.envint.2006.05.002.

24. Di Carlo, G., Mascolo, N., Izzo, A. A., & Capasso, F. (1999). Flavonoids: Old and new aspects of a class of natural therapeutic drugs. *Life Sciences, 65*(4), 337–353. https://doi.org/10.1016/S0024-3205(99)00103-1.

25. Fabrega, J., Luoma, S. N., Tyler, C. R., Galloway, T. S., & Lead, J. R. (2011). Silver nanoparticles: Behavior and effects in the aquatic environment. *Environment International, 37*(2), 517–531. https://doi.org/10.1016/j.envint.2010.10.012.

26. Falconer, I. R. (1998). Algal toxins and human health. In *Quality and Treatment of Drinking Water II* (Vol. 1, pp. 53–82). Springer, Berlin, Heidelberg. https://doi.org/10.1007/978-3-662-08072-5_4.

27. Fedtke, C. A. R. L., & Duke, S. O. (2005). Herbicides. In *Plant Toxicology* (4th edn., pp. 247–330).

28. Finney, D. J. (1971). Statistical logic in the monitoring of reactions to therapeutic drugs. *Methods of Information in Medicine, 10*(4), 237–245. https://doi.org/10.1055/s-0038-1634713.

29. Flora, S. J., Flora, G., & Saxena, G. (2006). Environmental occurrence, health effects and management of lead poisoning. In *Lead* (Vol. 1, pp. 158–228). Elsevier Science BV.

30. Fowler, D., Cape, J. N., Coyle, M., Flechard, C., Kuylenstierna, J., Hicks, K., & Stevenson, D. (1999). The global exposure of forests to air pollutants. *Water, Air, and Soil Pollution, 116*(1), 5–32. https://doi.org/10.1023/A:1005190706611.

31. Franssen, H. H., Van, E. A. C., & Stein, A. (1997). Use of spatial prediction techniques and fuzzy classification for mapping soil pollutants. *Geoderma, 77*(2–4), 243–262. https://doi.org/10.1016/S0016-7061(97)00055-4.

32. Frigerio, G., Mercadante, R., Polledri, E., Missineo, P., Campo, L., & Fustinoni, S. (2019). An LC-MS/MS method to profile urinary mercapturic acids, metabolites of electrophilic intermediates of occupational and environmental toxicants. *Journal of Chromatography B, 1117*, 66–76. https://doi.org/10.1016/j.jchromb.2019.01.016.

33. Gabathuler, R. (2010). Approaches to transport therapeutic drugs across the blood–Brain barrier to treat brain diseases. *Neurobiology of Disease, 37*(1), 48–57. https://doi.org/10.1016/j.nbd.2009.07.037.

34. Gianessi, L. P. (2013). The increasing importance of herbicides in worldwide crop production. *Pest Management Science, 69*(10), 1099–1105. https://doi.org/10.1002/ps.3517.

35. Gianessi, L. P., & Reigner, N. P. (2007). The value of herbicides in US crop production. *Weed Technology, 21*(2), 559–566. https://doi.org/10.1614/WT-06-171.1.

36. Giudice, L. C. (2016). Environmental toxicants: Hidden players on the reproductive stage. *Fertility and Sterility, 106*(4), 791–794. https://doi.org/10.1016/j.fertnstert.2016.07.1153.

37. Goldizen, F. C., Sly, P. D., & Knibbs, L. D. (2016). Respiratory effects of air pollution on children. *Pediatric Pulmonology, 51*(1), 94–108. https://doi.org/10.1002/ppul.23379.

38. Goldstein, B. D., & Carruth, R. S. (2003). Implications of the precautionary principle for environmental regulation in the United States: Examples from the control of hazardous air pollutants in the 1990 Clean Air Act amendments. *Law & Contemporary Problems, 66*(1), 247–265. https://doi.org/10.2307/1192575.

39. Gordon, C. J. (2003). Role of environmental stress in the physiological response to chemical toxicants. *Environmental Research, 92*(1), 1–7. https://doi.org/10.1016/S0013-9351(02)00069-8.

40. Grant, W. F. (1982). Cytogenetic studies of agricultural chemicals in plants. In *Genetic Toxicology* (pp. 353–378).

41. Guo, X., Wei, W., Li, Y., & Wang, L. Y. (2019). A study of different types of air pollutants on the efficiency of China's hotel industry. *International Journal of Environmental Research and Public Health, 16*(22), 4319. https://doi.org/10.3390/ijerph16224319.

42. Gupta, R. C., & Crissman, J. W. (2013). Agricultural chemicals. In *Haschek and Rousseaux's Handbook of Toxicologic Pathology* (Vol. 1, pp. 1349–1372). Academic Press. https://doi.org/10.1016/B978-0-12-415455-6.00053-2.

43. Gupta, R., Raza, N., Bhardwaj, S. K., Vikrant, K., Kim, K. H., & Bhardwaj, N. (2021). Advances in nanomaterial-based electrochemical biosensors for the detection of microbial toxins, pathogenic bacteria in food matrices. *Journal of Hazardous Materials, 401*, 123379. https://doi.org/10.1016/j.jhazmat.2020.123379.

44. Hallberg, G. R. (1987). Agricultural chemicals in ground water: Extent and implications. *American Journal of Alternative Agriculture, 2*(1), 3–15. https://doi.org/10.1017/S0889189300005654.

45. Hallberg, G. R. (1987). The impacts of agricultural chemicals on ground water quality. *GeoJournal, 15*(3), 283–295. https://doi.org/10.1007/BF00151892.

46. Handy, R. D., Von, D. K. F., Lead, J. R., Hassellöv, M., Owen, R., & Crane, M. (2008). The ecotoxicology and chemistry of manufactured nanoparticles. *Ecotoxicology, 17*(4), 287–314. https://doi.org/10.1007/s10646-008-0212-4.

47. Harkov, R. (1982). Toxic air pollutants—Assessing their importance. *Science of the Total Environment, 26*(1), 67–85. https://doi.org/10.1016/0048-9697(82)90053-6.

48. Harris, H. H., Pickering, I. J., & George, G. N. (2003). The chemical form of mercury in fish. *Science, 301*(5637), 1203. https://doi.org/10.1126/science.1087327.

49. Havlikova, M., & Kroeze, C. (2006). Evaluation of methods for quantifying agricultural emissions of air, water and soil pollutants. *Science of the Total Environment, 372*(1), 133–147. https://doi.org/10.1016/j.scitotenv.2006.09.017.

50. Havugimana, E., Bhople, B. S., Kumar, A. N. I. L., Byiringiro, E., Mugabo, J. P., & Kumar, A. R. U. N. (2017). Soil pollution-major sources and types of soil pollutants. *Environmental Science and Engineering, 11*(1), 53–86.

51. Henschler, D., & Lehnert, G. (1994). Biological exposure values for occupational toxicants and carcinogens. *Critical Data Evaluation for BAT and EKA Values* (Vol. 1, pp. 1–7).

52. Hirano, T., & Tamae, K. (2011). Earthworms and soil pollutants. *Sensors, 11*(12), 11157–11167. https://doi.org/10.3390/s111211157.

53. Hofmann, A. (1995). Fundamentals and possibilities of classification of occupational substances as developmental toxicants. *International Archives of Occupational and Environmental Health, 67*(3), 139–145. https://doi.org/10.1007/BF00513043.

54. Ibekwe, A. M., Papiernik, S. K., Gan, J., Yates, S. R., Yang, C. H., & Crowley, D. E. (2001). Impact of fumigants on soil microbial communities. *Applied and Environmental Microbiology, 67*(7), 3245–3257. https://doi.org/10.1128/AEM.67.7.3245-3257.2001.

55. Joint, F. A. O., Bend, J., Bolger, M., Knaap, A. G. A. C., Kuznesof, P. M., Larsen, J. C., & WHO Expert Committee on Food Additives. (2007). Evaluation of Certain Food Additives and Contaminants (No. 947, pp. 1–5). *World Health Organization Technical Report Series.*

56. Ju-Nam, Y., & Lead, J. R. (2008). Manufactured nanoparticles: An overview of their chemistry, interactions and potential environmental implications. *Science of the Total Environment, 400*(1–3), 396–414. https://doi.org/10.1016/j.scitotenv.2008.06.042.

57. Khan, M. N., Wasim, A. A., Sarwar, A., & Rasheed, M. F. (2011). Assessment of heavy metal toxicants in the roadside soil along the N-5, National Highway, Pakistan. *Environmental Monitoring and Assessment, 182*(1), 587–595. https://doi.org/10.1007/s10661-010-1777-0.

58. Khan, Z., Karataş, Y. U. S. U. F., Ceylan, A. F., & Rahman, H. (2021). COVID-19 and therapeutic drugs repurposing in hand: The need for collaborative efforts. *Le Pharmacien Hospitalier et Clinicien, 56*(1), 3–11. https://doi.org/10.1016/j.phclin.2021.01.001.

59. Kim, J. W., Park, S., Lim, C. W., Lee, K., & Kim, B. (2014). The role of air pollutants in initiating liver disease. *Toxicological Research, 30*(2), 65–70. https://doi.org/10.5487/TR.2014.30.2.065.

60. Kimbrough, D. E., Cohen, Y., Winer, A. M., Creelman, L., & Mabuni, C. (1999). A critical assessment of chromium in the environment. *Critical Reviews in Environmental Science and Technology, 29*(1), 1–46. https://doi.org/10.1080/10643389991259109.

61. Klaine, S. J., Alvarez, P. J., Batley, G. E., Fernandes, T. F., Handy, R. D., Lyon, D. Y., & Lead, J. R. (2008). Nanomaterials in the environment: Behavior, fate, bioavailability, and effects. *Environmental Toxicology and Chemistry: An International Journal, 27*(9), 1825–1851. https://doi.org/10.1897/08-090.1.

62. Knight, S. C., Anthony, V. M., Brady, A. M., Greenland, A. J., Heaney, S. P., Murray, D. C., & Youle, A. D. (1997). Rationale and perspectives on the development of fungicides. *Annual Review of Phytopathology, 35*(1), 349–372. https://doi.org/10.1146/annurev.phyto.35.1.349.

63. Koturbash, I., Beland, F. A., & Pogribny, I. P. (2012). Role of microRNAs in the regulation of drug metabolizing and transporting genes and the response to environmental toxicants. *Expert Opinion on Drug Metabolism & Toxicology, 8*(5), 597–606. https://doi.org/10.1517/17425255.2012.676930.

64. Krupa, S. V., & Legge, A. H. (2000). Passive sampling of ambient, gaseous air pollutants: An assessment from an ecological perspective. *Environmental Pollution, 107*(1), 31–45. https://doi.org/10.1016/S0269-7491(99)00184-2.

65. Kudsk, P., & Streibig, J. C. (2003). Herbicides–a two-edged sword. *Weed Research, 43*(2), 90–102. https://doi.org/10.1046/j.1365-3180.2003.00346.x.

66. Langford, N. J., & Ferner, R. E. (1999). Toxicity of mercury. *Journal of Human Hypertension, 13*(10), 651–656. https://doi.org/10.1038/sj.jhh.1000893.

67. Lawton, L. A., & Codd, G. A. (1991). Cyanobacterial (blue-green algal) toxins and their significance in UK and European waters. *Water and Environment Journal, 5*(4), 460–465. https://doi.org/10.1111/j.1747-6593.1991.tb00106.x.

68. Leshner, A. I., & Koob, G. F. (1999). Drugs of abuse and the brain. *Proceedings of the Association of American Physicians, 111*(2), 99–108. https://doi.org/10.1176/appi.ajp.111.2.99.

69. Levander, O. A. (1977). Nutritional factors in relation to heavy metal toxicants. In *Federation Proceedings* (Vol. 36, No. 5, pp. 1683–1687).

70. Lichtfouse, E. (2009). *Organic Farming, Pest Control and Remediation of Soil Pollutants* (Vol. 1, p. 418). Springer. https://doi.org/10.1007/978-1-4020-9258-4.

71. Loureiro, S., Tourinho, P. S., Cornelis, G., Van, D. B. N. W., Díez-Ortiz, M., Vázquez-Campos, S., & Van, G. C. A. (2018). Nanomaterials as soil pollutants. In *Soil Pollution* (Vol. 1, pp. 161–190). Academic Press. https://doi.org/10.1016/B978-0-12-814890-4.00009-2.

72. Mandal, B. K., & Suzuki, K. T. (2002). Arsenic round the world: A review. *Talanta, 58*(1), 201–235. https://doi.org/10.1016/S0039-9140(02)00268-0.

73. Mann, R. M., Hyne, R. V., Choung, C. B., & Wilson, S. P. (2009). Amphibians and agricultural chemicals: Review of the risks in a complex environment. *Environmental Pollution, 157*(11), 2903–2927. https://doi.org/10.1016/j.envpol.2009.05.015.

74. Manning, W. J., & Keane, K. D. (1988). Effects of air pollutants on interactions between plants, insects, and pathogens. In *Assessment of Crop Loss from Air Pollutants* (Vol. 1, pp. 365–386). Springer, Dordrecht. https://doi.org/10.1007/978-94-009-1380-8_18.

75. Mauderly, J. L., & Samet, J. M. (2009). Is there evidence for synergy among air pollutants in causing health effects? *Environmental Health Perspectives, 117*(1), 1–6. https://doi.org/10.1289/ehp.11608.

76. McNabb, P., Selwood, A. I., Holland, P. T., & Collaborators: Aasen, J., Aune, T., Eaglesham, G., Hess, P., Igarishi, M., Quilliam, M., Slattery, D., Van de Riet, J., Van Egmond, H., Van den Top, H., & Yasumoto, T. (2005). Multiresidue method for determination of algal toxins in shellfish: Single-laboratory validation and interlaboratory study. *Journal of AOAC International, 88*(3), 761–772. https://doi.org/10.1093/jaoac/88.3.761.

77. Meharg, A. A., & Hartley-Whitaker, J. (2002). Arsenic uptake and metabolism in arsenic resistant and nonresistant plant species. *New Phytologist, 154*(1), 29–43. https://doi.org/10.1046/j.1469-8137.2002.00346.x.

78. Menzer, R. E., & Nelson, J. O. (1991). Water and soil pollutants. In *Casaret and Doull's Toxicology: The Basic Science of Poisons* (4th ed., pp. 872–902). McGraw-Hill.

79. Milner, J., Vardoulakis, S., Chalabi, Z., & Wilkinson, P. (2011). Modelling inhalation exposure to combustion-related air pollutants in residential buildings: Application to health impact assessment. *Environment International, 37*(1), 268–279. https://doi.org/10.1016/j.envint.2010.09.012.

80. Moeller, M. R., Steinmeyer, S., & Kraemer, T. (1998). Determination of drugs of abuse in blood. *Journal of Chromatography B: Biomedical Sciences and Applications, 713*(1), 91–109. https://doi.org/10.1016/S0378-4347(98)00230-6.

81. Monn, C. (2001). Exposure assessment of air pollutants: A review on spatial heterogeneity and indoor/outdoor/personal exposure to suspended particulate matter, nitrogen dioxide and ozone. *Atmospheric Environment, 35*(1), 1–32. https://doi.org/10.1016/S1352-2310(00)00399-7.

82. Moreland, D. E. (1980). Mechanisms of action of herbicides. *Annual Review of Plant Physiology, 31*, 597–638. https://doi.org/10.1146/annurev.pp.31.060180.003125.

83. Morrison, H. I., Wilkins, K., Semenciw, R., Mao, Y., & Wigle, D. (1992). Herbicides and cancer. *JNCI: Journal of the National Cancer Institute, 84*(24), 1866–1874. https://doi.org/10.1093/jnci/84.24.1866.

84. Mostert, M. M., Ayoko, G. A., & Kokot, S. (2010). Application of chemometrics to analysis of soil pollutants. *TrAC Trends in Analytical Chemistry, 29*(5), 430–445. https://doi.org/10.1016/j.trac.2010.01.008.

85. Murphy, M. J. (2002). Rodenticides. *Veterinary Clinics: Small Animal Practice, 32*(2), 469–484. https://doi.org/10.1016/S0195-5616(02)00003-0.

86. Murphy, M. J. (2018). Anticoagulant rodenticides. In *Veterinary Toxicology* (pp. 583–612). Academic Press. https://doi.org/10.1016/B978-0-12-811409-0.00022-0.

87. Nazaroff, W. W., & Weschler, C. J. (2004). Cleaning products and air fresheners: Exposure to primary and secondary air pollutants. *Atmospheric Environment, 38*(18), 2841–2865. https://doi.org/10.1016/j.atmosenv.2004.02.040.

88. Nelson, M. E., Bryant, S. M., & Aks, S. E. (2014). Emerging drugs of abuse. *Emergency Medicine Clinics, 32*(1), 1–28. https://doi.org/10.1016/j.emc.2013.09.004.

89. Ng, C. Y., & Amini, F. (2021). Telomere length alterations in occupational toxicants exposure: An integrated review of the literature. *Exposure and Health, 13*(1), 119–131. https://doi.org/10.1007/s12403-020-00325-x.

90. Nicas, M., & Lomax, G. P. (1999). A cost-benefit analysis of genetic screening for susceptibility to occupational toxicants. *Journal of Occupational and Environmental Medicine, 1*, 535–544. https://doi.org/10.1097/00043764-199910000-00009.

91. Nielsen, E. G. (1987). *The Magnitude and Costs of Groundwater Contamination from Agricultural Chemicals: A National Perspective* (Vol. 576). US Department of Agriculture, Economic Research Service, Natural Resource Economics Division.

92. Nordstrom, D. K. (2002). Worldwide occurrences of arsenic in ground water. *Science, 296*(5576), 2143–2145. https://doi.org/10.1126/science.1075287.

93. Oremland, R. S., & Stolz, J. F. (2003). The ecology of arsenic. *Science, 300*(5621), 939–944. https://doi.org/10.1126/science.1081905.

94. Ostrosky-Wegman, P., & Gonsebatt, M. E. (1996). Environmental toxicants in developing countries. *Environmental Health Perspectives, 104*(suppl 3), 599–602. https://doi.org/10.1289/ehp.96104s3599.

95. Pinkerton, K. E., & Joad, J. P. (2006). Influence of air pollution on respiratory health during perinatal development. *Clinical and Experimental Pharmacology and Physiology, 33*(3), 269–272. https://doi.org/10.1111/j.1440-1681.2006.04315.x.

96. Piomelli, D., Giuffrida, A., Calignano, A., & De Fonseca, F. R. (2000). The endocannabinoid system as a target for therapeutic drugs. *Trends in Pharmacological Sciences, 21*(6), 218–224. https://doi.org/10.1016/S0165-6147(00)01573-1.

97. Piotrowski, J. K., Trojanowska, B., Wiśniewska-Knypl, J. M., & Bolanowska, W. (1974). Mercury binding in the kidney and liver of rats repeatedly exposed to mercuric chloride: Induction of metallothionein by mercury and cadmium. *Toxicology and Applied Pharmacology, 27*(1), 11–19. https://doi.org/10.1016/0041-008X(74)90182-0.

98. Pitt, J. I. (2000). Toxigenic fungi and mycotoxins. *British Medical Bulletin, 56*(1), 184–192. https://doi.org/10.1258/0007142001905491.

99. Preuss, R., Angerer, J., & Drexler, H. (2003). Naphthalene—An environmental and occupational toxicant. *International Archives of Occupational and Environmental Health, 76*(8), 556–576. https://doi.org/10.1007/s00420-003-0438-6.

100. Price, N. R. (1985). The mode of action of fumigants. *Journal of Stored Products Research, 21*(4), 157–164. https://doi.org/10.1016/0022-474X(85)90010-5.

101. Qu, R. Y., He, B., Yang, J. F., Lin, H. Y., Yang, W. C., Wu, Q. Y., & Yang, G. F. (2021). Where are the new herbicides? *Pest Management Science, 77*(6), 2620–2625. https://doi.org/10.1002/ps.6440.

102. Rai, D., Eary, L. E., & Zachara, J. M. (1989). Environmental chemistry of chromium. *Science of the Total Environment, 86*(1–2), 15–23. https://doi.org/10.1016/0048-9697(89)90120-4.

103. Rajkovic, A. (2014). Microbial toxins and low level of foodborne exposure. *Trends in Food Science & Technology, 38*(2), 149–157. https://doi.org/10.1016/j.tifs.2014.05.001.

104. Rech, M. A., Donahey, E., Cappiello, D. J. M., Oh, L., & Greenhalgh, E. (2015). New drugs of abuse. *Pharmacotherapy: The Journal of Human Pharmacology and Drug Therapy, 35*(2), 189–197. https://doi.org/10.1002/phar.1578.

105. Richard, J. L. (2007). Some major mycotoxins and their mycotoxicoses—An overview. *International Journal of Food Microbiology, 119*(1–2), 3–10. https://doi.org/10.1016/j.ijfoodmicro.2007.07.019.

106. Robinson, T. E., & Kolb, B. (2004). Structural plasticity associated with exposure to drugs of abuse. *Neuropharmacology, 47*(1), 33–46. https://doi.org/10.1016/j.neuropharm.2004.06.013.

107. Rositano, J., Newcombe, G., Nicholson, B., & Sztajnbok, P. (2001). Ozonation of NOM and algal toxins in four treated waters. *Water Research, 35*(1), 23–32. https://doi.org/10.1016/S0043-1354(00)00264-3.

108. Schatzmayr, G., Zehner, F., Täubel, M., Schatzmayr, D., Klimitsch, A., Loibner, A. P., & Binder, E. M. (2006). Microbiologicals for deactivating mycotoxins. *Molecular Nutrition & Food Research, 50*(6), 543–551. https://doi.org/10.1002/mnfr.200600060.

109. Schooltink, H., & Rose-John, S. (2002). Cytokines as therapeutic drugs. *Journal of Interferon & Cytokine Research, 22*(5), 505–516. https://doi.org/10.1089/10799900260162045.

110. Schrader, S. M., & Marlow, K. L. (2014). Assessing the reproductive health of men with occupational exposures. *Asian Journal of Andrology, 16*(1), 23. https://doi.org/10.4103/1008-682X.124807.

111. Schroeder, W. H., & Munthe, J. (1998). Atmospheric mercury—An overview. *Atmospheric Environment, 32*(5), 809–822. https://doi.org/10.1016/S1352-2310(97)00293-1.

112. Scow, K. M., & Johnson, C. R. (1996). Effect of sorption on biodegradation of soil pollutants. *Advances in Agronomy, 58*, 1–56. https://doi.org/10.1016/S0065-2113(08)60540-0.

113. Sharma, A., Tomer, A., Singh, J., & Chhikara, B. S. (2019). Biosorption of metal toxicants and other water pollutants by corn (maize) plant: A comprehensive review. *Journal of Integrated Science and Technology, 7*(2), 19–28. https://doi.org/10.25131/jist.019.07.02.19.

114. Sharma, G. K., Jena, R. K., Hota, S., Kumar, A., Ray, P., Fagodiya, R. K., & Ray, S. K. (2020). Recent development in bioremediation of soil pollutants through biochar for environmental sustainability. In *Biochar Applications in Agriculture and Environment Management* (Vol. 1, pp. 123–140). Springer, Cham. https://doi.org/10.1007/978-3-030-36571-1_6.

115. Shen, G. (2015). Quantification of emission reduction potentials of primary air pollutants from residential solid fuel combustion by adopting cleaner fuels in China. *Journal of Environmental Sciences, 37*, 1–7. https://doi.org/10.1016/j.jes.2015.01.001.

116. Shilo, M. (1967). Formation and mode of action of algal toxins. *Bacteriological Reviews, 31*(3), 180–193. https://doi.org/10.1128/br.31.3.180-193.1967.

117. Speijers, G. J. A., & Speijers, M. H. M. (2004). Combined toxic effects of mycotoxins. *Toxicology Letters, 153*(1), 91–98. https://doi.org/10.1016/j.toxlet.2004.03.005.

118. Stein, E. M., & Tallman, M. S. (2016). Emerging therapeutic drugs for AML. *Blood, The Journal of the American Society of Hematology, 127*(1), 71–78. https://doi.org/10.1182/blood-2015-09-665396.

119. Steiner, G., Suter, L., Boess, F., Gasser, R., De Vera, M. C., Albertini, S., & Ruepp, S. (2004). Discriminating different classes of toxicants by transcript profiling. *Environmental Health Perspectives, 112*(12), 1236–1248. https://doi.org/10.1289/ehp.7247.

120. Stuck, B. W. (1977). A new proposal for estimating the spatial concentration of certain types of air pollutants. *JOSA, 67*(5), 668–678. https://doi.org/10.1364/JOSA.67.000668.

121. Telisman, S., Azaric, J., & Prpic-Majic, D. (1986). Cadmium in blood as an indicator of integrated exposure to cadmium in the urban population. *Bulletin of Environmental Contamination and Toxicology, 36*(4), 641–646. https://doi.org/10.1007/BF01694963.

122. Tian, Y., Yao, X., & Chen, L. (2019). Analysis of spatial and seasonal distributions of air pollutants by incorporating urban morphological characteristics. *Computers, Environment and Urban Systems, 75*, 35–48. https://doi.org/10.1016/j.compenvurbsys.2018.12.008.

123. Van, D. F. M. (2000). Marine algal toxins: Origins, health effects, and their increased occurrence. *Environmental Health Perspectives, 108*(suppl 1), 133–141. https://doi.org/10.1289/ehp.00108s1133.

124. Van, E. H. P., Schothorst, R. C., & Jonker, M. A. (2007). Regulations relating to mycotoxins in food. *Analytical and Bioanalytical Chemistry, 389*(1), 147–157. https://doi.org/10.1007/s00216-007-1411-1.

125. Walker, R. (2002). Risk assessment of ochratoxin: Current views of the European scientific committee on food, the JECFA and the Codex Committee on Food Additives and Contaminants. *Mycotoxins and Food Safety, 1*, 249–255. https://doi.org/10.1007/978-1-4615-0115-2_20.

126. Watt, B. E., Proudfoot, A. T., Bradberry, S. M., & Vale, J. A. (2005). Anticoagulant rodenticides. *Toxicological Reviews, 24*(4), 259–269. https://doi.org/10.2165/00139709-200524040-00003.

127. Winner, W. E., Coleman, J. S., Gillespie, C., Mooney, H. A., & Pell, E. J. (1991). Consequences of evolving resistance to air pollutants. In *Ecological Genetics and Air Pollution* (Vol. 1, pp. 177–202). Springer, New York, NY. https://doi.org/10.1007/978-1-4615-0901-0_10.

128. Zawadzki, J., Szuszkiewicz, M., Fabijańczyk, P., & Magiera, T. (2016). Geostatistical discrimination between different sources of soil pollutants using a magneto-geochemical data set. *Chemosphere, 164*, 668–676. https://doi.org/10.1016/j.chemosphere.2016.09.016.

129. Zhang, Q., Zhang, Z., Lu, T., Yu, Y., Penuelas, J., Zhu, Y. G., & Qian, H. (2021). Gammaproteobacteria, a core taxon in the guts of soil fauna, are potential responders to environmental concentrations of soil pollutants. *Microbiome, 9*(1), 1–17. https://doi.org/10.1186/s40168-021-01155-3.

130. Zhang, T., & Zhang, H. (2022). Microbial consortia are needed to degrade soil pollutants. *Microorganisms, 10*(2), 261. https://doi.org/10.3390/microorganisms10020261.

131. Zhukova, A. G., Ulanova, E. V., Fomenko, D. V., Kazitskaia, A. S., & Iadykina, T. K. (2011). Specificity of cellular response to various occupational toxicants. *Meditsina Truda i Promyshlennaia Ekologiia, (7)*, 23–26. https://doi.org/10.31089/1026-9428-2011-7-23-26.

132. Zuccato, E., Calamari, D., Natangelo, M., & Fanelli, R. (2000). Presence of therapeutic drugs in the environment. *The Lancet, 355*(9217), 1789–1790. https://doi.org/10.1016/S0140-6736(00)02261-1.

Chapter

TOXICOLOGY OF FOOD AND FOODBORNE DISEASES

6

Contents

Introduction

The ancient scientific field of toxicology seeks to characterize and comprehend how substances affect living things. The study of physiology—the normal functioning of the body—chemistry—the properties and quantification of potentially harmful substances—and pathology—the investigation of the genesis and progression of disease—are all integrated into the field of toxicology. Food toxicology studies the potential health risks associated with natural and contaminant-containing foods. Knowing how these substances are transformed into so-called metabolites in the body and environment is crucial to comprehending the health effects of all these chemicals, both natural and man-made. Chemicals' ultimate effects on health are often influenced by both the parent molecules and their metabolites.

Orientation and Directional Terms

Term	Definition	Illustration
Food toxicology	Food toxicology studies how natural or synthetic poisons and toxicants in diverse food products cause harmful, detrimental, or adverse side effects in living organisms.	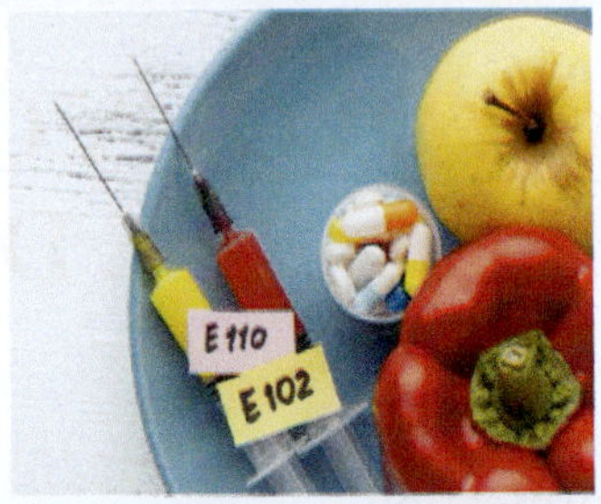
Chromatography	An important biophysical technique that enables the separation, identification, and purification of the components of a mixture for qualitative and quantitative analysis.	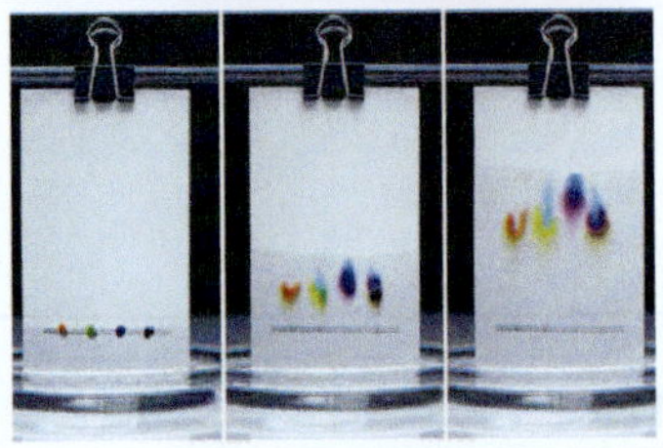
Immunoassays	A biochemical test that measures the presence or concentration of a macromolecule or a small molecule in a solution through the use of an antibody or an antigen.	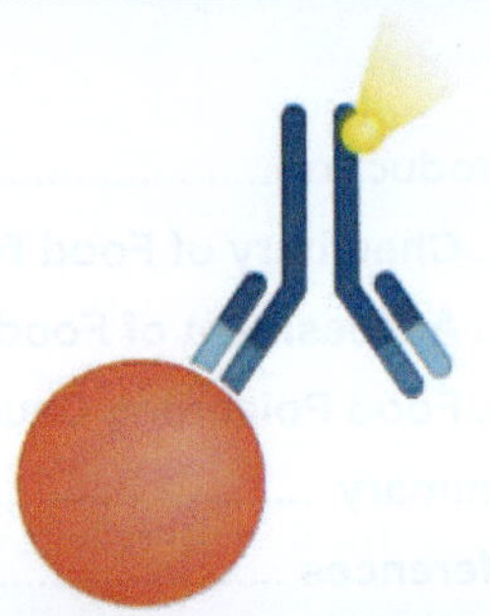
Molecular targets	A term used to describe certain genes, proteins, and other molecules that are involved in the growth, spread, and survival of cancer cells and may be used as targets for cancer treatment.	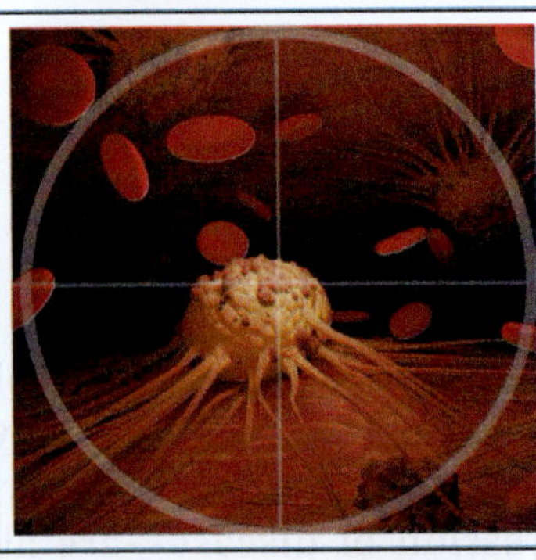
Cellular pathways	A chain of reactions transmits signals from the cell surface to a variety of intracellular targets—a process called intracellular signal transduction.	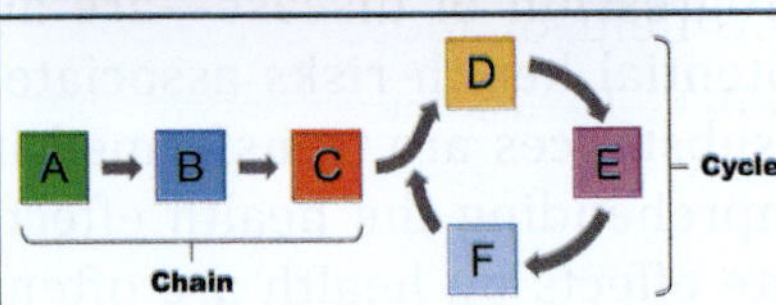

6.1. Chemistry of Food Toxicology

The study of the interactions between chemical compounds found in food and the human body is known as food toxicology. The goal of this field is to understand better how these interactions can affect human health and have toxic effects. The study of food toxicants' mechanisms of action and toxicological effects, as well as their identification, characterization, and quantification, are all included in the broad field of food toxicology. The analysis of food contaminants, which can include naturally occurring toxins, environmental pollutants, food additives, pesticides, heavy metals, and microbial toxins, is a fundamental area of food toxicology. To ensure food safety and regulatory compliance, analytical chemistry techniques like mass spectrometry, spectroscopy, chromatography, and immunoassays are used to identify and quantify these contaminants in food matrices at trace levels.

Comprehending the chemical characteristics of toxicants is imperative in evaluating their conduct within food systems and forecasting their destiny throughout food processing, storage, and arrangement. Solubility, stability, reactivity, and partition coefficients are a few examples of factors that affect how toxicants are distributed and bioavailable in food matrices, as well as how the body absorbs and processes them. The study of chemical reactions that take place during food preparation, cooking, and storage that may result in the formation of hazardous or toxic compounds is included in the field of food toxicology chemistry. For instance, in heat-processed foods like baked goods or fried potatoes, the Maillard reaction—a sequence of non-enzymatic browning reactions between reducing sugars and amino acids—can produce acrylamide, a known carcinogen.

Additionally, food toxicology studies the mechanisms of action through which harmful substances affect human health. This includes understanding the elements influencing an individual's susceptibility to toxicity, such as genetic polymorphisms or underlying medical conditions, as well as clarifying the molecular targets, cellular pathways, and physiological processes impacted by toxicants. Essential to food toxicology are risk assessment and risk management, which determine possible health risks from exposure to foodborne toxicants and create plans to reduce those risks. To protect public health, this entails determining safety thresholds and regulatory limits, assessing the risks posed by particular toxicants, and estimating population exposure levels.

6.1.1. Toxicology Models and Toxicological Dose Descriptors

In the early days of toxicological research, the mechanism of toxicity of chemicals was studied using tissue fragments, isolated cells, or subcellular fractions. Of course, these in vitro studies have limited human relevance. It is believed that using animals yields more pertinent data. Through examining the detrimental effects of substances in vivo, the toxicologist can also look into how the breakdown products contribute to the overall toxic response. As a metabolic organ, the liver is significant in this regard. Ultimately, population research or the collection of exposure data sheds more light on the applicability of the detected in vitro toxicity. Modern toxicology uses co-cultures of different kinds of cells. The toxicological read-out parameters have also improved in recent years. It is possible to observe real-time intracellular changes in parameters like pH and calcium, thanks to imaging techniques. Furthermore, there has been a significant advancement in computer-aided toxicity prediction, leading to the addition of in silico techniques to complement in vitro and in vivo models. Positive new approaches are starting to surface. Growing tiny organ systems on a chip with flow transport of compounds across the chip through so-called microfluidics is becoming more and more feasible. The mechanistic adverse biochemical pathways are being studied in more detail. It is anticipated that all of these advancements will culminate in a "virtual human" that can be used to test and forecast a compound's toxicity.

Toxicologists use dose descriptors to characterize the relationship between the effect of a chemical compound and the dose or concentration at which it occurs. These descriptors are important in assessing risk and quantifying chemical hazards. One commonly known dose descriptor is the LD50, which represents the dose at which 50% of exposed animals will die. However, the use of LD50 has limitations as it does not provide information on the mode of action of the chemical and requires animal testing to determine. Additionally, factors such as duration and route of exposure play a crucial role. The unit of LD50 is mg/kg bw/d, indicating the amount of substance administered per kg bodyweight per day. In inhalation toxicology, the LC50 is used to measure the concentration-dependent death of an animal through compounds administered via the air. The unit of LC50 is mg/l, indicating the concentration of the chemical in the air, sometimes using the unit ppm (Table 6.1).

Table 6.1. *Toxicology Models*

Early Toxicology	Current Toxicology	Future Toxicology
Tissue, cells, subcellular fractions, genes	Organo-typic cell culture (coculture, organ function)	Human on a chip (multi-organ models with micro fluidics)
Animal models	Cell culture + omics or image analysis	Toxicity mechanisms (adverse outcome pathways, 'human toxome')
Human (population-based studies, human exposure data)	Integrated test strategies (combined tests) In silico prediction (structure-activity relationships)	Systems toxicology (virtual human)

Source: https://www.wageningenacademic.com/doi/pdf/10.3920/978-90-8686-933-6_13.

When an exposure level (a dose or a concentration) is attained at which there is no indication of a rise in the severity of an adverse effect between the exposed species and the appropriate, i.e., unexposed, in charge. This toxicological dose descriptor is typically obtained through 28-day or 90-day repeated dose studies, which are indicated as subchronic or chronic toxicity studies with animals, respectively. The most sensitive animal's long-term NOAEL is used, among other things, to determine the Acceptable Daily Intake (ADI). A compound's acceptable daily intake (ADI) is the highest amount that can be consumed for the rest of one's life without posing a significant risk to one's health. To achieve this, a safety or uncertainty factor is applied (typically 100), accounting for the interindividual variations among humans as well as the difference in sensitivity between animal species and humans (a factor 10). Thus, the long-term NOAEL divided by 100 yields the ADI.

The Lowest Observed Adverse Effect Level (LOAEL) can be used to determine threshold safety exposure levels in humans if a NOAEL cannot be reached. Obviously, stricter safety regulations need to be implemented. For chemical risk assessment, the benchmark dose (BMD) is utilized in addition to the NOAEL. The term is not totally accurate since the BMD can also refer to a concentration as opposed to a dose. Actually, a BMD is the concentration or dose that causes an adverse effect's response rate to alter in a predictable way. The benchmark response (BMR) is the name given to the predetermined response itself. The default BMR for a negative effect is typically set to 5% or 10%. The BMD is not affected by the doses chosen for the experiment, but the NOAEL is. Unlike the BMD, the NOAEL does not account for the shape of the dose response curve. Regretfully, obtaining the NOAEL is relatively simple, but determining a BMD requires a significant amount of time. Lastly, compared to the BMD, the NOAEL is more well-known.

6.1.2. Food Toxicology

The study of substances present in food that may be harmful when consumed is known as food toxicology. It is simple to conclude that one of the earliest scientific fields is food toxicology because access to safe food is necessary for human survival. The gathering of food was essential to our ancestors' survival, and they needed to know what was safe and unsafe to eat. Sadly, a lot of this ancient wisdom has been lost. Nowadays, very few people in the West go wild to forage for food. The crop plants are cultivated by modern humans, therefore, the amount of endogenous toxins found in wild varieties is decreased. These days, we depend on the safety and quality of the goods we purchase. Therefore, the modern consumer assumes that the food is completely safe. This has resulted in the application of the "better safe than sorry" (also known as the precautionary principle) in the EU in cases of scientific uncertainty. The European Food Safety Authority (EFSA), the EU agency responsible for food safety, attempts to control the uncertainty surrounding food safety, which has become increasingly difficult to accept. Regretfully, achieving complete safety is unattainable and will inevitably result in failure. Simply put, it is impossible to be aware of every ingredient in our food. Thousands of compounds, the majority of which lack chemical characterization and unknown bioactivity, are found in a typical diet. Furthermore, even though we primarily utilize farmed crop plants, there are still a lot of endogenous. These plants contain naturally occurring, possibly hazardous substances. The traditional method used in toxicology to estimate a health risk involves defining the substance's hazard and the extent of exposure to it.

$$\text{Risk} = \text{Hazard} \times \text{Exposure}$$

The amount of substances found in food that have been characterized is extremely small. This makes ensuring complete safety more difficult. Food products can, at most, have an estimated risk/benefit ratio; the risk and benefit of any given food product are only approximations and not guarantees. Risk assessment is still considered a scientific endeavor, but one should not overvalue the scientific method. As mentioned, there are a lot of unknowns concerning the individual substances as well as the combinations of compounds that make up the food matrix. This makes it more difficult to identify and characterize hazards effectively. Characterizing the hazards of man-made chemicals is simpler. Research is made easier by the chemical's widespread availability in large quantities and pure form. The exposure needs to be ascertained for scientific risk assessment. Understanding the administration route (for food, primarily oral), single dose or multi-hit (for food, primarily a single daily exposure), sensitization, absorption (uptake via the intestine), distribution throughout the body or even within specific organs, metabolism, and excretion are all included in exposure. These procedures establish the concentration and, consequently, the risk at the site of toxic action. The scientific toolbox of toxicology is also utilized in risk assessment to determine the probability of the risk, or how likely it is that an adverse event will occur. Additionally, the risk's outcomes are known, i.e., what is the anticipated harm?

6.1.2.1. Risk Management

Decisions about risk management are primarily based on policy, control opportunities over the risks, and legal considerations. The choices made regarding risk management will also be influenced by a number of other social and economic factors. A comparative risk analysis will consider the relationship to other risks. Questions concerning the intended degree of reduction will be included in issues regarding potential risk reduction. Risk management will include topics on risk reduction strategies. Naturally, the available budget will be important. How much money should be spent, and what kind of financial commitment is there?

6.1.2.2. Risk Perception

The ability of citizens to perceive risks is poor. Facts that have been distorted by the media (especially social media) or by past incidents affect how people evaluate risks. The risks associated with new discoveries seem greater because they are typically viewed with suspicion. Conversely, the familiar causes one to underestimate the risks. When risks are unintentionally imposed or seen as needless, they are typically regarded as significant. Furthermore, how unfairly risks are distributed will affect how people perceive risks. Better public education about risks is therefore required. Effective risk communication will result from an interactive exchange of ideas and information. (Figure 6.1).

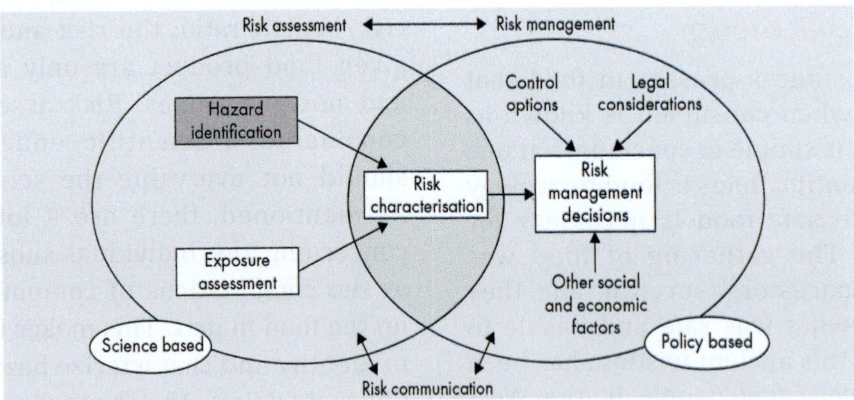

Figure 6.1. *The risk analysis framework with the elements risk assessment, risk management and risk communication.*

Source: https://www.wageningenacademic.com/doi/pdf/10.3920/978-90-8686-933-6_13.

Usually, food specialists and non-specialists have different concerns regarding food safety, given the disparity in their perceptions of food risk. A recent study conducted in Japan examined how risk perception changed over a 15-year span. The public's concern over chemical contamination and pesticide residues peaked in 2004, but it has since declined. The risk of food poisoning by dangerous microorganisms was not well known in 2004, but it was ranked as the highest risk in 2018. According to food experts, contaminants are still on the public list even though they do not pose a threat to food safety in 2018. The 2011 survey was conducted shortly after the Fukushima nuclear accident, which may have contributed to the highest concern scores for radioactive materials. The difference between food experts and the general public can be seen in their comparison. It also demonstrates the difficulty in providing sufficient risk communication in the area of food safety.

6.1.3. Natural Toxins

6.1.3.1. Phytotoxins

Plants use thorns or a bitter taste to defend themselves against herbivores. Furthermore, a vast range of toxins, or phytotoxins, are found in many plants. These poisons serve as an organism's natural defense against insects, predators, and microbes. Essentially, plants produce their own insecticides. According to calculations, 99.99% (by weight) of the pesticides we eat are naturally occurring (Ames et al., 1990). It is simple to examine the toxicological significance of exposure to synthetic chemicals from a different angle when considering the massive exposure to these naturally occurring chemicals, or phytotoxins. Human perception of potential hazards varies depending on one's ability to compare the toxic load of synthetic chemicals like pesticides with naturally occurring chemicals. Figure 6.2 effectively illustrates this distinction by contrasting the degree of concern that consumers and food experts have regarding pesticide residues in food.

Level of concern	2004		2011		2018	
	Specialists	Others	Specialists	Others	Specialists	Others
Very concerned	Contaminants	Pesticide residues	Radioactive materials	Radioactive materials	Food poisoning	Food poisoning
	Food poisoning	Contaminants	Food poisoning	Food poisoning	Health foods	Antimicrobial resistance
	Pesticide residues	Antimicrobial resistance	Contaminants & Health foods[1]	Pesticide residues	Antimicrobial resistance	Contaminants
	Antimicrobial resistance	Food additives		Antimicrobial resistance & Food addit.[2]	Mycotoxin	Mycotoxin
Somewhat concerned	BSE	Genetically modified food	Pesticide residues		Allergen	Health foods & Radioactive materials[3]

[1] Both at 3rd level of concern. [2] Both at 4th level of concern. [3] Both at 5th level of concern (somewhat).

Figure 6.2. *Ranking order of concern level on food safety-related hazards conducted in 2004, 2011 and 2018 and comparing food specialists and the general public (others). The five levels of concern vary from very concerned (level 1) to somewhat concerned (level 5).*

Source: https://www.wageningenacademic.com/doi/pdf/10.3920/978-90-8686-933-6_13.

6.1.3.2. Cyanogenic Glycosides

The paralytic illness known as konzo, which affects rural populations in Africa, is most likely brought on by eating inadequately processed cassava. These populations have especially low dietary intakes of sulfur amino acids. These amino acids play a crucial role in cyanide detoxification and subsequent excretion in the urine. Cyanide comes from the bitter cassava, which makes up a large portion of their diet, and its high cyanogenic glycoside content. Combining a high intake of cyanogenic glycosides with a low intake of sulfur amino acids is harmful.

6.1.3.3. Lectins

Although they can also be found in bacteria or animals, plants are the main source of lectins. Antinutrients are another term for lectins. One popular example is the phytohaemagglutinin found in raw beans, which is eliminated during cooking. While some lectins, like those found in potatoes, are non-toxic, others have a higher heat resistance. Another lectin is the extremely poisonous ricin found in beans made from the castor oil plant (*Ricinus communis*). Protein synthesis is inhibited by ricin. The toxicity, which is primarily gastrointestinal, may not show symptoms for several hours. Fever and cough are the initial signs following inhalation. Because lectins bind to specific saccharides, they can be used as affinity reagents in laboratory research (Table 6.2).

Table 6.2. *Natural Toxins in Food: Source and Adverse Health Effect*

Toxin	Source	Adverse Health Effects
Cyanogenic glycosides	Cassava, sorghum, stone fruits, and almonds.	Cyanide poisoning potentially leads to decreased blood pressure, headache, vomiting, cyanosis, death.
Furocoumarines	Parsnips, celery, citrus plants such as lime, lemon, grapefruit, and bergamot.	Gastrointestinal effects (e.g., interaction with biotransformation of drugs), phototoxic (phytophotodermatitis, severe skin reactions under sunlight).
Lectins	Several types of beans, in particular red kidney beans. Boiling destroys lectins.	Vomiting, diarrhea, nutritional deficiencies, and immune reactions.
Mycotoxins	Certain moulds that grow on cereals, dried fruits, nuts, spices.	Severe illness, even death.
Solanines and chaconine	Solanaceae plants, potatoes, tomatoes and eggplants.	Nausea, diarrhea, vomiting and eventually coma and convulsion.
Poisonous mushrooms	A variety of toxins produced by the fungus	Vary from vomiting, diarrhea, confusion, hallucinations to death.
Pyrrolizidine alkaloids	Many plants, frequently weeds, that contaminate food crops	Acute toxicities, such as hepatotoxicity and DNA-damaging effects.
Marine toxins	Produced during blooms of certain algae. Shellfish like mussels, scallops and oysters can contain these toxins	Diarrhea, vomiting, tingling, and paralysis.

Source: https://www.wageningenacademic.com/doi/pdf/10.3920/978-90-8686-933-6_13.

6.1.3.4. Mycotoxins

Certain kinds of molds (fungi) produce mycotoxins. In food processing, many mycotoxins do not degrade chemically. In warm, humid environments, molds can grow on or within food. Illness and cancer are among the long-term consequences of exposure. When *Aspergillus flavus* and *Aspergillus parasiticus* produce mycotoxins, the result is called aflatoxins. Items that are susceptible to infection include corn, peanuts, rice, pistachios, hazelnuts, and different spices. As a result, derivative goods like beer, peanut butter, and peanut flour bread may also include aflatoxins. Food tainted with aflatoxin spreads to animals through milk, eggs, and meat, among other foods. An animal's kidneys can be poisoned by the mycotoxin ochratoxin. For a class of structurally related mycotoxins, the single term "ochratoxin" is used. Numerous other names for mycotoxins are comparable to this. In addition to grains, coffee beans, dried fruit, wine, and beer, ochratoxin is primarily produced by Aspergillus and Penicillium.

Apples and apple juice produced from contaminated fruit are the main dietary sources of the mycotoxin patulin. Fusarium fungi can grow on a range of different cereal crops and produce other significant mycotoxins, such as deoxynivalenol (DON), nivalenol (NIV), and zearalenone (ZEN). There have been numerous reports of cattle exposed to the pneumotoxin 4-ipomeanol. Fusarium solani, a mold that grows on rotting sweet potatoes fed to cows, is the source of this toxin. In multiple cases, it resulted in cow deaths.

6.1.3.5. Solanines and Chaconine

Potato, tomato, and eggplant (aubergine) belong to the nightshade family, Solanaceae, which produces the so-called glycoalkaloids, solanines, and chaconine. Both green tomatoes and potato sprouts synthesize high amounts. Stress results in the formation of the phytotoxins (e.g., following bruising or UV light exposure). These alkaloids possess strong fungicidal and insecticidal effects. It is important to remember that newly developed potato cultivars can release harmful amounts of alkaloids. Lenape, a potato cultivar from the 1960s, is a prime example. It seemed that this potato was extremely resistant to illness. Unfortunately, because of its high alkaloid content, it was also unfit for human consumption and caused nausea and vomiting. As a result, it was taken off the market in 1970.

6.1.3.6. Mushroom Poisoning

The public is always quite interested in learning about mushroom poisoning. It is likely more dangerous for animals than for humans to be exposed to toxic mushrooms, although this is still underreported. In fact, human toxicity can be totally avoided by properly identifying edible mushrooms. Furthermore, foods and pharmaceutical products may benefit from the immune-modulating properties of beta-glucans from mushrooms.

6.1.3.7. Pyrrolizidine Alkaloids

Pyrrolizidine alkaloids are produced by thousands of plants as a defense against insect damage. How to keep these plants out of the food chain is a big worry. Furthermore, it is becoming more widely known that pyrrolizidine alkaloids may be present in certain therapeutic herbs or somewhat unusual teas. Remarkably, compared to humans, sheep, goats, and occasionally cattle can withstand far higher levels of pyrrolizidine alkaloids. This is most likely due to the protective effects of the rumen microbiota.

6.1.3.8. Marine Toxins

A handful of marine toxin families are known to exist, including okadaic acid, dinophysistoxins, saxitoxins, brevetoxins, domoic acid, azaspiracids, pinnatoxins, yessotoxins, pectenotoxins, and cyclic imines. Most of these toxin families are global in distribution. They don't taste or smell, and freezing or cooking won't get rid of them. Another toxin, tetrodotoxin (TTX), is discovered in certain foods, such as mussels. Algae and bacteria produce this neurotoxin. These toxins are concentrated in the bodies of mussels and oysters because they filter a lot of seawater. Until the precise source of the TTX found in mussels is determined, the Netherlands has a very strict safety norm for TTX in shellfish meat: 44 micrograms/kg. One well-known instance is the puffer fish, which contains TTX, and is considered a delicacy in Japan. Only highly trained chefs are permitted to prepare the fish in order to avoid the dining patrons becoming fatally intoxicated with TTX.

Ciguatera is a foodborne illness linked to marine toxins that is most frequently reported worldwide. Ciguatoxin, a lipid-soluble polyether ($C_{60}H_{86}O_{19}$), is the toxin in question. To date, a large number of natural analogs have been found. Dinoflagellates are the source of them. Typically, a circumglobal belt that includes Hawaii, the South Pacific, Australia, the Caribbean, and the Indo-Pacific experiences chikungunya outbreaks. But cases have also been reported in Northern Europe and North America as a result of the transportation of tainted fish. There is no known specific treatment for the toxicity's neurological symptoms. However, mannitol given intravenously or anticonvulsant medication may lessen the severity of the poisoning. Natural toxin levels typically remain below the threshold for human toxicity in a balanced diet. Other strategies to reduce the risk of phytotoxins to health include telling people:

- Not to assume that natural is synonymous with safe;
- Not to eat food that does not smell or taste fresh or has an unusual taste;
- To throw away bruised, damaged or discolored or mouldy food;
- To only eat wild plants or mushrooms that have been identified as nonpoisonous.

Over ten thousand years have passed since humans have successfully created food plants with ever-improving performance. The majority of the crops grown today are the product of traditional plant breeding techniques, which produced edible wild form varieties that at first had unfavorable high concentrations of natural toxins. Breeders can now further optimize crop production by balancing crop disease resistance and human safety by maximizing the level and timing of biosynthetic generation of natural toxins, thanks to the current state of genomic knowledge. Interesting situations can occur when a zero tolerance is recommended for a compound in food products where the compound also occurs naturally.

Chloramphenicol is an antibiotic that exhibits a wide range of activity. It is employed in veterinary medicine for both preventative and therapeutic purposes. Determining an Acceptable Daily Intake (ADI) is hampered by the absence of scientific data. As such, the establishment of a maximum residue limit (MRL) was not feasible. This was then converted into a zero-tolerance policy that was based on the food's achievable detection limit. The maximum residue limit is currently set at 0.0003 mg/kg. As analytical technological capabilities grow, the detection limit gets progressively smaller. This essentially indicates that the zero tolerance level decreases to progressively lower exposure levels. Food products become ever "cleaner" as a result of enhanced detection capabilities. The ecological background level is crossed at a particular point. In the case of chloramphenicol, this is true. *Streptomyces venezuelae* is a species of actinobacteria, which are prokaryotic organisms that are thought to be an intermediate group between bacteria and fungi. This species was recently found in a marine setting as well. Large batches of shrimp have been thrown out due to detectable levels of chloramphenicol. This is the result of applying a zero-tolerance policy. However, a detection limit as part of the approval process disregards the relevance of toxicology.

A so-called Minimum Required Performance Limit (MRPL) was introduced in response to this discussion in an effort to harmonize the analytical methodology used to measure substances. The Threshold of Toxicological Concern (TTC), which takes into account fresh toxicological knowledge, is a better criterion for ensuring safety (vide infra).

6.1.4. Pesticides

Hundreds of pesticide products have been approved for use. There are various ways to classify all these products. One way is via the pest they address or the effect they cause, as shown in Figure 6.3. It illustrates the huge variety in available pesticide products.

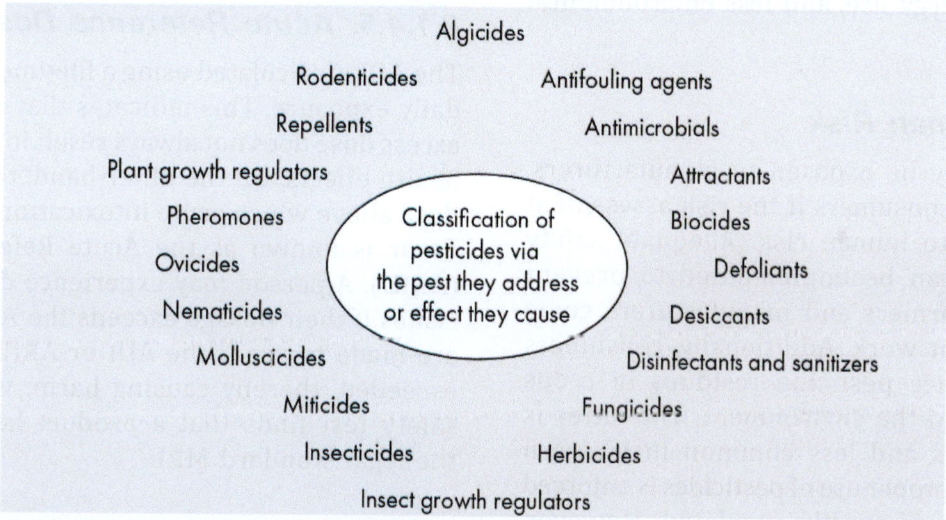

Figure 6.3. *A possible classification of pesticides.*

Source: https://www.wageningenacademic.com/doi/pdf/10.3920/978-90-8686-933-6_13.

6.1.4.1. Benefits

The ideal pesticide (1) is selective, i.e., other organisms should not be affected; (2) is effective in its action on the target; (3) is metabolized in nature, i.e., after the harvest, no residues are detected; and (4) remains active after long-term usage, i.e., resistance to the pesticide does not occur. There is no emergence of pesticide resistance. No pesticide satisfies all four requirements. The toxicologist can help with that. In addition to the target organism, other organisms that are affected by pesticide use include the environment (environmental toxicology) and humans (human toxicology).

This means that to determine the risk, both the hazard and the exposure must be measured because human beings can become exposed to the breakdown products of pesticides, which can also be toxic. Research should ideally look into both the parent compound and its metabolites. These advantages and disadvantages should eventually be balanced. Numerous advantages include increased yields, better aesthetics, safety, extended shelf life, less labor-intensive physical work, reduced fuel consumption for weeding, less disturbance of the soil, and fewer pest outbreaks. Furthermore, invasive species are managed, and pests are geographically contained. According to Cooper and Dobson, these main advantages result in a wide range of remarkable secondary benefits, such as enhanced food safety and human health, decreased energy use, and less environmental degradation.

6.1.4.2. Human Risk

Pesticides may be exposed to manufacturers, farmers, and consumers if the risk assessment is restricted to human risk. Adequate safety precautions can be implemented to prevent exposure if farmers and manufacturers come into contact at work. Additionally, consumers may experience pesticide residues in crops or exposure to the environment. The latter is becoming less and less common in Western counties. The proper use of pesticides is enforced and their use is strictly regulated. However, a critical analysis of the literature identifies a number of shortcomings with reference to exposure assessment and the characterization and quantification of health outcomes.

6.1.4.3. Acceptable Daily Intake

Various factors determine the toxicological limits. An Acceptable Daily Intake (ADI) has been established for every pesticide. The amount of pesticide (ADI) that a person can consume every day of their life without experiencing any negative side effects is known. The ADI is typically derived from animal experiments. A safety factor is used to translate the data from animals to humans, and another safety factor is applied to make sure that the ADI holds true for those who are sensitive.

6.1.4.4. Maximal Residue Level

A Maximum Residue Level (MRL) is set for each pesticide. This represents the maximum amount of pesticide residue that can exist in a product. The mean daily consumption, environmental toxicity, political and economic ramifications, and mean daily consumption are all considered in this MRL human toxicity data.

6.1.4.5. Acute Reference Dose

The ADI is calculated using a lifetime of constant daily exposure. This indicates that a single ADI excess dose does not always result in detrimental health effects. On the other hand, the pesticide dose above which acute intoxication issues may occur is known as the Acute Reference Dose (ARfD). A person may experience direct health issues if their dosage exceeds the ARfD. Checks are made to see if the ADI or ARfD have been exceeded, thereby causing harm, when a food safety test finds that a product has exceeded the legal standard MRL.

6.1.4.6. Threshold of Toxicological Concern

It's critical to acknowledge that the majority of toxicological knowledge relates to specific compounds. The combinations of compounds are less well understood. The Threshold of Toxicological Concern (TTC) method might be useful in this situation. The TTC is a rather practical approach that works on the premise that the body can withstand substances up to a point at which a dose is reached that causes concern. Even in the absence of a complete toxicity database, a TTC can be established for compounds with comparable structural properties based on their chemical structure. Many years after making this recommendation, EFSA cautiously released a guideline on the application of the TTC in food safety evaluation. The TTC value for pesticides in the carbamate and organophosphate categories is 18 μg/person per day. A TTC value of 0.3 μg/kg body weight per day is thus obtained.

The public is afraid of synthetic chemicals. This so-called "chemophobia" appears to be related to the pesticides sprayed on crops. Given the real risk these chemicals pose when used properly, it seems excessive that many consumers will go to considerable measures to avoid them. Many people don't seem to feel that the many benefits of using modern pesticides correctly outweigh the risk. Pesticides are essential to the long-term, sustainable production of nutritious food. The highly persistent pesticides of the past are no longer in use, which raised serious concerns because they built up in the food chain.

6.1.5. Low-Dose Toxicity

The standard idea in toxicology, which also applies to food toxicology, is that the health risk estimate's parameters assume linearity in response. Put another way, increased toxicity results in increased harm to health. This idea has a very long history. Considered the father of toxicology, Paracelsus, was the first to propose linearity. He is credited with coining the proverb "everything is poison and nothing without poison; the dosage alone makes that a thing is no poison.". It became apparent to him that everything can become toxic at a sufficiently high dose. This is, in actuality, pure linearity. His full name was Philippus Aureolus Theophrastus Bombastus von Hohenheim, and he was a doctor and theologian. He used minerals and novel remedies containing mercury, sulfur, iron, and copper sulfate while traveling through the South German and Swiss regions. While administering these metals and salts to patients, he most likely observed that raising the dosage of his compounds did, in fact, cause toxicity.

A number of physiological models have had their results attempted to be linearized. We now understand that in toxicology and physiology, linearity is not a descriptive reality. Understanding the effects of compounds has been made possible by the reductionist approach to toxicological research. On the other hand, applied abstraction can quickly result in inappropriate concreteness. In the fields of physiology and toxicology, we are not merely recipients of the thousands of substances that have the potential to cause havoc with our bodies; conversely, we adjust. This adaptive response, also referred to as hormesis, is an attempt to restore homeostasis by a moderate overcompensation for a chemical disturbance of the organism's homeostasis. Research on low-dose exposure to substances commonly regarded as toxic chemicals demonstrates that the dose-response curve is bell-shaped rather than linear.

Hormesis can be defined as an adaptive reaction to low levels of stress, toxicity, or damage that gives some physiological systems a temporary boost in robustness. According to Paracelsus and the most recent toxicology models, a compound has harmful, grade-bad characteristics. More compounds are more harmful. We are able to calculate an ADI and an ARfD as a result. There are more than just "bad" or "good" compounds in the more realistic hormesis (adaptive) model. The biological organism's plasticity determines a compound's effect. In this hormesis model, the challenge for toxicology is to convert a risk assessment into risk-reduction measures because, as we all know, not all bad things are bad. It will undoubtedly make risk communication even more difficult. There is a clear "enhanced homeostasis" in the hormetic zone. It's also been referred to as enhanced resilience. This process has been elucidated in cell models. In fact, a small amount of toxicity may even be beneficial. (Figure 6.4).

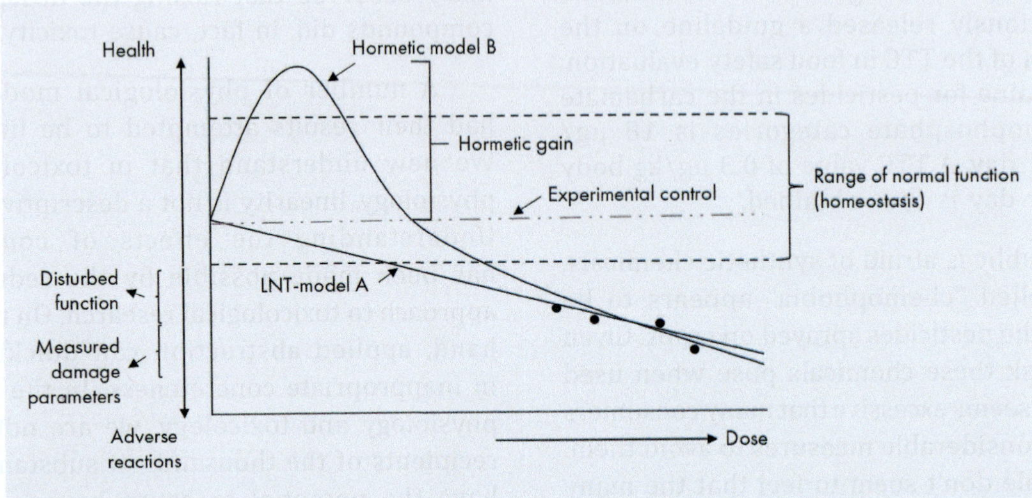

Figure 6.4. *Illustration of (A) a linear dose-response curve; and (B) a biphasic or hormetic bell-shaped dose response curve.*

Source: https://www.wageningenacademic.com/doi/pdf/10.3920/978-90-8686-933-6_13.

A static state is described by the WHO's definition of health, which is "a state of complete physical, mental, and social well-being and not merely the absence of disease or infirmity.". Furthermore—and maybe not surprisingly—the definition implies absoluteness with the word "complete" coming before the word "well-being" in the wake of World War II. The phrase "complete well-being" inadvertently brought up the issue of society becoming more and more medicalized. As of right now, "the ability to adapt" is a better definition of health. Thus, enhanced adaptive responses are a crucial component of health. Toxic compounds (in small doses) may promote adaptability and are therefore considered beneficial to health. This is true not only for natural toxins found in food but also for industrial chemicals. There are a growing number of examples that support this idea. Flavonoids, which are present in fruits and vegetables, promote adaptability. Actually, flavonoids may have some beneficial effects on health as a result of their harmful interactions with proteins.

6.2. Assessment of Food Toxicology

Food toxicity may have had its beginnings when Hippocrates said, "Let food be thy medicine and medicine thy food," more than two millennia before modern science was developed. Food toxicants have been identified and characterized thanks to advancements in modern biochemistry, molecular biology, cell culture methods, computer science, and bioinformatics. Improved food safety has resulted from mechanistic insights obtained through food toxicity assessment using various models, including in vitro biochemical, cell-based in vitro, animal in vivo, and clinical settings. Measurement of toxicants and toxicity in food involves two related areas: (1) actual toxicant effects measurements in various models, such as in vitro biochemical systems, cell-based in vitro systems, animal in vivo models, or clinical settings analyzing systemic or organ-specific toxicity; and (2) assessment and/or prediction of potential toxicants in food. The identification of additional possible toxicants in food can be facilitated by the mechanistic knowledge obtained from the assessment of toxicant effects. This is why these two are related. Pharmacology is the field that developed most food toxicology assessment systems. Since many of the most widely used medications in the world are derived from natural products—as the term "nutraceutical" illustrates—pharmacology and nutritional science have common roots.

The mechanisms underlying the effects of toxicants are complex, involving both internal and external interactions with important molecules that are crucial to metabolism, gene expression, signaling pathways, cell integrity, and translation. Their effects seem to be concentrated on the production of electrophilic species (ES) for a range of toxicants, which causes oxidative stress and persistent inflammation. Toxicants cause oxidative reactions that accumulate damaged macromolecules, which damage tissues, organs, and cells. Thus, toxins may be key players in degenerative diseases like Alzheimer's, Parkinson's, and Huntington's, as well as cell death, chronic inflammation, aging, multiple sclerosis, myocardial infarction, arteriosclerosis, diabetes, rheumatoid arthritis, sterility, cataracts, and many other conditions. Numerous biochemical systems have been developed for in vitro assessment to analyze detrimental effects on the integrity or activity of important biomolecules. These molecules have a role in translation and expression of genes, metabolism, signaling pathways, and cell integrity. Enzymes, receptors, membrane lipids, nucleic acids, and/or factors involved in gene expression are among the many molecules that are impacted. Numerous viability assays are frequently employed at the cellular level to measure the effects of putative food toxicants to extrapolate the range of dosages that are used for maximal tolerated concentrations in both clinical and in vivo animal models. Many cell-based in vitro systems were created in addition to targeted in vitro analyses that concentrate on important enzymes that are unique to individual cells and receptor-dependent pathways to gain further mechanistic insights. The gold standard for toxicity assessment still seems to be in vivo rodent models; however, these conventional testing methods have several drawbacks, including high costs, low throughput readouts, inconsistent responses, moral dilemmas, and worries about human extrapolation. As a result, novel tactics have been created, and the conventional toxicological paradigm has shifted from an apical endpoint approach based on animal models to a mechanism-based approach utilizing in silico techniques.

Many high-throughput and high-content screening technologies are used in silico screening systems, which combine computer-based algorithms with targeted in vitro cell-based models. Toxicogenomics, toxicoproteomics, or toxicometabolomics, in that order, can be used to measure cell-specific biomarkers on gene, protein, or metabolite levels. Food toxicology data acquired from in vitro biochemical, cell-based, in vivo animal models, and in silico systems have been integrated, resulting in the identification and application of particular surrogate biomarkers in clinical settings as well as a mechanistic understanding of systemic or organ-specific toxicity in humans. While intricate in vitro cell culture systems combined with in silico systems offer distinct mechanistic insights into in vivo toxicology that are more applicable to humans, they can never fully replicate the intricate interplay among various pathways found in an intact organism. The use of substitute lower hierarchy animal models, such as nematodes (*Caenorhabditis elegans*), fruit flies (*Drosophila melanogaster*), or zebrafish (*Danio rerio*), is another improvement in toxicity assessment. Compared to conventional rodent models, these models have advantages in terms of high throughput, genetic modification, and ethical considerations. The startling finding of the high level of gene homology between humans and zebrafish, fruit flies, or nematodes demonstrated the importance of using alternative sub-mammalian vertebrate and invertebrate models.

In general, the advancements in food toxicology have greatly increased the rate of drug and food safety prediction to levels that were unthinkable just ten years ago. The predictability and robustness of in vitro cell-based toxicity models have improved due to a deeper understanding of the molecular mode of action on important targets of biological pathways, improving food safety. Furthermore, stem cell-based screening and three-dimensional organotypic models, while still in the early stages of development, will improve the predictivity of acute toxicity, aid in the resolution of basic biological queries, and/or allow for the testing of innovative therapeutic strategies. Notwithstanding these successes, raising the rate of predictivity in a number of areas, including endocrine disruption, neurotoxicity, genotoxicity, carcinogenicity, immunotoxicity, food allergies, and reproductive and developmental toxicity, remains extremely difficult at the moment.

6.2.1. Molecular Effects of Toxicants

While there are many different factors that contribute to toxic effects in humans, most of them seem to center around the production of free radicals. Nearly all biomolecules can be oxidized by various electrophilic species (ES), such as reactive nitrogen species (RNS) and reactive oxygen species (ROS). While some toxicants directly cause ES, others cause a secondary reaction that triggers immunocompetent leukocytes—which are essential to the inflammatory cascade—to produce ES indirectly. By interfering with transcription factors and/or DNA, ES are also involved in the modulation of gene expression, which can result in mutations and the development of cancer. The breakdown of cells, tissues, and organs is caused by the buildup of damage to membrane lipids, cellular proteins, carbohydrates, and nucleic acids. These and other findings support the theory that chronic inflammation and oxidative stress caused by toxicants are major contributors to aging, degenerative diseases, and cell death.

ROS comprise differently reduced oxygen species such as the superoxide anion radical ($\bullet O_2^-$), hydrogen peroxide (H_2O_2), and the highly reactive hydroxyl radical ($\bullet OH$). Dismutation of these radicals leads to hydrogen peroxide as a fairly stable ROS member. Heavy metals (iron, but also copper, chromium or vanadium), as an important group of toxicants, can generate the highly toxic hydroxyl radical by way of the Fenton reaction ($H_2O_2 + Fe^{2+} \rightarrow {}^{\bullet}OH + OH^- + Fe^{3+}$). Therefore, the amount of hydroxyl radicals formed in a cell depends on endogenous ROS generation, but also on the amounts of reduced metal ions for the Fenton reaction to occur. The other highly reactive group of molecules consists of reactive nitrogen species (RNS). The signal molecule nitric oxide (NO) exists as NO^+, $NO^{\bullet}$ and NO^- while the peroxynitrite ion ($ONOO^-$) is generated by the reaction of NO with the superoxide anion radical.

Numerous degenerative diseases can arise as a result of the oxidation of lipids, proteins, nucleic acids, and carbohydrates, which produces a range of harmful breakdown products. When lipid-containing cell structures undergo lipid peroxidation, a variety of hazardous compounds, such as alcohols, ketones, alkanes, aldehydes, and ethers, are produced. These compounds may exacerbate cell damage, necrosis, or apoptosis. The most sensitive ES targets for proteins are the thiolgroups of cysteine residues. Structure/function alterations and protein aggregation may result from redox-dependent modifications of intra- and intermolecular disulfide bonds. Enzymes, transporters, signal transducers, or structural proteins may all malfunction as a result of these combined ROS-induced damages. ES specifically targets nucleic acids, which can result in mutations. Single and double-strand breaks, DNA–DNA, DNA–protein, and DNA–lipid adducts, as well as a variety of base modifications like 8-hydroxy-deoxyguanosine, 5-hydroxylmethyluracil, 8-hydroxydeoxyadenine, and thyminglycol, can all be caused by ES damage to nucleic acids. Because mitochondrial DNA (mtDNA) lacks corresponding histones, the mitochondrial DNA repair system is not fully functional, and electron leakage from the respiratory chain produces free radicals, mtDNA is especially vulnerable to oxidative damage. It is interesting to note that carbohydrate oxidation may also contribute to DNA damage. This is because free radical damage to DNA can lead to oxidation and fragmentation of deoxyribose fragments, which are thought to be a major cause of mutations by inhibiting the actions of DNA polymerase and DNA ligase.

6.2.2. In Vitro Biochemical Assessment of Toxicity

Numerous in vitro biochemical assessment systems are centered around measuring primary or secondary products originating from proteins, nucleic acids, carbohydrates, and oxidized lipids, or they measure the integrity or activity of a range of important biomolecules that are crucial for cell integrity, metabolism, signaling pathways, gene expression, and translation. Measuring a chemical's ability to alter an enzyme's activity or its affinity for a specific receptor or other biomolecule is the most straightforward approach to obtain a mechanistic understanding of how a chemical acts at the molecular level. Various biochemical in vitro assays are available to analyze various aspects such as drug or neurotransmitter metabolism, binding and activity of different receptors, integrity or mutation of DNA and RNA, membrane lipids, and many more. Given their strong association with carcinogenesis, DNA-reactive toxicants in food present a particularly interesting target for genotoxicity risk assessment. Traditional use of the Ames bacterial reverse mutation test is to assess the potential genotoxic activity of food compounds that may cause mutations. The growth of multiple histidine-dependent Salmonella strains with distinct mutations in different histidine operon genes serves as the foundation for the Ames test.

Numerous enzyme and receptor-binding assays have been created to investigate particular molecular mechanisms of action of various receptors (e.g., ion channels, nuclear receptors, tyrosine kinases, -protein coupled receptors, signaling transduction enzymes, phosphodiesterases, kinases, proteases, phosphatases), and drug-metabolizing enzymes (e.g., monooxygenases of cytochrome P450) or neurotransmitters (e.g., cholinesterase (acetyl)). The human ether-a-go-go-related gene (hERG) potassium ion channel or the acetylcholinesterase activity assay are commonly used as in vitro prescreening tools for a comprehensive evaluation of cardiotoxicity or neurotoxicity, respectively. Additional assays track possible toxicant effects that could conflict with anti-inflammatory medications. A high-throughput screening for microsomal prostaglandin E synthase activity may be used for these.

When developing novel drug candidates, xenobiotic metabolism is a frequent issue that may also arise with food-borne toxins.

The cytochrome P450 (CYPs) monooxygenase drug-metabolizing phase I enzymes are by far the most significant class of metabolic enzymes. However, there are a number of other classes of biotransformation enzymes, which are referred to as phase II enzymes, such as uridine diphosphate glucuronosyltransferases (UGTs), glutathione S-transferases (GSTs), N-acetyltransferases (NATs), sulfotransferases (SATs), and methyltransferases (MTs). Most studies on inhibition use fluorescent or luminescent substrates, recombinant CYPs and UGTs, as well as different kinases. They use protein-based microarrays in high-throughput formats. Alternative methods make use of recombinant CYP450s metabolizing enzyme toxicology assay chips (MetaChips), which work in conjunction with cell-based screening to enable cell-specific screening while evaluating the toxicity of the metabolites produced. It makes sense that there are so many in vitro biochemical testing platforms available for CYP450 enzymes because in vivo the liver depends on these enzymes for xenobiotic detoxification. Nearly all of the relevant human xenobiotic metabolizing enzymes in this family are not functionally expressed in many hepatoma-derived HepG2 cell lines used for hepatotoxicity screening.

In many different biochemical in vitro assays, lipid peroxidation—characterized by radical chain reactions with the production of a variety of breakdown products—serves as a marker for oxidative stress and inflammation. The thiobarbituric acid test uses the identification of generated aldehydes—named "thiobarbituric reactive substances" (TBARS)—especially malondialdehyde, to ascertain the extent of lipid peroxidation. This method is thought to be the first worldwide measurement of lipid peroxidation in a range of chemical and biological materials due to its simplicity and sensitivity. Additionally, F2-isoprostanes, which are produced during lipid peroxidation, are dependable and stable markers of oxidative stress. The detection of oxidative damage linked to pathological or experimental conditions in subcellular fractions, tissue homogenates, or various organs has also been effectively achieved through the use of tert-butyl hydroperoxide-initiated chemiluminescence.

6.2.3. Cell-Based in Vitro Assessment of Toxicity

Comparing basic biochemical assays with the use of cellular models reveals a much higher level of complexity. Numerous human cell lines are accessible, and numerous cell-based in vitro assays have been created to screen for food toxins. Generally, two main methods are used: (1) a target-organ-based method that uses a panel of various cell types with more specialized functions, such as representative cell lines from different organs like the liver, heart, kidney, lung, brain, or others; and (2) a universal screening method that uses one or a few cell lines to assess cell viability.

6.2.3.1. Viability Assays

Several cellular bioassays that integrate various cytotoxicity endpoints, such as membrane leakage or cellular activity, are routinely used for the general assessment of cytotoxicity. An indirect measure of cell viability is typically performed. Certain assays for viability, like the neutral red, alamar blue, or MTT assay, are metabolic measurements of cellular activity, while others, like the trypan blue, propidium iodide, crystal violet, or lactate dehydrogenase assay, analyze membrane integrity based on exclusion. When testing on humans and animals, the inhibitory concentrations (IC values) discovered through viability assays are subsequently utilized to determine the starting dosage. With the use of assay systems that employ a range of particular multiplexed panels, inhibitory effects on cell viability as a measure of cytotoxicity due to necrosis, apoptosis, or autophagy can be further distinguished. The trypan blue exclusion method, which uses the ratio of stained to unstained cells in a sample as a reflection of membrane damage, is a well-known and repeatable technique to assess cell viability. Traditionally, the technique is carried out by counting cells, but trypan blue staining has been presented as a sophisticated quantitative measure. The crystal violet assay, like the trypan blue exclusion assay, is based on the growth rate reduction reflected by stained cells as a result of crystal violet's reaction with negatively charged cell components like peptidoglycans or nucleic acids. Apart from dye measurements, an established method for assessing membrane integrity is enzyme activity analysis. Thus, the release of intracellular enzymes into the extracellular medium, such as lactate dehydrogenase (LDH) or others, is used as a marker for cell membrane damage.

The alamar blue assay, MTT, and neutral red (NR) assays are a few other commonly used viability assays that quantify cellular activity. The MTT viability assay is based on mitochondrial activity and uses the yellow tetrazolium salt MTT (3,(4,5-dimethylthiazol-2-yl)-2,5,-diphenyl-tetrazoliumbromide) to form a blue formazan product by mitochondrial dehydrogenase activity. In contrast, the NR assay gauges cell viability by endocytic uptake of neutral red into lysosomes of uninjured cells. Redox reactions transform blue, oxidized resazurin into reduced resorufin, which is red and extremely fluorescent, in the alamar blue assay, which is similar to the MTT method. Different antioxidants may cause different cell types to exhibit false-positive results when using the MTT method, which is based on intracellular redox reactions. Hence, it seems prudent to incorporate additional viability tests in addition to MTT-as well as the alamar blue technique for cell-based toxicity investigation. The central nervous system, liver, kidney, heart, muscle, and other organs are all highly toxic when there is damage to the mitochondria, and a growing number of degenerative diseases are linked to mitochondrial dysfunction. Thus, a crucial consideration for toxicity assessment is how toxicants affect mitochondria.

6.2.3.2. Genotoxicity, Nutrigenomic and Immunotoxicity Testing

Given that many toxicants have the ability to produce electrophilic species, it is not surprising that many of them cause oxidative damage and RNA or DNA oxidation, which can result in genotoxicity. Finding potentially cancer-causing food ingredients is one of the goals of genotoxicity testing because there is a strong correlation between genotoxicity and carcinogenicity. Furthermore, persistent inflammation is commonly acknowledged to play a significant role in the development of cancer and a number of other degenerative illnesses, such as diabetes, arthritis, Alzheimer's disease, and cardiovascular disease. Thus, nutrigenomic screening—a field that examines the impact of nutritional compounds on gene expression—has been used to develop cell-based models that assess the effect of food ingredients on inflammation.

Different exploratory genetic toxicity assays are used to quantify chromosomal damage in eukaryotic cells for cell-based genotoxic screening. The Comet assay, the micronucleus clastogenicity assay, the Chinese hamster ovary (CHO) chromosomal aberration assay, and the mouse lymphoma tk gene mutation assay are commonly used models. Interestingly, genotoxicity testing has a high false positive rate (low specificity), which may be related to the recent finding of non-covalent DNA interaction and toxicant interference with essential DNA metabolizing proteins like DNA polymerases and topoisomerase. The micronucleus test, which is used for genotoxic screening of chromosomal damage in bone marrow polychromatic erythrocytes, clearly illustrates the connection between cell-based in vitro, ex vivo, and in vivo evaluation. Moreover, there are multiple ex vivo test models available for immunotoxicity. Functional immunological tests measure natural killer cell activity, T- and B-cell immune responses, and macrophage activity. Regarding additional human organ-based ex vivo tissue or organ toxicology research on the liver, kidney, lung, heart, or brain, there is a benefit to comparing and extrapolating data from in vitro to in vivo studies.

6.2.3.3. Complex Cellular Toxicity Assays

One cell line is typically used for viability, genotoxicity, immunotoxicity, or nutrigenomic testing. Recently, new and sophisticated in vitro human cell-based systems have been used more frequently to model mammalian tissues holistically. Single-cell measurements can be made for a wide range of characteristics, including major signaling pathways, gene and protein expression levels, receptor activity, cytoskeletal and membrane integrity, energy status, organelle morphology, cell motility, cell cycle status, and cell differentiation. Complex human in vitro cell-based models are well suited to deconstruct complex toxicological pathways of specific organs by predicting the in vivo response through comparison throughout the panel of different cells by quantitative in vitro to in vivo extrapolation. Complex cell-based in vitro models that do not have problems with interspecies extrapolation have a high predictivity and robustness thanks to correlation analysis with animal and clinical studies. Thus, high content and high throughput complex cellular in vitro models are frequently employed, with an emphasis on organ-specific toxicity, including neurotoxicity, cardiotoxicity, hepatotoxicity, and respiratory toxicity. Three-dimensional organotypic models achieve an even greater level of complexity. Even though they are still in their infancy, organotypic systems have the potential to predict acute toxicity very well, provide answers to basic biological questions, and allow the testing of novel therapeutic approaches—often using cells derived from patients.

6.2.4. In Vivo Toxicity Assessment in Animals

Although intricate cell culture systems can offer distinctive perspectives on in vivo toxicology, they can never fully replicate the higher order interactions found in an entire organism. As a result, in vivo toxicology—which involves giving a specific molecule or complex food ingredient to animals to assess acute, subacute, and chronic effects—has been the gold standard for toxicity assessment. Many specific high-content animal models have been developed as a result of a substantial body of data regarding their responses. These models may be able to replicate the genetic heterogeneity of the human population and assess potential toxicity to reproduction and development, neurotoxicity, genotoxicity, carcinogenicity, immunotoxicity, food allergies, and endocrine disruption.

Rats make up the majority of the animals used, and the pharmaceutical industry estimates that 7000 animals and tens of millions of dollars are needed for each test compound in order to obtain statistically significant results. The quantity of compounds or food ingredients that need to be tested, as well as the expenses associated with the current in vivo assessment systems, are skyrocketing despite the fact that the number of animals used in food toxicity screening is declining. In addition to low-throughput readouts, traditional in vivo toxicity testing raises ethical questions about the use of such large numbers of animals from animal protection organizations. Finally, there are disagreements over whether the data is easily applicable to humans because of variations in species sensitivity as well as the diversity of the human population, which is demonstrated by a continuous rise in reports of unfavorable occurrences. Concerns about extrapolability, low throughput readouts, high costs, and ethical issues have prompted calls for different approaches to toxicity testing techniques.

With a roughly 50% decrease in the number of animals needed for toxicological testing, the paradigm surrounding the widespread use of rodents for in vivo toxicity testing has changed recently. Because mechanisms are now better understood, this was accompanied by a targeted use of particular animal models. Rats don't seem to be the best model for studying cholesterol levels, but the knowledge we have about the effects of toxicants on lipids, for instance, comes from the fact that mini pigs and humans have similar lipid metabolism. More genetic diversity in vivo high-content models that replicate human genetic heterogeneity, transgenic animals that model common diseases, and/or genetic polymorphisms that take into account specific groups in the general population that might be particularly at risk after exposure to a food component were also used to achieve higher specificity.

The important discoveries of homologous genes related to development, immune response, cancer, or related pathways in humans demonstrated the value of using alternative sub-mammalian vertebrate and invertebrate models in addition to improving the specificity of traditional animal models. Three model organism test platforms in particular, are well-suited for high-throughput screening. Among them are the nematode C. elegans and the fruit fly D. melanogaster and the zebrafish D. rerio. Compared to traditional rodent models, the use of these and other alternative lower hierarchy surrogate animal models offer an advantage in terms of ease of ethical concerns regarding high throughput and genetic manipulation. Alternative in vivo models do, however, have the extrapolation problems associated with species differences, just like any other animal model.

For more than a century, researchers studying genetics and developmental biology have used the fruit fly D. melanogaster as a model organism. A functional homolog of nearly 75% of human disease-causing genes exists in D. melanogaster, according to the genome's complete sequencing. Fruit fly genetics can be altered through extensive genetic manipulation using RNA interference (RNAi) to cause knockout or knockdown. The high degree of orthologs linked to genes known to be involved in neurodegenerative diseases makes fruit flies an intriguing candidate for chemical toxicity screens, especially for neurotoxicity. Nematode C. elegans is frequently utilized in biomedical research due to its ease of lab culture. Functional orthologs of over 50% of human genes exist in C. elegans and each of the 959 somatic cells of the worms have undergone lineage-specific characterization. With regard to D. melanogaster, numerous transgenic strains that are well-suited for a differential toxicity screening by high-throughput genomic studies are readily available thanks to a range of molecular techniques. C. elegans is an excellent model for testing neurotoxicity because it exhibits basic learning abilities and has a high degree of neurotransmitter conservation. The D. rerio zebrafish has been employed as a vertebrate model organism for a range of studies, including toxicology and drug discovery, in more recent times. Because of their significant physiological, anatomical, and genetic similarities to humans, zebrafish and humans have remarkably similar toxicity profiles, which is reflected in the growing use of zebrafish as in vivo model systems. In addition to being cheap, easy to manipulate genes, and having a short generation time, the zebrafish model is particularly useful for microarray and proteomic research, high-throughput screening, and other related applications. Zebrafish larvae are transparent, which makes them perfect for more in-depth investigations using immunohistochemistry or in situ hybridization, as well as studies on organ morphology using in vivo imaging techniques.

6.3. Food Poisoning Caused by Bacteria (Food Toxins)

There are pollutants in the environment that can react negatively in people when they enter the body in a variety of ways, including through ingestion, inhalation, injection, or absorption. Chemical compounds, poisons, toxic gases, and bacterial toxins are some of the primary pollutants. Their effects are contingent upon exposure duration and dose, and they are found in various locations. Toxins produced by bacteria or other toxic substances in food can cause foodborne diseases (FBDs), which can lead to severe diarrhea, toxic shock syndrome, debilitating infections like meningitis, and even death. In addition, FBDs can cause disability. Food contaminated with pathogenic microorganisms that possess multiple factors of virulence, which allow them to cause an infection, is the means by which food-borne bite-back disease is spread. Certain bacterial genres can produce toxins directly in food, but other genres can produce toxins once they reach the intestine. Salmonella species is one of the pathogens linked to foodborne illnesses (FBDs) that is also regarded as toxic. *Listeria monocytogenes*, *Bacillus cereus*, *Clostridium botulinum*, *Clostridium perfringens*, *Vibrio parahaemolyticus*, and *Vibrio cholerae* have all been identified. It is possible to avert foodborne illnesses, acute diarrhea syndromes, fever, and even dehydration death, particularly in young children and individuals with compromised immune systems.

Toxins from bacteria, chemicals, hazardous gases, and poisons can all be considered the primary pollutants. Poisoning can result in acute poisoning or chronic illnesses like cancer, among other diseases that humans can contract from consuming various types of pollutants. Toxins produced by bacteria or other toxic substances found in food can also lead to foodborne diseases (FBDs), which can be crippling. The fact that poisoning is the leading cause of morbidity and mortality globally should not be overlooked. Intoxication can be of two types: (a) intoxication brought on by chemicals (such as drugs, pesticides, heavy metals, gases, and solvents), where the patient comes into direct contact with the toxic substance; and (b) food poisoning, where the food contaminated with pathogens or chemical products is the means of transmission. Of the six million chemicals known today, 80,000 to 100,000 are frequently found in various everyday products, making chemical poisoning a health concern. As of 2006, the World Health Organization (WHO) estimated that chemical exposure was responsible for over 25% of poisoning cases and 5% of cancer, neuropsychiatric disorders, and vascular diseases worldwide. Because a detailed medical history including the patient's exposure routes, dosage, and timing of the chemical exposure is necessary, diagnosing chemical poisoning is challenging. On the other hand, there exist protocols that make the diagnosis and treatment of chemical poisoning incidents easier.

Moreover, foodborne illness, also known as food poisoning, is one of the major issues facing public health globally. As per the WHO, 1 in 10 individuals globally, or 600 million people, contract foodborne illnesses annually as a result of contaminated food. Due to this population's susceptibility to diarrheal illness, 420,000 of these individuals pass away, including 125,000 children under the age of five. Approximately 43% of FBDs occur in these patients. Approximately 70% of FBDs are caused by food that has been tainted by microbes. Toxins that can be produced in food or after the pathogen has colonized the digestive tract are among the virulence factors that bacteria possess, which enable them to cause a disease and are responsible for foodborne illness disorders (FBDs). Note that the purpose of this chapter is to provide information on the main foodborne pathogens that cause toxins, their symptoms, treatment options, and diseases they can cause. It also aims to identify the main sources of contamination in street markets and restaurants.

6.3.1. Types of Bacterial Toxins

A bacterial toxin is a macromolecule mainly of protein origin, which can cause toxic damage in a specific organ of the host. Toxins can be divided in endotoxins and exotoxins:

- The most significant antigen found in Gram-negative bacteria are endotoxins, also known as lipopolysaccharides (LPS), which are parts of the outer membrane that are released into the medium following various bacterial processes like lysis and cell division. Endotoxic shock and tissue damage are possible outcomes of this endotoxin.
- LPS are formed by three regions:
- Lipid A is a type of glycolipid that is created when fatty acids—typically capric, lauric, myristic, palmitic, and stearic acids—are bound to a disaccharide called glucose. These fatty acids are then inserted into the bacterial outer membrane.
- The nucleus a heteropolysaccharide derived from hexoses and heptoses.
- Lipid A and the nucleus are bound by the sugar acid 2-keto-3-deoxyoctanate (KDO).
- The O chain is a repeating unit polymer of 1–8 glycosidic residues; this polymer is highly variable among bacterial species and genus.

Apart from the endotoxin's pyrogenicity, the bacterial adherence mechanism to the host cell has also been found to play a significant role. This is because earlier research has shown that alterations or inhibitions in LPS expression can affect the adherence of the bacteria to the cell.

- **Exotoxins.** These are the macromolecules of protein origin, which are produced and later released to the medium by the microorganism. Depending on their mechanism of action, exotoxins are divided as follows:
- **Toxins Type I.** These toxins modify the host's cells without internalizing in the cells; for example, the superantigens produced by Staphylococcus aureus and Streptococcus pyogenes.
- **Toxins Type II.** Hemolysins and phospholipases are among the toxins in this group; they are distinguished by their ability to cause pore formation and/or rupture host cell membranes. This virulence factor, such as aerolysin and GCAT protein produced by Aeromonas spp., allows the pathogen to invade the host cell.
- **Toxins Type III.** Its binary structure gives these toxins the name A/B. As an example, the Shiga toxin produced by Escherichia coli O157:H7, the Cholera toxin (Ctx) produced by V. cholerae, and the Anthrax toxin produced by Bacillus

anthracis are examples of toxins that cause damage to cells. Fraction B is responsible for binding to the cell's receptor, while fraction A is the unit with enzymatic activity.

The pathophysiology of diarrheal disease is significantly influenced by the exotoxins of Gram-negative enteropathogenic bacteria, which cause excessive liquid secretion without destroying or killing intestinal mucosal cells. These toxins are distinct from cytotoxins and are collectively referred to as enterotoxins. Additionally, there are two other categories of toxins: those with neurotoxic activity and those that modify the cytoskeleton. Some toxins exhibit activity that falls into more than one of the groups listed in Table 6.3.

Table 6.3. *Classification of Enteric Toxins*

Toxin Type	**Definition**
Enterotoxin	In vitro tests show that it causes a net secretion in ligated intestinal segments without causing damage to nonerythrocytic cells or exhibiting histological evidence of intestinal lesion. It causes the using chamber's short circuit current (Isc) and potential difference (PD) to rise without showing any signs of intestinal damage; this leads to the release of (active) electrogenic anions. Additionally, a toxin may hinder the absorption of electrically neutral NaCl, leading to net ion secretion.
Cytoskeleton-altering toxin	It has been repeatedly demonstrated to be caused by the rearrangement of F-actin, and it modifies the cellular form. The toxin is not fatal, but it can cause only minor cell damage. It may or may not be linked to intestinal epithelial cells' evidence of net secretion in *in vitro* or *in vivo* disease models.
Cytotoxin	It causes cell or tissue damage, usually ending with cell death. The toxin may or may not be associated with net secretion in *in vivo* or *in vitro* disease models in intestinal epithelial cells.
Neurotoxins	It involves the release of one or more neurotransmitters from the enteric nervous system. It alters the activity of smooth muscle in the intestine.

Source: https://www.intechopen.com/chapters/56521.

Toxins produced by pathogens involved in foodborne diseases are as follows:

Cholera toxin (Ctx) (Vibrio cholerae), Thermolabile toxin (LT) Thermostable toxin (ST) (Enterotoxigenic E. coli), Shiga Toxin (Shigella dysenteriae and E. coli O157:H7) Botulinum toxin (BTX) (Clostridium botulinum), CPE Enterotoxin (Clostridium perfringens), Alpha-Toxin, Beta-Toxin, Epsilon-Toxin and Iota-Toxin (C. perfringens), Toxin A/Toxin B (Clostridium difficile), Enterotoxins (A, B, C1, C2, D and E, G, H, I, J), Toxic Shock Syndrome Toxin (TSST-1), Cereulide, and hemolysin BL (HBL), nonhemolytic enterotoxin (NHE) (S. aureus), Citotoxin K or CytK (Bacillus cereus).

6.3.2. Risk Factors and Prevention Measures Associated with Food Poisoning

Food contamination by pathogenic bacteria that produce toxins is the main risk factor for bacterial food poisoning. This contamination can happen at any time, either from the crop (vegetables, for example) or right before eating due to consumer manipulation. As a result, food poisoning can affect anyone on the planet. Food poisoning is, therefore, a global public health concern, with children, the elderly, pregnant women, and those with compromised immune systems typically being the most affected. As would be expected, a person's age, gender, place of residence, and socioeconomic status are important factors in the development and acquisition of food poisoning. Food contamination can happen at any stage of the production process, from primary to final consumer. As a result, the risks associated with it vary depending on the practices used at each stage, including farming, raising livestock, and fishing; industrializing the production of processed foods; marketing the product at points of sale; and shipping the finished product to homes, public dining areas, and restaurants. Producers should take precautions against pollution from air, water, or natural fertilizers during primary production, taking into account the unique features of the area in which they raise, breed, and reproduce livestock. Unsafe agricultural practices, such as using sewage for irrigation and using manure as natural fertilizer, pose the greatest risk of contamination in primary production. These practices go against the fundamental principle of avoiding the contamination of raw materials with feces at all costs.

Aside from that, proper temperature and time management during food preparation, processing, cooling, and storage is another crucial component in guaranteeing food safety and quality. It is vital to take into account the physical, chemical, and microbiological properties of every kind of food, such as water activity, pH, and type, as well as the initial population of microorganisms present, to effectively control these parameters. Likewise, other factors must be considered, like usage and shelf life, or whether the food is packaged, raw, processed, or ready to eat. Ready-to-eat food must be kept apart from raw or unprocessed food in terms of both space and time, as microbiological contamination can happen through direct contact as well as through the air, utensils, contact surfaces, or the handler's hands. Furthermore, the latter needs constant washing or disinfection. Water is necessary at every stage of the food chain, so it may be the primary cause of contaminated food. Water used for food handling must be drinkable and meet the physical, chemical, and microbiological requirements indicated by its name. As such, control and monitoring of the type and source of water used at each stage are then imperative. Systems that guarantee the upkeep, cleaning, and sanitation of facilities must be established and closely watched over. These systems also come with sufficient waste management and efficient pest control. These pose a risk of contamination of any kind, which is why it's imperative to put in place precautions against pest entry and prevention measures against their nesting and proliferation. The last requirement is that any physical, chemical, or biological method of pest eradication that does not pose a risk to human health or food safety must be used.

Food transportation is crucial in the food chain for preventing contamination and the growth of microorganisms in food, so it is important to think about ways to prevent contamination of any kind and to create an environment that inhibits the growth of pathogenic microorganisms and the generation of bacterial toxins. Temperature, direct sunlight exposure, humidity, and airflow are some crucial variables to consider when transporting food. At this point, the kind of packaging and containers that are used are also crucial; the latter two, along with the transportation conditions, should be selected according to the qualities of the food being transported. The information that manufacturers and suppliers provide to consumers about the properties and safe handling of prepackaged foods is another crucial factor. For this reason, food must typically be packaged and labeled so that the consumer has the knowledge necessary to handle, store, and prepare the products safely without endangering their health. To facilitate quick identification and market recalls of goods that may be harmful to human consumption, labels should also include a batch number.

Microorganisms, and specifically bacteria, are found in all types of environments because they can multiply in a wide range of conditions. Although bacteria are adept at adapting to their surroundings, some circumstances are more conducive to bacterial growth than others. FATTOM (Food, Acidity, Time, Temperature, Oxygen, and Moisture) is the acronym for these conditions, which include food, humidity, acidity, temperature, time, and oxygen. Food poisoning, bacterial infections, and bacterial growth can all be avoided by being aware of these ideal conditions. Most foods are perishable because they provide the nutrients needed for microbial growth, making them easy targets for microorganism development. Controlling the growth of microorganisms under specific conditions and the conditions used to prevent food spoilage to extend the period that physicochemical and organoleptic characteristics must be maintained within minimum acceptance parameters are necessary to lessen food degradation and prevent foodborne illnesses. There are two categories of factors that influence the rate of microorganism proliferation: extrinsic and intrinsic.

6.3.2.1. Intrinsic parameters

The internal features of food products and how these features support or influence the growth of microorganisms are the more relevant intrinsic factors influencing the rate of proliferation. Examples of these factors are water activity, pH, oxidation-reduction potential, nutrient content and type, biological structures, and inhibiting substances.

- Water activity

According to its definition, it is the volume of water available for microbial growth; a decrease in water availability also results in a decrease in microbial proliferation. The amount of water available for metabolic activity, not the total moisture content, determines the extent of microbial growth. Water activity (Aw) is a unit of measurement used to describe the amount of water required by microorganisms. It is calculated by dividing the water vapor pressure of food substrate by the water vapor pressure of pure water at the same temperature. Relative humidity (RH), or RH = 100 × Aw, is related to this idea. For most microorganisms, an approximate optimal Aw of 0.99 is required for growth, whereas an Aw greater than 0.91 is required for most bacteria. Compared to Gram-positive bacteria, Gram-negative bacteria need higher values. Aw of 0.99 or higher is found in most natural food products. In general, the requirements of water activity are highest for bacteria, lowest for fungi, and intermediate for yeasts. While fungi and yeasts can grow on partially dehydrated surfaces with an Aw of 0.80 or less, most bacteria that break down food do not grow on surfaces with an Aw lower than 0.91. Halophytes have the lowest recorded value for bacteria in food, at 0.75, whereas xerophilic fungi and osmophilic yeasts have grown at Aw values of 0.65 and 0.61, respectively.

- P^{H}

As a unit of measurement to determine the acidity or alkalinity levels of a substance, in this case food, pH is defined as the negative logarithm of hydronium ions concentration. The measurement of pH is based on the quantity of free hydrogen ions (H^+). At least two aspects of the microbial cell are impacted by adverse pH: the movement of nutrients into the cell and the efficiency with which its enzymes function. H^+ and OH^- ions are largely unable to pass through the cytoplasmic membrane of microorganisms, and their concentration in the cytoplasm stays relatively constant even in the face of large fluctuations in the pH of the surrounding medium. Because essential elements like DNA or ATP require a neutral medium, the ability of microorganisms to multiply in environments that are either above or below the neutral level depends on their capacity to adjust the pH of the surrounding medium to a more suitable range.

Most microorganisms grow best at a pH that is near neutrality, which is between 6–7. While they can survive in values between 1.5 and 8.5, yeasts can grow in an acidic environment and flourish in an intermediate range (4.0–4.5). Although fungi can withstand a broad pH range (0–11), they typically grow more quickly in an acidic environment (too acidic for bacteria and yeast). pH values that are closer to neutral are typically more conducive to bacterial growth. However, the growth of acidophilic bacteria is limited to substrates with a pH of up to 5.2, below which the growth ceases completely. Generally speaking, fungi and yeasts can break down fruits, vinegars, and wines because their pH levels are lower than those needed for bacterial growth. Vegetables are more susceptible to bacterial or fungal decomposition because they typically have pH values lower than fruits. On the other hand, most meats and seafood have pH values of 5 or higher, which means that bacteria, fungi, and yeasts can break them down.

- Oxidation-reduction potential

An indicator of a substrate's ability to oxidize and reduce is its oxidation-reduction potential (O/R). Put another way, O/R potential can be broadly defined as the ease with which a substrate gains or loses electrons (a food product is reduced when it gains electrons, but oxidizes when it loses them; consequently, a food product that easily gives electrons is a good reducing agent and the one that receives electrons is a good oxidizing agent). Certain microorganisms need reducing conditions, while others need oxidizing conditions, to grow to their maximum potential. When electrons are transferred from one compound to another, a potential difference is created between the two compounds; this difference can be measured and expressed as millivolts [mV]). This difference can be used to express the O/R potential of a system. An electrical potential is more positively correlated with the degree of oxidation of a substance and more negatively correlated with its degree of reduction. There is no electrical potential when the oxidant and reducer concentrations are equal.

Aerobic saprophytes are those that can transfer hydrogen as H^+ and e- (electron) to molecular oxygen; in other words, anaerobic microorganisms grow best in environments with negative Eh values (reduced), while aerobic microorganisms grow best in those with positive Eh values (oxidized). Any of the conditions can support the growth of facultative microorganisms. The lowest and maximum Eh values (in mV) required for both aerobic and anaerobic growth must be considered as they may be fatal to the opposing group. Food ingredients like ascorbic acid, reducing sugars in fruits and vegetables, and the -SH groups in meats all aid in maintaining reducing conditions. Certain aerobic bacteria, referred to as microaerophiles, like Lactobacillus and Campylobacter, thrive in conditions that are somewhat less oxygenated.

Although some tend to be facultative anaerobes, most yeasts and fungi found in food are aerobic. Given that vegetables, especially juices, typically have Eh values between +300 and +400 mV, it is not shocking to learn that aerobic bacteria and fungi are frequently responsible for the decomposition of these kinds of products. Eh values in meats are typically −200 mV, while in ground meats, they are typically +200 mV. The Eh values of different kinds of cheese range from -20 to -200 mV.

- Content of nutrients

The majority of microorganisms have nutritional needs, and since these can be met by eating food, they will flourish given the correct circumstances. These needs include nitrogen, energy, minerals, vitamins, and related growth factors. The least demanding microorganisms on nutrients are generally fungi, then yeasts, Gram-negative bacteria, and finally, Gram-positive bacteria. Amino acids are the main sources of nitrogen that heterotrophic microorganisms use. Many different kinds of organisms may use a large number of different nitrogen compounds for this purpose. For instance, whereas some of them are able to use peptides and proteins, others are able to use free nucleotides and amino acids. Most organisms will typically use simpler substances like amino acids before going after more complex ones like high molecular weight proteins. Lipids and polysaccharides are comparable in this regard.

Food microorganisms typically use sugars, alcohols, and amino acids as energy sources. Because fungi have enzymes that can hydrolyze proteins, complex carbohydrates, and lipids into simpler components, they are the most efficient users of these materials. Many bacteria can also do this, but most yeasts need simpler molecules. Minerals are necessary for all microorganisms, while their vitamin needs differ. Some bacteria and fungi are able to produce enough B vitamins on their own, but others require a source of these nutrients, and food products are a great way to provide them. Gram-positive bacteria require one or more of these substances to grow because they have a lower capacity for synthesis. On the other hand, because they can synthesize most, if not all, of their requirements, gram-negative bacteria and fungi can grow in food products that have low B vitamin contents.

6.3.2.2. Extrinsic parameters

Microorganisms develop primarily due to food factors, which can be either extrinsic or external. This phrase refers to environmental elements that influence the rate at which microorganisms grow; these elements include temperature, relative humidity, oxygen availability, and the existence and activity of other microorganisms.

- Storage temperature

Microorganisms can only grow within a certain range, which includes both minimum and maximum temperatures. As a result, in addition to determining the rate of proliferation, ambient temperature also influences the genera of microorganisms that will proliferate and the level of microbial activity that is observed. A few degrees difference in temperature will promote the growth of entirely different organisms, which will lead to a distinct kind of food decomposition and/or foodborne illness. These qualities make thermal treatment a useful tool for managing microbial activity. While certain genera develop below 0°C and other genera grow at temperatures above 100°C, most microorganisms proliferate best at temperatures between 14 and 40°C. Nevertheless, when choosing a storage temperature, food quality must be considered. While it may seem ideal to store all food items at temperatures that are comparable to or lower than those of refrigeration, this is not the best way to preserve the desired quality of some food items, like bananas, whose quality is best preserved in storage at 13–17°C rather than 5–7°C. Similarly, many vegetables—including potatoes, celery, cabbage, and many others—benefit from temperatures close to 10°C. In all situations, the success of the storage temperature is largely dependent on the relative humidity and the existence or absence of gases like ozone and carbon dioxide.

- Oxygen availability and presence of other gases in the environment

The microorganisms that will be active are determined by oxygen availability, just like by temperature. Some can only grow in the complete absence of oxygen, while others can grow in both the presence and absence of the gas. Microorganisms classified as aerobic are those that need free oxygen to grow, anaerobic are those that can survive without it, and facultative microorganisms are those that can grow in both conditions. The most significant atmospheric gas for managing food microbes is carbon dioxide. It is used in food packaging with a modified atmosphere along with oxygen. Another antimicrobial gas found in the atmosphere is ozone, which has been used for decades to extend the shelf life of some food varieties. It works well against a wide range of microorganisms, but because it is a strong oxidizer, it should not be used in food products that contain a lot of fat because it may hasten rancidity. Normal air ozone levels range from 0 to 5 parts per million, which inhibits the growth of yeast and some bacteria that break down food.

- Relative humidity in the environment

Regarding the water activity of a food item and the development of microorganisms on surfaces, the relative humidity (RH) of the surrounding air is crucial. Temperature is one extrinsic factor that influences microbial growth. Microorganisms require a high concentration of water to grow and function. When a food product's A_w is set at 0.60, it's critical that it be stored in relative humidity (RH) conditions that prevent it from absorbing humidity from the air. This prevents the food from increasing its own A_w from the surface and subsurface to a point where microbiological growth can occur. Food, equipment, walls, and ceilings can all experience humidity condensation because of high relative humidity. Wet surfaces from condensation encourage microbial growth and breakdown. Lower relative humidity inhibits the growth of microorganisms. Food products that have low relative humidity (A_w) absorb moisture until they reach equilibrium when they are placed in high RH environments. Similar to this, food items with a high A_w lose moisture when exposed to low relative humidity. RH and temperature have a relationship that needs to be considered when choosing the right storage conditions for food products. In general, RH decreases with increasing temperature and vice versa.

- Presence and activities of other microorganisms

Hydrogen peroxide, organic acids, bacteriocins, antibiotics, and other substances that can inhibit or kill other organisms are produced by certain organisms that are found in food. The lactic acid-producing bacteria that produce bacteriocins, which are found in meat and other food products, are highly sought-after. Gram-positive bacteria produce bacteriocins, which are physiologically active proteins with bactericidal properties. These bacteria produce certain bacteriocins that inhibit a range of food pathogens, such as *B. cereus*, as well as *Listeria* spp., *A. hydrophila* as well as *S. aureus*. Food products typically find their way to the final customer through restaurants, community dining rooms, or homes. At these places, precautions against food poisoning should be taken, especially in areas where large amounts of food are distributed, like vacuum cooking, cold chain, frozen chain, and hot chain. In the hot chain, such as a buffet, food is kept at temperatures above 65°C and should be consumed within a maximum of 12 h. Similarly, in the frozen chain, food is gradually lowered to −18°C and defrosted at temperatures higher than 65°C at the time it will be served to the customer (not earlier).

The use of chemical or physical food preservation techniques is another crucial precaution. Traditional or industrial pasteurization, dehydration, preservation in a modified atmosphere, and radiation are examples of physical methods. Microbial markers can be used to ensure proper quality control and reduce the risk of food poisoning. While many of these markers do not pose a health risk, they do point to deficiencies in the hygienic and sanitary quality of food products, which can also shorten their shelf life and be linked to the presence of pathogenic microorganisms. Enterococci, total coliforms, fecal coliforms, aerobic mesophilic, and *E. coli* are the primary microbial markers, as well as *S. aureus*. Following the identification of risk factors, a system that prevents and reduces each one must be put in place. To do this, a method known as Hazard Analysis and Critical Control Point (HACCP) was developed, which has a scientific foundation and a systematic profile. A microbiological approach should take into account the kind of microorganism or metabolite (toxins) that pose a health risk to humans, the analytical techniques for identifying and quantifying it, the quantity of samples that must be collected, the dimensions of the analytical unit, and the microbiological limits that are thought to be sufficient at particular food chain points.

6.3.3. Foodborne Diseases

A variety of toxins, including those caused by bacteria, fungi (mycotoxins), plants, algae, and metals, as well as hazardous chemicals (pesticides, zinc, and copper) and physical contaminants, can be found in food products and result in the well-known "foodborne diseases" that affect those who consume them.

Foodborne diseases can be classified into two groups: poisoning and infection.

- **Poisoning** is caused by the intake of chemical or biological toxins; or toxins produced by pathogens, the latter can be found in food, even if the bacterium is not there.
- **Infection** is caused by the intake of food containing viable pathogens. Furthermore, a toxic infection (toxicoinfection), formerly known as a toxin-mediated infection, is caused by eating food with bacteria that grow and produce a toxin inside the body.

Microorganisms in food thrive in the right conditions and release toxins. Toxins are absorbed through the intestinal epithelial lining when contaminated food is consumed, resulting in local tissue damage. Toxins can potentially cause harm when they get to organs like the kidney or liver, the central nervous system, or the peripheral nervous system. Diarrhea, vomiting, headaches, nausea, pain, fever, diarrhea with mucus and blood (dysentery), and rectal tenesmus are the most typical clinical symptoms of foodborne illnesses. Tables 6.4 to 6.6 list some of the microorganisms that can result in foodborne illnesses through poisoning, intoxication, or toxicoinfection. These illnesses are typically identified by looking at the clinical history or symptoms of the patient.

Table 6.4. *Pathogens that Cause Infection*

Bacteria	Disease/Medical Complications	Food Products Involved
Salmonella enterica serovar Typhi and *Salmonella enterica serovar Paratyphi*	Typhoid and paratyphoid fever.	Undercooked pork, beef and poultry, contaminated eggs, and milk.
Salmonella spp.	Salmonellosis (*Salmonella* Typhimurium, *Salmonella* Enteritidis).	Undercooked poultry, cauliflowers, and tomatoes.
Vibrio vulnificus	Septicemia in people with underlying diseases or people who are taking immunosuppressive drugs or steroids.	Seafood, usually oysters.
Mycobacterium bovis	Cervical lymphadenopathy, intestinal lesions, and chronic cutaneous tuberculosis.	Contaminated milk.
Mycobacterium avium, subspecies *paratuberculosis*	Crohn's disease.	Pasteurized milk.
Listeria monocytogenes	Meningitis, encephalitis, sepsis in pregnant women, intrauterine or cervical infection that can lead to miscarriage or birth of a dead child.	Raw beef, pork, poultry, vegetables and milk, cheese, ice cream, smoked fish, and raw fish.

Source: https://www.intechopen.com/chapters/56521.

Table 6.5. *Pathogens that Cause Intoxication*

Bacteria	Disease/Medical Complications	Food Products Involved
Clostridium botulinum	Paralysis of arms, legs, trunk, and respiratory muscles.	Mixture of oil and nonacid garlic, potatoes cooked at high temperatures, and stews.
Bacillus cereus	Fried rice syndrome.	Rice cooked at high temperatures, sauces, soups, and puddings.
Staphylococcus aureus	Toxic shock syndrome.	Meat and meat products cooked at high temperatures, poultry, and salads with mayonnaise.

Source: https://www.intechopen.com/chapters/56521.

Table 6.6. *Pathogens that Cause Toxico-Infection*

Bacteria	Disease/Medical Complications	Food Products Involved
Escherichia coli 0157:H7	Hemorrhagic colitis, Hemolytic *uremic syndrome in children.*	Hamburgers, nonpasteurized milk, contaminated water, spinach, and lettuce.
Shigella spp.	Hemolytic Uremic Syndrome.	Salads, lettuce, raw vegetables, and milk.

Aeromonas spp.	Meningitis, peritonitis, myocarditis, hemolytic uremic syndrome, necrotizing fasciitis in wounds.	Meat (beef, sheep, pork and chicken), vegetables, eggs, fish, seafood, and prepared food.
Cronobacter sakazakii	Permanent neurological or developmental deficits; death.	Powdered infant formula.
Vibrio parahaemolyticus	Gastroenteritis, septicemia and wound infection. Severe infections in immunocompromised people.	Raw or undercooked seafood, usually oysters.
Clostridium perfringens	Clostridial necrotizing enteritis.	Meat juice, stews, cooked beans, meat cooked at high temperatures.
Campylobacter spp.	Campylobacteriosis, arthritis, meningitis, *Campylobacter jejuni* can cause Guillain-Barré Syndrome.	Cheese made with raw milk and chicken meat.
Yersinia enterocolitica	Yersiniosis, enterocolitis, pseudoappendicitis, mesenteric lymphadenitis, infections in wounds, joints and the urinary tract, and Reiter's syndrome.	Nonpasteurized milk, tofu, nonchlorinated water, undercooked meat, oysters and fish.
Vibrio cholerae serogroup O1 or serogroup O139	Cholera.	Contaminated water and raw seafood.
V. cholerae serogroup no-O1	Less severe than cholera; gastrointestinal infections, sepsis.	Raw, semicooked or recontaminated fish and shellfish after cooking.

Source: https://www.intechopen.com/chapters/56521.

Toxins produced by pathogens involved in foodborne diseases have different characteristics, some of them are shown in Table 6.7.

Table 6.7. *Main Toxins Produced by Pathogens Involved in Foodborne Diseases and their Biological Effect*

Name	Biological Effect
Cholera toxin (Ctx) (A-5B)	It activates the adenylyl cyclase; increases the levels of intracellular cAMP promoting fluid, and electrolytes secretion in the intestinal epithelium, causing diarrhea. It is a potent exotoxin.
Thermolabile toxin (LT) (A-5B)	Similar effect as the Cholera toxin.
Thermostable toxin (ST)	The binding of ST to the guanylyl cyclase receptor results in an increase of cyclic GMP, affecting the flow of electrolytes. It promotes water and electrolytes secretion from the intestinal epithelium by causing diarrhea.
Shiga toxin (A-5B)	Inactivates the ribosomal subunit 60S and inhibits protein synthesis causing the death of susceptible cells.
Botulinum toxin (A/B)	It is a neurotoxin consisting of a heavy and a light chain linked by a disulfide bond. It is a Zn^{++}-dependent protease. It inhibits the presynaptic release of acetylcholine from peripheral cholinergic neurons, resulting in flaccid paralysis. The neurotoxin exists in seven different serotypes (A-G).

CPE enterotoxin	Lethal, cytotoxic, and enterotoxic activity. Stimulates the adenylyl cyclase allowing the increase of cAMP in epithelial cells, which causes diarrhea.
Alpha-toxin	It produces gas gangrene. It has phospholipase (PLC), sphingomyelinase, hemolytic, and dermonecrotic activities. The mature protein is organized into two domains; the amino-terminal, which contains the PLC activity, and the carboxyl-terminal binding, which depends on calcium. Depending on the lipid composition of the cell membrane, the alpha-toxin may be hemolytic in the presence of calcium.
Beta-toxin	It forms selective pores for monovalent cations in lipid bilayers and sensitive cells membranes, so it functions as a neurotoxin capable of producing arterial constriction.
Epsilon-toxin	Produced and secreted by a prototoxin that, when it suffers a specific proteolytic cleavage, it acquires its maximum biological activity. Activation can be catalyzed by proteases such as trypsin, chymotrypsin, and a zinc-dependent metalloproteinase.
Iota-toxin	It has dermonecrotic, cytotoxic, enterotoxic activities, and it causes intestinal histopathological damage. This toxin is binary and consists of a binding peptide (Ib) and an enzymatic peptide (ADP-ribosyltransferase) (Ia). The first one is necessary to internalize the second one. The Iota-toxin requires proteolytic removal of a propeptide fragment, which allows the Ib unit to be inserted into the membrane and to interact with the Ia portion to form a heptameric pore that allows the K^+ and Na^+ ions to escape; in addition to the Ia portion entrance into the cell where it ribosylates the G-actin to depolymerize the actin filaments, with the consequent destruction of the cytoskeleton. The Iota-toxin is generally activated by the effect of the proteases present in the intestinal tract.
Toxin A/Toxin B	It modifies the Rho, a subfamily of GTP-binding proteins that regulate cytoskeletal actin. The deamination of the glutamine residue at position 63 of Rho to a glutamic acid produces a dominant-active Rho protein incapable of hydrolyzing the GTP, resulting in cellular necrosis and bloody diarrhea associated with colitis.
Enterotoxins (A, B, C1, C2, D and E, G, H, I, J)	Enterotoxins are thermostable; they differ in toxicity. Staphylococcal enterotoxins are superantigens that cause massive activation of the immune system, including lymphocytes and macrophages; the exact role in emesis is not known.
Toxic Shock Syndrome Toxin (TSST-1)	Superantigen that acts on the vascular system causing inflammation, fever, and shock.
Cereulide	Thermostable peptide, toxic for the mitochondria when acting as a potassium ionophore.
HBL, NHE, Citotoxin K or CytK	HBL is a three-component hemolysin; two protein subunits, L2 and L1 (cytolytic components), and a B protein (favors binding to the host cell), apart from the hemolytic effect, it is cytotoxic, dermonecrotic and causes vascular permeability. NHE also consists of three components (NheA is a cytolytic component and NhB and NheC favor binding to cells of small intestine). Both toxins are organized into operons (*hbl* and *nhe*), where the genes encoded the NHE components are transcribed together. CytK forms pores in the epithelial cells membrane, and it has necrotizing and cytotoxic activity.

Note: A-5B indicates that the subunits are separately synthesized but associated by noncovalent bonds during secretion and binding to target. 5B indicates that the binding domain of the protein is composed by five identical subunits. A/B denotes a toxin synthesized as a simple polypeptide divided into domains A and B that can be separated by proteolytic cleavage. HBL: hemolysin BL, NHE: nonhemolytic enterotoxin.

Source: https://www.intechopen.com/chapters/56521.

6.3.3.1. Foodborne diseases caused by bacterial toxins

This section will be addressed to some diseases caused by consuming food contaminated with bacterial toxins or microorganisms that produce them. Among some of the most important diseases are the ones transmitted by *V. cholerae, S. aureus, B. cereus C. perfringens, C. botulinum and Listeria monocytogenes.*

- Vibrio cholerae

V. cholerae has a free life cycle, is common in aquatic environments, and can persist in its virulence without proliferating in both fresh and saltwater for extended periods. They can be isolated in fish and seafood and are more common in temperate waters. Serogroups *V. cholerae* O1 and O139 are the most noteworthy species that cause the disease. The remaining strains of the species, including non-O1, also frequently result in extraintestinal infections, but their diarrheal syndromes are not as severe as cholera. V's primary virulence factor is the CTX toxin, also known as the Cholera toxin, cholerae O1 (Ogawa, Inaba, and Hikojima serotypes, Classical and El Tor biotypes) and O139; following an incubation period of two to five days, it contributes to the development of profuse diarrhea; the stools have the consistency of rice water, and there is an electrolyte imbalance and dehydration that can be fatal. Since the pathogen can spread to other people, about 75% of infected individuals do not exhibit the previously listed symptoms. Despite this, the pathogen is excreted in their feces for 7–14 days, making it a very serious source of contamination. The most susceptible demographics are adults, children, and HIV-positive individuals.

The existence of the ctxAB gene identifies this toxin. V. Although the ctx gene is present in cholerae no-O1, it is rarely expressed. Despite this, there is currently no quicker test available, and the WHO is working to validate new rapid diagnoses. Using laboratory techniques, the bacteria can be separated and identified from stool samples. The key to effective treatment is timely rehydration with intravenous or oral solutions. Antibiotics should only be used in cases of severe dehydration. Enough sanitation, a steady supply of clean drinking water, and food security are necessary to stop the spread of cholera. Furthermore, the need for vaccine administration has arisen from the inadequacy of control measures to prevent contamination; oral vaccines have been developed as a means of averting outbreaks. In places where the disease is endemic, these vaccinations are administered to more susceptible populations. Experience with various mass vaccination campaigns in nations like Mozambique, Indonesia, Sudan, and Zanzibar makes it abundantly evident that vaccination cannot be improvised at the last minute; rather, it requires careful and early planning and preparation. The Cholera Toxin Subunit B (CTB) is a relatively easily manageable adjuvant due to its lack of toxicity, stability, and ease of expression. The application potential of proteins is further expanded by their ability to be expressed in a wide range of organisms. Currently, CTB is utilized in vaccinations like the *V. cholerae* vaccine Dukoral made up of recombinant CTB and dead bacteria. Given its great adjuvant effect, this protein has been approved for use as a vaccine adjuvant in both Europe and Canada. As a result, it is expected to play a significant role in vaccine formulation going forward.

- Staphylococcus aureus

One of the most prevalent illnesses that *S. aureus* contracts is a foodborne Staphylococcus infection. This is one of the diseases that public health programs around the world are most concerned about; it is caused by bacteria producing one or more toxins while growing at permissive temperatures; however, the amount of toxin consumed determines how long the disease takes to incubate. The disease can be brought on by small doses of enterotoxins; large outbreaks have been reported to be brought on by a concentration of 0–5 ng/mL in contaminated chocolate milk. *S. aureus* generates a range of toxins. The nine thermostable enterotoxin serotypes that make up the Staphylococcal enterotoxin family are part of a larger family of pyrogenic toxins, or superantigens. Immunosuppression and nonspecific T-cell proliferation can be brought on by pyrogenic toxins. Because enterotoxins are so stable, they can withstand freezing and drying temperatures, which makes them ideal for use in industrial settings. Additionally, they can remain completely active in the digestive tract following infection because they are resistant to the proteolytic enzymes trypsin and pepsin at low pH. The exact mechanism through which poisoning occurs is still unknown. On the other hand, it has been noted that enterotoxins directly impact the vagus nerve and the intestinal epithelium, stimulating the emetic center. According to estimates, humans can become poisoned by staphylococci by consuming 0–1 µg of enterotoxins. In addition to poisoning, because *S. aureus* produces enterotoxin type B and toxic shock syndrome toxin 1 (TSST-1), it can also cause toxic shock syndrome.

Nausea, vomiting, cramps in the abdomen, salivation, and diarrhea may or may not be present are among the symptoms. The most typical symptoms are the first three. It is typically a self-limiting illness that resolves in 24 to 48 h, but it can worsen, particularly in young children, the elderly, and those with weakened immune systems. High fever, hypotension, erythematous rash (similar to scarlet fever), skin peeling during recovery, flu-like symptoms, vomiting, and diarrhea are the hallmarks of toxic shock syndrome.

The staphylococcal enterotoxin in the food or the recovery of at least 105105 *Staphylococcus aureus* per gram derived from food waste are used to diagnose the illness. . Numerous techniques, including molecular biology, immunological methods, and bioassays, can be used to detect the enterotoxin. Pulsed-field electrophoresis and multilocus sequences from the spa or SCCmec gene can be used to genetically characterize the isolated strains. When food products were involved in outbreaks, that's where S. Meat and its byproducts, poultry and eggs, milk and its byproducts, salads, and bakery goods (cream-filled cakes and stuffed sandwiches) are stores at room temperature, which allows aureus to grow at its best.

The rise of methicillin-resistant strains, which can be found in food (primarily in meat and milk), is another factor that needs to be considered. It is crucial to remember that many isolates recovered from outbreaks are not examined for antibiotic susceptibility; nevertheless, given the range of issues these strains can cause, the test ought to be carried out. They have been implicated as the cause of blood infection outbreaks and wounds in hospitalized immunocompromised patients. The foodborne disease caused by *S. aureus* might be avoidable. Food products could be cooked above 60°C and refrigerated below 5°C since it is known that the temperature range between 6 and 46°C is acceptable for the growth and production of the enzyme. Thus, keeping the food cold chain in place can stop the microorganism from growing. By employing hygienic and safe manufacturing procedures, the contamination by *S. aureus* is possible to stop.

- Bacillus cereus

B. cereus is a common environmental microorganism that can easily contaminate any system used in the processing or production of food because it forms endospores. Both pasteurization and cooking procedures will not harm the bacteria. Three enterotoxins, hemolysin BL (HBL), nonhemolytic (NHE), and cytotoxin K (CytK), which cause the emetic syndrome and diarrhea, as well as three phospholipases, phosphatidylinositol hydrolase, phosphatidylcholine hydrolase, and hemolytic sphingomyelinase, have been shown to be produced by this microorganism. Cereulide is a thermostable cyclic peptide that binds to the serotonin receptor to stimulate the afferent vagal pathway, which in turn induces vomiting. Over time, the toxin builds up in food and is produced by the microorganism during its stationary growth phase. The toxin's structural makeup accounts for its resistance to food processing techniques. The proteins that form enterotoxins, binding and lithic factors, cannot pass through the gastric barrier intact, which is why it is thought that preformed or extracellular enterotoxins in food are not involved in the pathogenesis of the bacterium. In contrast, the thermolabile enterotoxins, HBL and NHE, produced inside the host's small intestine during the exponential phase of the bacterium's vegetative growth, are the cause of diarrheal syndrome. The spores that germinate reaches the small intestine are thought to be the cause of diarrhea, as is the growth and concurrent production of the enterotoxin. Three components make up HBL, a hemolysin that causes vascular permeability and has hemolytic, cytotoxic, and dermonecrotic effects. The two protein subunits (L2 and L1) and the one B protein make up HBL. Three additional components make up NHE: NheA, NheB, and NheC. It's been shown that strains that produce emetic toxins don't also produce enterotoxins. The cytotoxin K is similar to the Alpha-toxin of *S. aureus* and the Beta-toxin of *C. perfringens*.

In addition, the 45 kDa polypeptide known as enterotoxin FM (EntFM), which is encoded by the bacterial chromosome's entFM gene, has been described. Although it hasn't been directly linked to food poisoning, the gene has been found in strains that spread diarrhea; in mice and rabbit experiments, it causes vascular permeability. The vomiting and nausea associated with the emetic syndrome are akin to those caused by S. poisoning by Aureus. Soon after eating food contaminated with the preformed toxin, symptoms start to manifest. Poisoning typically starts with mild symptoms that go away after a day or two, but more serious cases need to be hospitalized. The diarrhea resulting from of the secretory variety, much like the kind that V produces. cholerae. Pain from colic is comparable to that from *C. perfringens* poisoning. It is a self-limiting syndrome. By looking for these gene (nonribosomal production of cereulide); by detecting the hblD, hblC, and hblA genes encoding the L1, L2, and B protein components of the HBL toxin, respectively; or by detecting the nheA, nheB, and nheC genes of the NHE toxin components, enterotoxins can be identified by immunoassays or molecular biology (conventional PCR and multiplex PCR). A real-time PCR test can be used to search for the 16S ribosomal gene.

In addition to resulting in food poisoning, *B. cereus* can also result in systemic and local infections in patients who are immunocompromised, in neonates, in drug users, in patients who have had surgery or trauma, or in patients who are catheterized. Foods high in starch content, such as flours, meats, milk, cheese, vegetables, fish, and rice and its derivatives, are the most likely to become contaminated. While there have been studies showing that the emetic toxin can be found in a variety of food products, the strains that produce diarrheagenic toxins thrive in a wide range of food products, from vegetables to sauces and stews. The strains that produce emetic toxin grow well in rice dishes (fried and cooked) and other starchy products. Strains obtained from infections are susceptible to gentamicin, vancomycin, clindamycin, erythromycin, and streptomycin; however, they are resistant to β-lactam antibiotics, such as third-generation cephalosporins. The main causes of food poisoning by *B. cereus* are inadequate cooking temperatures, contaminated equipment, and unhygienic conditions at the locations where food is processed and prepared. cereus and its toxins; for this reason, it is advised to cook food at temperatures higher than 100°C or to store it at temperatures lower than 4°C. Food should also be quickly warmed or cooled to reduce the likelihood of potential poisoning and to prevent prolonged exposure to temperatures that promote spore germination.

- Clostridium perfringens

The anaerobic bacterium *C. perfringens* produces spores that can live in soil, sediments, and places where animal and human waste can contaminate surfaces. It is widely dispersed throughout the environment and is regularly discovered in the intestines of both domestic and wild animals, including humans. Because *C. perfringens* produces four distinct toxins (alpha, beta, epsilon, and iota), it is categorized into five groups (A, B, C, D, and E). Each of the five groups produces the alpha-toxin. The beta-toxin acts as a neurotoxin that can constrict blood vessels by creating specific pores in lipid bilayers for monovalent ions. After tetanus and botulinum neurotoxins, the epsilon-toxin is the most potent clostridial toxin (BoNTs). It is created and secreted by a prototoxin that requires a particular proteolytic cleavage to reach its peak biological activity. Trypsin, chymotrypsin, and a zinc metalloprotease can all catalyze this process.

Though its exact nature is unknown, the toxin receptor is known to be a surface protein that is secured by glycosylphosphatidylinositol. Its primary biological activity is the generation of edema; it is hemolytically non-lethal. Since the binding peptide (Ib) required for the internalization of the enzymatic peptide (Ia; ADP-ribosyltransferase) forms the Iota-toxin, it belongs to the family of binary toxins. Ib cannot be inserted into the membrane and cannot interact with Ia without the proteolytic removal of a propeptide fragment. Once inside the cell, Ia is ribosylated by G-actin, which depolymerizes Actin filaments by breaking down the cytoskeleton of the cell. Ib, when inserted into the membrane, forms a heptameric pore that permits the exit of K+ and Na+ ions and the entry of Ia. Iota-toxin causes enterotoxic, cytotoxic, dermonecrotic, and histopathologically-damaging effects on the intestinal tract. But this bacterium's virulence isn't just caused by these four toxins; Type A strains of the bacteria also produce 15 other toxins, among which the CPE enterotoxin, which causes diarrhea in humans and animals, is found. The NetB toxin is often linked to necrotic enteritis in birds, and the Beta2-toxin is reportedly linked to enteritis. This toxin is associated with 5 or 15% of gastrointestinal diseases in humans, distinct from food poisoning, such as diarrhea brought on by antibiotics. Sporotization is linked to the digestive tract's toxin production. Only one case has raised the possibility of poisoning from the preformed toxin, indicating that the disease is foodborne.

C. perfringens is responsible for causing food poisoning, which is characterized by severe abdominal cramps and diarrhea occurring 8–22 h after consuming contaminated food. The illness typically lasts for 24 h, but in some cases, symptoms can persist for 1–2 weeks. In more severe cases, ingestion of food containing type C strains of the bacteria can lead to necrotic enteritis, also known as pig-bel disease, which can be fatal. Deaths from necrotic enteritis are often caused by intestinal infection, necrosis, and septicemia, with elderly individuals being at higher risk. Diagnosis of the disease involves detecting the presence of toxins in the stools of patients, using traditional culture methods or molecular techniques to identify specific genes like cpe, plc, and etx.

Meat and products derived from it are among the principal food products in question. If the food is cooked correctly, it can prevent the disease; however, there is a chance of cross-contamination if the cooked food comes into contact with raw or contaminated ingredients or contaminated surfaces. For infections brought on by the toxins of the bacteria, there is no known treatment or remedy. Intravenous fluids, oral rehydration salt solutions, and pain and fever medication are examples of supportive care. The surgical debridement and removal of the affected tissue, along with the high doses of antibiotics, are the mainstays of treatment for gas gangrene. Penicillin G, metronidazole, or chloramphenicol are the systemic treatments for necrotizing enterocolitis; a segmental jejunum resection is the surgical procedure of choice in 50% of cases. The antibiotics that are active against anaerobic bacteria are effective; however, since some strains of bacteria are resistant to penicillin and clindamycin, antimicrobial susceptibility testing should be done, particularly on patients who need long-term care or who have severe illnesses.

- Clostridium botulinum

C. botulinum is a spore-forming microorganism that can remain viable for long periods in unfavorable environmental conditions. There are four groups of *C. botulinum*, with seven antigenic variants of botulinum neurotoxins (A–G). Groups I and II are the main causes of botulism in humans, while Group III causes botulism in several animal species, and Group IV is not associated with the disease in either humans or animals. Group I, also known as *C. botulinum*-proteolytic, forms highly heat-resistant spores, while Group II, known as *C. botulinum*-non-proteolytic, forms moderately heat-resistant spores. Different groups produce different neurotoxins, with some being more common in causing disease in animals than in humans. Botulinum toxins are metalloproteins with endopeptidase activity that require zinc for function. The toxins have a general structure with two chains, one heavy and one lighter, each with specific functions in causing botulism.

C. botulinum is a bacteria known for producing the botulinum toxin. Group II strains can have varying numbers of genes that code for different neurotoxins, with possibilities ranging from one to three genes producing one to three neurotoxins. Some strains may have both active and inactive toxins. In Type F strains, the toxin can have characteristics of Type B and Type E neurotoxins. The neurotoxins form complexes with accessory proteins that protect and help them enter the host cells. Some strains have been found to produce multiple botulinum toxins, such as F4, F5, and A2. The significance and evolutionary consequences of producing multiple toxins are still unclear. Evidence suggests horizontal gene transfer plays a role in toxin production, but the differences between Group I and Group II strains remain unclear. Research on toxins isolated from various *C. botulinum* groups is ongoing.

A serious illness with a high death rate is botulism. Common symptoms include flaccid muscle paralysis; occasionally, blurred vision precedes an acute symmetrical decrease of bilateral paralysis, which can progress to respiratory and cardiac muscle paralysis if left untreated. After months or even years, the patient's condition may improve if the severe case is not fatal. Foodborne botulism, wound botulism, and intestinal botulism in infants and adults are the three varieties of botulism. The first type, known as infant/adult intestinal botulism, is an infection linked to the growth of microorganisms and the formation of neurotoxins in the intestines; the second, known as wound botulism, is an infection linked to the growth of cells and the formation of toxins in the wound, frequently acquired following drug abuse; and the third, known as foodborne botulism, is a poisoning brought on by ingesting neurotoxins produced in food. Toxin concentrations as low as 30 ng are sufficient to induce illness and occasionally even death. The onset of symptoms is usually between 2 and 8 days following the consumption of tainted food, though they can also sometimes happen between 12 and 72 h.

Only clinical symptoms can be used to diagnose botulism, and it can be challenging to distinguish it from other illnesses. The best and most straightforward method for verifying the condition in a lab setting is to show that the toxin is present in the patient's serum, feces, or food items. Neutralization in a rodent is one of the most sensitive and popular ways to find the toxin. The culture of the specimens takes five to seven days, and the test takes 48 h. The diagnosis of infant botulism is made by looking for the microbe and botulinum toxins in children's feces. Among the documented cases, 90% are linked to the consumption of homemade preserved foods, particularly veggies; industrial meat and fish preparation is hardly ever linked to botulism. A variety of food items, including canned corn, pepper, soups, beets, asparagus, ripe olives, spinach, tuna chicken, chicken liver, ham, sausages, stuffed eggplants, lobster, and honey, have the bacteria or botulinum toxin spores present. It is essential to take the proper precautions when handling and processing food to reduce the risk of contracting botulism, particularly when new or modified technologies are involved. In the current industry, the "botulinum cook" method makes canned goods possible. Chlorine and chlorinated compounds are useful for sanitizing areas where food is handled industrially. Moreover, ozone and ethylene oxide can be used to deactivate spores.

6.3.3.2. Listeria Monocytogenes

L. monocytogenes is a facultative intracellular microorganism widely distributed in nature, capable of surviving both in the soil and the cytosol of a eukaryotic cell. Considering somatic (O) and flagellar (H) antigens, this bacterium can be classified into 13 serotypes (1/2a, 1/2b, 1/2c, 3a, 3b, 3c, 4a, 4b, 4b, 4c, 4d, 4e, 7), but only the serotypes 1/2a, 1/2b, and 4b are responsible for more than 98% of the cases of human listeriosis. Furthermore, it has also been grouped into four lineages (I, II, III, and IV), where lineage I (serotypes: 1/2b, 3b, and 4b) and lineage II (serotypes: 1/2a, 1/2c, 3a, and 3c) include most strains isolated from clinical cases; lineage I strains have a greater pathogenic potential. Lineages III and IV include strains of serotypes 4a, 4c, and an atypical 4b.

L. monocytogenes expresses multiple virulence factors, which allow to enter and survive in several nonphagocytic cells. Following cellular internalization, the bacteria escape from the endocytic vesicle into the cytoplasm, where they divide and submit the F-actin in accordance with their mobility to spread from cell to cell. This process is mediated by listeriolysin O (LLO) and two phospholipases. The cholesterol-dependent toxin known as LLO, which is encoded by the hly gene, can create holes in phagosome membranes that let L. monocytogenes to evade the inner and outer vacuoles. A phosphatidylinositol phospholipase C (PI-PLC), which has phosphatidylinositol as its substrate, and a phosphatidylcholine phospholipase C (PC-PLC), a lecithinase with enzymatic activity over phosphatidylcholine, phosphatidylserine, and phosphatidylethanolamine, both increase the cytolytic activity of LLO. Since zinc-dependent metalloprotease Mpl is necessary for the maturation of PC-PLC, which is expressed as a protoenzyme, the bacterium can obtain the nutrients it needs for intracellular multiplication once it is freed in the cytosol. Research has indicated that LLO plays a crucial role in invasion processes by breaking through the host cell's plasma membrane and initiating the bacterium's internalization in human hepatocytes. Additionally, other research has demonstrated that LLO is unable to mediate L's intracellular survival. monocytogenes in neutrophils, whereupon early degranulation triggers the release of proteases, including matrix metalloproteinase-8, which eliminates LLO and prevents membrane perforation.

L. monocytogenes causes a severe infection known as listeriosis, which is usually acquired after the intake of food contaminated with the microorganism. It is uncommon for the disease to strike anyone who is not in one of the aforementioned categories because it primarily affects pregnant women, newborns, the elderly, and immunocompromised individuals. In pregnant women, listeriosis is a mild disease; however, in fetuses and newborns, it is severe. Immunocompromised individuals and those over 65 are at risk of developing bloodstream infections (sepsis) or brain infections (encephalitis or meningitis). The infection can occasionally impact the abdomen, thorax, joints, and bones. Rarely is listeriosis diagnosed, although it can cause fever and diarrhea similar to other foodborne microorganisms. Listeria pregnancy symptoms include fever, exhaustion, and soreness in the muscles. The organism can result in early labor, stillbirth, miscarriage, and infection in the fetus during pregnancy. The symptoms in the other risk groups include headaches, stiff necks, dizziness, loss of balance, seizures, fever, and sore muscles. Although symptoms have been reported 70 days after exposure or even the day of the poisoning, invasive listeriosis usually manifests 1 to 4 weeks after eating food contaminated with the bacterium. The bacterium is typically cultured from tissues or fluids, such as blood, cerebrospinal fluid, or placenta, in order to diagnose the illness. This microbe can be identified from food products using a variety of techniques, including the use of chromogenic media, immunological techniques (some of which are nonspecific), molecular techniques (hybridization, PCR, and real-time PCR), microarrays or biosensors, and particular commercial techniques. The plcA virulence gene, which codes for PI-PLC, is typically found and used to distinguish between hemolytic and nonhemolytic strains. The hemolysin or PI-PLC activities of different Listeria species can be used to distinguish between pathogenic and nonpathogenic species.

L. monocytogenes is a microorganism that can be present in many food products, mainly in dairy products, soft cheeses, cheeses made with unpasteurized milk, celery, cabbage, ice cream, hot dogs, and processed meats. Infection with *L. monocytogenes* can be treated with antibiotics such as ampicillin, although penicillin is more effective. In cases of meningitis and endocarditis, as well as in individuals with weakened immune systems, such as neonates, certain medical professionals advise using gentamicin. Ampicillin is reserved for isolated listerial bacteremia in pregnant patients. Trimethoprim-sulfamethoxazole and vancomycin are additional antibiotics that are useful. Because they are ineffective against the microorganism, cephalosporins should not be used to treat listeriosis. Similar to the recommendations for other foodborne pathogens, there are general guidelines to prevent listeriosis. High-risk individuals are advised against eating soft cheeses like Feta, Brie, and Camembert, blue cheeses, or Mexican-style cheeses (white, fresh, or panela), unless they are made with pasteurized milk; they should also refrain from eating smoked seafood, pâté, or chilled meat spreads, hot dogs, processed meats, or cold cuts, unless they have been reheated at a high temperature.

6.3.4. Strategies for Disease Prevention

The risk of contamination and, as a result, food poisoning among consumers is increased by a number of factors related to the sourcing, handling, and preparation of food. It is vital to understand the steps that can be taken to prevent or avoid contracting a disease caused by food poisoning related to bacterial toxins, given the significance of foodborne diseases, the frequency of cases reported, and their severity. By means of cross-contamination, toxic microorganisms from the environment or, in the case of animals, the normal microbiota are introduced into food products. The microorganisms settle down in the intestines after the contaminated food is consumed, colonize, and, if the strain is toxic, produce the toxins that cause harm. Similarly, a period of incubation is required before the onset of symptoms. Therefore, all food sectors, including restaurants, manufacturing, and distribution companies, pay special attention to hygiene measures for food handling to prevent food handlers from inoculating the bacteria they carry on the skin on their hands. Health care measures, especially those related to hand hygiene of food handlers, should be implemented to prevent the occurrence of such diseases. They also need to guarantee food safety, so the food industry will set up procedures and policies to guarantee the highest standards of quality and food safety along the entire food supply chain (from production and procurement to consumption).

A portion of these standards are outlined and managed by the Codex Alimentarius, which is tasked with developing and establishing international food standards alongside the World Health Organization and the Food and Agriculture Organization of the United Nations. Their goals are to safeguard human health, guarantee the quality of food products, and ensure that these standards are applied correctly and equitably. For food products that are processed, semi-processed, or raw, the Codex Alimentarius standards are relevant. Apart from all the elements involved in food processing, food quality standards aim to guarantee that food items are manufactured in a sanitary manner while maintaining their nutritional value. Microbiological procedures pertaining to the use of food additives, pesticide use and control, and the allowable limits of medications or hormones used in animal production are among the primary standards.

Toxic bacteria cannot contaminate food when food is handled properly unless facilities, supplies, tools, and equipment are kept available for the cleaning and disinfection process. Cleaning processes will involve removing food residues and other contaminants as effectively as possible; these processes need to be ongoing because cleaning with soap and water alone is insufficient because some microorganisms have the capacity to settle on these surfaces and form biofilm, which allows them to survive in unfavorable conditions. The techniques can be physical, using heat, turbulent washes, or vacuum washes, or chemical, using alkaline and acidic detergents. Moreover, dirt can be removed with brushes or sponges; however, proper usage technique must be considered to guarantee effectiveness, and the same cleaning tool should not be used in areas containing processed and unprocessed food. Depending on the type of surface and the product's presentation (liquid, solid, or semisolid), the manufacturer will recommend specific conditions for the concentration and duration of action when using detergents or disinfectant substances. These cleaning procedures will be recorded, along with the areas that were cleaned and the cleaner, and will be subject to routine quality control and monitoring. Using a cleaning solution and sponges or brushes to remove residues from smooth surfaces is sufficient; this is done in situ, unlike with disassembled equipment that needs to be cleaned piece by piece. The cleaning technique will be determined by what needs to be cleaned. For the proper and effective application of cleaning techniques, all the aforementioned information about the establishment's cleaning must be provided in writing to the staff members in charge of this duty.

In this industry, pest control is another crucial factor. Sites where food is produced are home to a variety of pests, which require extra caution because they frequently serve as carriers of pathogens and toxic bacteria that can harm consumers' health. The three most prevalent pests are cockroaches, flies, and rodents. Food facilities should stay away from air vents and cracks to keep pests out. Food products should be stored high up and in sealed containers or bags to keep rodents from sniffing them. To effectively control pests, it is important to continuously monitor insects using techniques like electric lamps to deter flying insects and catch patches that may contain pheromones to attract them. Fly infestations are the most prevalent type of insect pest in food establishments and are a major cause of foodborne illness and other types of food poisoning. Adhesive traps can be used in restaurants, kitchens, and other locations where food is prepared to help food establishments get rid of flies and prevent any contamination of food products. To control rodent pests, traps are utilized; however, careful planning is required to decide how many traps to set up and where. Other pest prevention measures include caulking air vents, avoiding cracks, and storing food high up, in sealed containers, or in bags to keep rodents from sniffing it. To guarantee quality and food safety, it is now crucial to clean the work areas, particularly the kitchen and any surfaces that come into contact with food.

The preservation of food products' quality without the presence of chemical, physical, or biological pathogens, or any other undesired alterations that could have an impact on the health of the consumer, is known as food safety, and it is a human right that all governments are required to uphold. To guarantee this quality, it is necessary to implement appropriate measures such as identifying and managing possible sources of contamination within the establishment, storing food properly by keeping raw and processed food separate, and handling food items according to their animal or vegetable origin. Installation of drainage systems and proper waste management must be considered. Raw food should be kept apart from previously processed food, and similar surfaces should not be exposed when it comes to design, equipment distribution, and food preparation areas. To prevent the contamination of food, staff restrooms should be located at a distance from areas where food is prepared. Ensuring a work environment that promotes food processing and minimizes the risk of food poisoning caused by toxic bacteria requires the use of appropriate uniforms and footwear, as well as attention to ventilation, temperature control, and air quality. The seven basic principles of the HACCP system guarantee food safety by identifying hazards and preventive measures, identifying critical control points, establishing limits, monitoring critical control points, using corrective measures, verifying processes, and registering the applied processes. An effective and systematic alternative to prevent toxico-infection is the HACCP system, which identifies specific hazards and develops control measures to solve them.

As a preventive measure to avoid food contamination and foodborne diseases, WHO proposes the five keys for food safety.

- **Keep clean:** It refers to washing hands before and during food preparation; after going to the toilet; washing and sanitizing surfaces and equipment for food preparation, and to keep them away from insects and animals.
- **Separate raw and cooked food:** Prepare in different surfaces raw and cooked food and use different equipment for each type of food.
- **Cook thoroughly:** Food cooked thoroughly allow the removal of bacteria and other pathogens; toxins produced by bacteria and pathogens can also be destroyed.
- **Keep food at safe temperatures:** Do not leave cooked food at room temperature for more than 2 h to avoid bacteria proliferation, and try not to store frozen food for long periods of time.
- **Use safe water and raw materials:** Safe treated water must be used when preparing food; use fresh food products and wash adequately. Pre-processed products such as pasteurized milk, should be used as directed and not be used beyond their expiry dates.

A Closer Look

Foodborne Pathogens and Toxins

Contamination of food and water sources is a significant concern in food toxicology, posing serious threats to public health. Foodborne pathogens include a variety of microorganisms, such as bacteria, viruses, and parasites that can cause illness when ingested. Bacterial pathogens like *Salmonella*, *Escherichia coli* (E. coli), *Listeria monocytogenes*, and *Clostridium botulinum* are among the most notorious. These bacteria can contaminate a wide range of foods, including meats, dairy products, vegetables, and prepared foods. For instance, *E. coli* O157:H7 is commonly associated with undercooked beef and can cause severe gastrointestinal illness, kidney failure, and even death. *Salmonella* can contaminate eggs, poultry, and other foods, leading to symptoms such as diarrhea, fever, and abdominal cramps. *Listeria* is particularly dangerous for pregnant women, newborns, and the immunocompromised, potentially causing meningitis and septicemia.

Viruses like norovirus and hepatitis A are also critical foodborne pathogens. Norovirus is highly contagious and can spread rapidly through contaminated food and water, as well as from person to person, causing acute gastroenteritis characterized by vomiting, diarrhea, and stomach pain. Hepatitis A virus, typically transmitted through the consumption of contaminated food or water, can lead to liver inflammation, jaundice, fatigue, and abdominal pain. The long incubation period and potential for severe liver damage make hepatitis A a significant concern in food safety.

Parasitic pathogens such as *Toxoplasma gondii*, *Cryptosporidium*, and *Trichinella spiralis* also contribute to foodborne illnesses. *Toxoplasma gondii*, found in undercooked meat and contaminated water, can cause toxoplasmosis, which is particularly severe for pregnant women and individuals with weakened immune systems. *Cryptosporidium* can contaminate drinking water and cause cryptosporidiosis, characterized by watery diarrhea, stomach cramps, and dehydration. *Trichinella spiralis* is associated with undercooked pork and wild game, causing trichinellosis, which can lead to gastrointestinal symptoms followed by muscle pain and swelling.

In addition to pathogens, foodborne toxins produced by microorganisms, plants, and marine organisms pose serious health risks. Bacterial toxins such as botulinum toxin from *Clostridium botulinum* and staphylococcal enterotoxins from *Staphylococcus aure*us can cause severe food poisoning. Botulinum toxin, one of the most potent toxins known, can lead to botulism, characterized by muscle paralysis and potentially fatal respiratory failure. Staphylococcal enterotoxins cause rapid onset of vomiting and diarrhea.

Marine biotoxins, such as ciguatoxins, saxitoxins, and domoic acid, are produced by algae and can accumulate in fish and shellfish. Consumption of contaminated seafood can result in ciguatera fish poisoning, paralytic shellfish poisoning, and amnesic shellfish poisoning, respectively, with symptoms ranging from gastrointestinal distress to neurological impairment and even death.

Effective control of foodborne pathogens and toxins requires rigorous food safety practices, including proper cooking, handling, and storage of food, as well as thorough hygiene practices among food handlers. Public health initiatives and regulatory measures are crucial in monitoring and managing foodborne risks to protect consumers and reduce the incidence of foodborne illnesses. By understanding the sources, transmission, and effects of foodborne pathogens and toxins, efforts can be made to enhance food safety and safeguard public health.

Summary

- Toxicology is an old scientific discipline that tries to describe and understand the effect of compounds on life forms.
- The chemistry of food toxicology explores the interactions between chemical compounds present in food and the human body, with a focus on understanding how these compounds can exert toxic effects and impact human health.
- The chemistry of food toxicology also encompasses the study of chemical reactions that occur during food processing, cooking, and storage, which can lead to the formation of toxic or potentially harmful compounds.
- Food toxicology focuses on substances found in food that, when consumed, may cause harm. Because acquiring safe food is an essential part of human survival, it is easy to conclude that food toxicology is one of the oldest scientific disciplines.
- Risk management is mainly policy based and control opportunities over the risks and legal considerations govern risk management decisions. Several other economic or social factors will have an influence on the risk management decisions.
- Eating insufficiently processed cassava is probably the cause of a paralytic disease that occurs in rural populations in Africa which is known as konzo. The diet in these populations is particularly low in sulphur amino acids.
- Lectins are primarily found in plants but also occur in animals or bacteria. Lectins are sometimes referred to as anti-nutrients. A well-known example is phytohaemagglutinin in raw beans which is destroyed by cooking.
- Mycotoxins are produced by certain type of moulds (fungi). Many mycotoxins are chemically stable and survive food processing. Moulds grow on/in food under warm, damp and humid conditions. Long-term effects of exposure include cancer and immune deficiency.
- Mushroom poisoning always receives quite a lot of public attention. However, exposure to toxic mushrooms is probably a greater risk for animals than for humans, which remains underreported. In fact, detailed identification of edible mushrooms can completely prevent human toxicity.
- Hundreds of pesticide products have been approved for use. There are various ways to classify all these products.
- The toxicological boundaries are set by different parameters. For each pesticide, an Acceptable Daily Intake (ADI) has been determined. The ADI is the dose of the pesticide that can be ingested daily for a lifetime without an adverse effect.
- The ADI is based on lifelong continuous daily exposure. This means that a single excess dose of the ADI does not immediately lead to a negative health effect.
- It is important to realise that most toxicological knowledge is for individual compounds. Less is known about combinations of compounds. In this case the Threshold of Toxicological Concern (TTC) approach may be helpful.

- The usual concept in toxicology, also in food toxicology, is that the parameters used to estimate a health risk assume linearity in response. In other words, more toxin leads to more health damage. This notion goes back a long time.

References

1. Abe, A., Koyama, K., Uehara, C., Hirakawa, A., & Horiguchi, I. (2020). Changes in the risk perception of food safety between 2004 and 2018. *Food Safety, 8*, 90–96.
2. Barlow, S. M., Greig, J. B., Bridges, J. W., Carere, A., Carpy, A. J., Galli, C. L., et al. (2002). Hazard identification by methods of animal-based toxicology. *Food and Chemical Toxicology, 40*(2), 145–191. https://doi.org/10.1016/S0278-6915(01)00140-4.
3. Bast, A. (2002). The risk to eat: Natural versus man-made toxins. In G. Voss & G. Ramos (Eds.), *Chemistry of crop protection* (pp. 63–68). Wiley-VCH.
4. Bast, A., & Hanekamp, J. C. (2014). 'You can't always get what you want'–Linearity as the golden ratio of toxicology. *Dose Response, 12*(4), 664–672. https://doi.org/10.2203/dose-response.13-043.Bast.
5. Bast, A., Semen, K. O., & Drent, M. (2021). Pulmonary toxicity associated with occupational and environmental exposure to pesticides and herbicides. *Current Opinion in Pulmonary Medicine, 27*, 274–283. https://doi.org/10.1097/MCP.0000000000000763.
6. Clemson Food Safety Education Program. (2012). Section 2: Foodborne bacterial pathogens [Internet]. Available from: www.foodsafetysite.com (accessed on 3 August 2024).
7. Hanekamp, J. C., & Bast, A. (2015). Antibiotics exposure and health risks: Chloramphenicol. *Environmental Toxicology and Pharmacology, 39*, 213–220. https://doi.org/10.1016/j.etap.2014.12.012.
8. Hanekamp, J. C., Bast, A., & Kwakman, J. H. J. M. (2012). Of reductionism and the pendulum swing: Connecting toxicology and human health. *Dose Response, 10*, 155–176. https://doi.org/10.2203/dose-response.11 037.Hanekamp.
9. Iriarte, M. J., Ugarte, J. C., & Salazar, L. (2001). Utility of the airborne endotoxins assay in different occupational environments as a risk indicator by biological agents. *Mapfre Medicina, 12*(4), 234–240.
10. Kaiser, D., Douches, D., Dhingra, A., Glenn, K. C., Reed Herzig, P., Stowe, E. C., & Swarup, S. (2020). The role of conventional plant breeding in ensuring safe levels of naturally occurring toxins in food crops. *Trends in Food Science & Technology, 100*, 51–66. https://doi.org/10.1016/j.tifs.2020.03.013.
11. Kirk, M. D., Pires, S. M., Black, R. E., Caipo, M., Crump, J. A., Devleesschauwer, B., Döpfer, D., Fazil, A., Fischer-Walker, C. L., Hald, T., Hall, A. J., Keddy, K. H., Lake, R. J., Lanata, C. F., Torgerson, P. R., Havelaar, A. H., & Angulo, F. J. (2015). World Health Organization estimates of the global and regional disease burden of 22 foodborne bacterial, protozoal, and viral diseases, 2010: A data synthesis. *PLoS Medicine, 12*(12), e1001921. https://doi.org/10.1371/journal.pmed.1001921.
12. Kroes, R., Renwick, A. G., Cheeseman, M., Kleiner, J., Mangelsdorf, I., Piersma, A., Schilter, B., Schlatter, J., Van Schothorst, F., Vos, J. G., & Würtzen, G. (2004). Structure-based thresholds of

toxicological concern (TTC): Guidance for application to substances present at low levels in the diet. *Food and Chemical Toxicology, 42*, 65–83. https://doi.org/10.1016/j.fct.2003.08.005.

13. Nauta, M. J., Andersen, R., Pilegaard, K., Pires, S. M., Ravn-Haren, G., Tetens, I., & Poulsen, M. (2018). Meeting the challenges in the development of risk-benefit assessment of foods. *Trends in Food Science & Technology, 76*, 90–100. https://doi.org/10.1016/j.tifs.2018.04.008.
14. O'Brien, P. J. (2014). High-content analysis in toxicology: Screening substances for human toxicity potential, elucidating subcellular mechanisms and in vivo use as translational safety biomarkers. *Basic & Clinical Pharmacology & Toxicology, 115*(1), 4–17. https://doi.org/10.1111/bcpt.12126.
15. Ospina, M. M. L., Martínez, D. M. E., Pacheco, G. O. E., & Quijada, B. H. (2016). Vigilancia y análisis de riesgo en salud pública. Protocolo de Vigilancia en Salud Pública. Intoxicaciones por sustancias químicas. Instituto Nacional de Salud. PRO-R02.006 (Versión 02), 1–75.
16. Paustenbach, D. J. (2000). The practice of exposure assessment: A state-of-the-art review. *Journal of Toxicology and Environmental Health, Part B: Critical Reviews, 3*(3), 179–291. https://doi.org/10.1080/10937400009547766.
17. Ramachandran, G. (2014). Gram-positive and Gram-negative bacterial toxins in sepsis: A brief review. *Virulence, 5*(1), 213–218. https://doi.org/10.4161/viru.27489.
18. Ramírez-Peña, E. O. (2014). Etiology of acute diarrheal disease: An improved system for monitoring outbreaks of foodborne diseases in Peru. *Revista Cuerpo Médico HNAAA, 7*(1), 54–61.
19. Romero, H. S., & Iregui, C. A. (2010). El lipopolisacárido. *Revista de Medicina Veterinaria, 19*, 37–45.
20. Sears, C. L., & Kaper, J. B. (1996). Enteric bacterial toxins: Mechanisms of actions and linkage to intestinal secretion. *Microbiology and Molecular Biology Reviews, 60*(1), 167–215. https://doi.org/10.1128/MMBR.60.1.167-215.1996.
21. Todar, K. (2008–2012). *Todar's Online Textbook of Bacteriology: Bacterial protein toxins.* Available from: http://textbookofbacteriology.net/proteintoxins.html (accessed on 3 August 2024).
22. Van der A, J. G., & Sijm, D. T. H. (2021). Risk governance in the transition towards sustainability: The case of bio-based plastic food packaging materials. *Journal of Risk Research, 24*, 1639–1651. https://doi.org/10.1080/13669877.2020.1770832.
23. Van Steenwijk, H. P., Bast, A., & De Boer, A. (2021). Immunomodulating effects of fungal beta-glucans: From traditional use to medicine. *Nutrients, 13*(4), 1333. https://doi.org/10.3390/nu13041333.
24. Vrolijk, M., Deluyker, H., Bast, A., & De Boer, A. (2020). Analysis and reflection on the role of the 90-day oral toxicity study in European chemical risk assessment. *Regulatory Toxicology and Pharmacology, 117*, 104786. https://doi.org/10.1016/j.yrtph.2020.104786.
25. Weseler, A. R., & Bast, A. (2012). Pleiotropic-acting nutrients require integrative investigational approaches: The example of flavonoids. *Journal of Agricultural and Food Chemistry, 60*(36), 8941–8946. https://doi.org/10.1021/jf301295c.
26. Weseler, A. R., & Bast, A. (2017). Masquelier's grape seed extract: From basic flavonoid research to a well-characterized food supplement with health benefits. *Nutrition Journal, 16*, 5. https://doi.org/10.1186/s12937-017-0233-2.

27. Wiedenfeld, H., & Edgar, J. (2011). Toxicity of pyrrolizidine alkaloids to humans and ruminants. *Phytochemistry Reviews, 10*(1), 137–151. https://doi.org/10.1007/s11101-010-9204-6.

28. World Health Organization. (2015). *Informe estimación de la carga mundial de las enfermedades de transmisión alimentaria*. Ginebra. Available from: http://www.who.int/mediacentre/news/releases/2015/foodborne-disease-estimates/es/ (accessed on 3 August 2024).

Chapter

7

GERIATRIC TOXICOLOGY

Contents

Introduction

A subspecialty of toxicology called "geriatric toxicology" is concerned with the harmful effects of drugs on the elderly. Because aging brings with it unique physiological and pharmacokinetic changes that can affect how drugs and other toxic substances are metabolized and eliminated, this area of toxicology is especially important. Renal and hepatic function generally decline with age and are essential for many substances' detoxification and elimination. Adverse drug reactions (ADRs) and drug interactions are more common in elderly patients due to their multiple comorbidities and frequent prescription of multiple medications. The concurrent use of multiple medications, or polypharmacy, is prevalent in this population and can result in complicated interactions that are not fully understood.

Older adults are more susceptible to toxicity even at lower dosages because of their decreased physiological reserve, which also means that they are less able to counteract the harmful effects of substances. Furthermore, the distribution of lipophilic drugs can be impacted by changes in body composition, such as an increased fat-to-lean body mass ratio, which can result in a prolonged action and the buildup of toxic substances. The risk of unintentional overdoses or incorrect medication use can be increased by cognitive decline, which is common in the elderly. Since older adults often use these more frequently, geriatric toxicology also takes into account the effects of environmental toxins, supplements, and over-the-counter (OTC) medications. Another factor is the altered sensitivity to recreational drugs and alcohol, which can have stronger effects because of the physiological changes mentioned earlier. A multidisciplinary approach is necessary for assessing and managing toxicity in the elderly. This includes carefully reviewing the patient's medical history, current medications, and general state of health. To reduce the risks, it also calls for the creation of guidelines and therapeutic interventions tailored to each age group. To improve the safety and effectiveness of pharmacotherapy in the aging population and ultimately improve their quality of life, healthcare providers must have a solid understanding of the fundamentals of geriatric toxicology.

Orientation and Directional Terms

Term	Definition	Illustration
Adverse drug reactions	An adverse drug reaction is a "response to a drug which is noxious and unintended and which occurs at doses normally used in man for prophylaxis, diagnosis, or therapy of disease or for the modification of physiologic function."	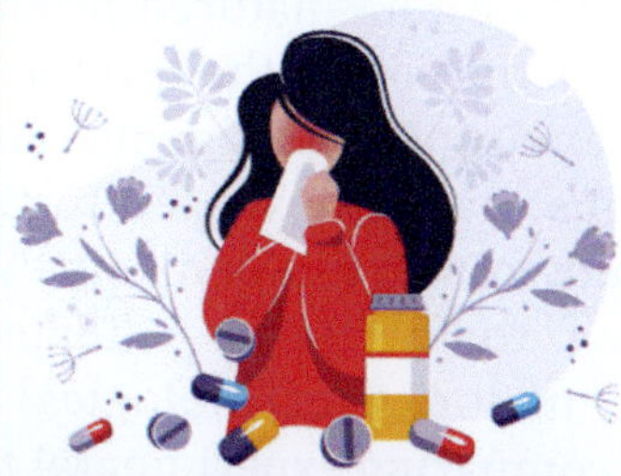
Chemical toxicity	The ability of a substance to cause harmful health effects. These effects can strike a single cell, a group of cells, an organ system, or the entire body.	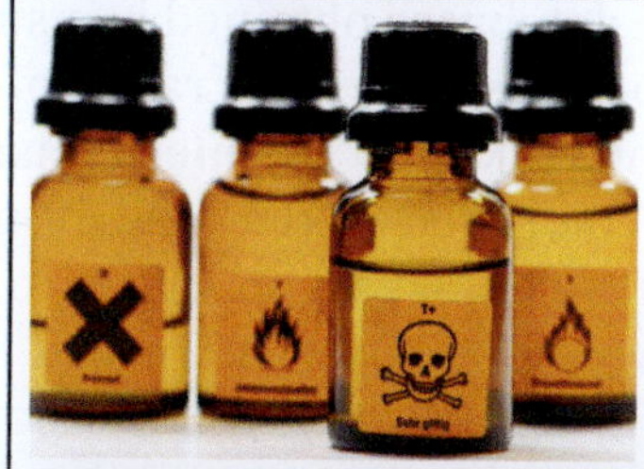
Pharmacogenetics	A field of medicine that investigates how a person's genetic makeup may affect how their body processes certain medications.	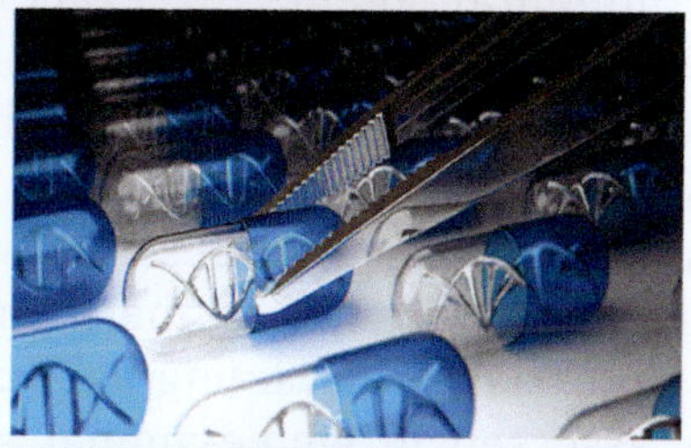
Biomarkers	A biological molecule found in blood, other body fluids, or tissues that is a sign of a normal or abnormal process, or of a condition or disease.	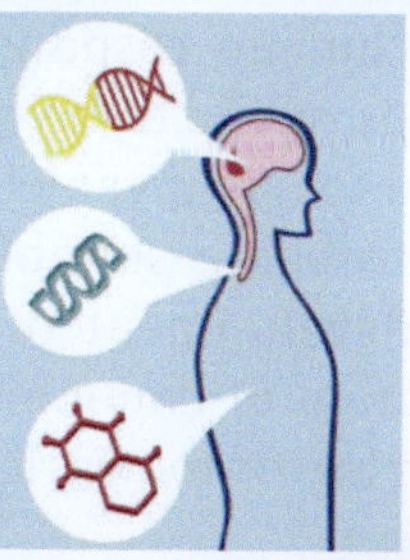
Toxicity testing	Toxicology testing is the process of determining the degree to which a substance of interest negatively impacts the normal biological functions of an organism, given a certain exposure duration, route of exposure, and substance concentration.	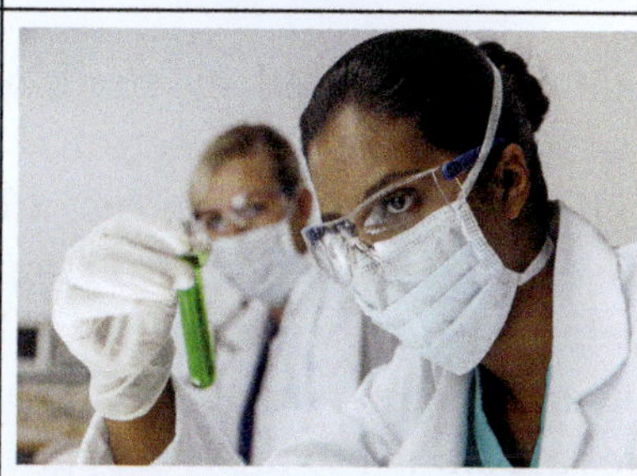

7.1. Principles of Toxicology in the Context of Aging

Toxicology is a dual-natured science. It is the empirical definition of the level of toxicity and risk that environmental agents pose to human populations that are exposed to them, as well as the study of the mechanisms by which they exert their toxic effects. * Toxicology, more than the majority of biological disciplines, relies on comparing experimental findings with extensive databases obtained by using standard test procedures on a wide range of substances and radiation kinds. The mechanisms of aging must be compared to the toxicity mechanisms of known toxic agents in order to investigate both the potential for increased toxicity for elderly individuals and the potential for environmental agents to exacerbate aging processes. Furthermore, it will be necessary to identify tests that will enable the screening of environmental agents for their potential to interact with aging processes or to pose a greater risk to the elderly. After the identification of such potentially interacting agents, they need to be assessed in whole-animal systems that serve as suitable human response surrogates. The chosen species needs to be representative of human reaction to any given chemical under test, in addition to being suitable in terms of aging. Both the development of test systems and the identification of common mechanisms must occur within the framework of the current databases.

Aging is perceived by some as a harmful process, and certain functional alterations associated with aging do resemble harmful processes. It is evident that changes in organ and cellular integrity as well as homeostasis are linked to aging; in fact, many aging-related changes are similar to those brought on by toxins. Therefore, changes in metabolic states that cause the body to produce harmful molecules or changes in the regular regulation of the body's concentrations of different natural substances may be linked to aging. According to toxicologic research, if a substance's concentrations differ significantly from normal, even the most improbable substances may be connected to tissue damage. The usefulness of viewing aging as a toxic end point is highlighted by nutrition. For instance, neurologic damage can result from both an excess or a deficiency in vitamin B6 (and these changes superficially resemble those accompanying aging). The fact that aging is either the main cause of or a contributing factor in all age-related diseases is another reason that aging can be helpfully investigated as a toxic process in and of itself. Moreover, aging occurs during all whole-animal experiments and is not easily stopped. Therefore, any toxic processes brought about by outside factors have the potential to interact with aging processes. The potential impact of such an interaction would be higher in the case of chronic exposures or toxic effects whose latency spans a significant portion of a person's life.

Is it possible to replicate the harmful effects of aging through chemical or physical agents? While the complete answer would take up much of this discussion, the short answer is that many environmental agents can, in high enough concentrations, cause some pathologic alterations and physiologic deteriorations that resemble those seen in the elderly. This type of imitation is restricted since an agent typically causes a single tissue to age in one or two ways at most. Particularly harmful substances that affect the entire body include ionizing radiation. An important finding that shouldn't be overinterpreted is that toxic agents don't universally mimic the signs of aging, even in a particular tissue. Molecular lesions resembling those caused by aging may be produced by a poisonous substance. In the field of toxicology, however, it has been observed that the expression of cellular or molecular damage at the tissue level is not strictly related to the toxic agent. It is sometimes the case that different agents that are thought to cause similar types of damage at the cellular or molecular level cause different types of tissue damage. On the other hand, different toxicants can occasionally produce pathologic effects that are similar to one another; in other words, different agents can cause different processes to manifest the same effects.

Aging causes deterioration in all tissues. A similarly comprehensive toxicologic approach is necessary to observe the extent of aging's effects. An extra focus needs to be placed on assessing data bases for long-term whole-animal bioassays, since these toxicologic assessments are a key instrument for quantitative risk assessment and have been used to assess the effects of prolonged exposure to toxic agents at low concentrations, including agents that are important to the environment. Immunotoxicology and neurotoxicology ought to be highlighted as well. Unknown etiology of some neurologic and immunologic deficits are observed in a significant percentage of the elderly population, and the majority of environmental agents have not been screened for neurotoxic and immunotoxic effects. When examining how aging and the environment are related, two common issues raise the most concerns from a toxicologic standpoint. First, toxicologic methods of identifying disruptions in the fundamental biology of the aging processes are not easily practicable since the mechanisms of aging are unknown. The second reason the empirical approach fails is that no test designed to identify agents that specifically impact aging or the elderly has comparative data to support it. Finding agents that specifically affect aging or the elderly while also understanding the mechanisms of aging is one way to tackle the two issues. While much work has been put into the former, the latter would require significant resources. This report aims to provide the most cost-effective and scientifically sound solution for the two problems.

In addition to aspects of conventional toxicology that appear most relevant to the relationship of chemical toxicity and aging, three new types of questions must be addressed:

- If the standard long-term bioassay could detect large age-associated pathologic changes, how can agents that might interact with the aging processes to increase or hasten the appearance of pathologic effects or reduced resilience in the aged are identified? It is unclear whether the bioassay can mimic exposures that are inherent in the human environment and absent from the clean laboratory environment of the surrogate animal.
- For example, in multistage carcinogenesis, exposure to a cancer initiator can sensitize animals to later exposure to a cancer promoter. How can acute or subacute exposures in utero, during development, or during maturity that sensitize the exposure to other agents be identified? It is very challenging to address whether comparable pathways cause any of the diverse range of pathologic effects seen in the elderly using conventional toxicologic testing methods.
- The question of whether testing done on young animals can predict the response of older animals is more specific because most toxicity is measured in young animals; that is, how can environmental agents, especially pharmaceuticals,

that hold increased hazard for the aged be identified? When two age groups of animals react to an agent in qualitatively similar but quantitatively different ways, the application of a safety factor may allow the use of young animal data to predict risk in older age groups. Such extrapolation would be impossible if the mechanisms of action were different, necessitating testing on older animals, which would come with associated costs and the lack of comparable data.

The general ideas of toxicology are outlined in the remaining portion of this chapter (i. e., distribution, metabolism, and excretion), how chemicals affect the body as we age, toxicity mechanisms at different physiologic organization levels, and the significance of pharmacogenetics, biomarkers, and toxicity testing.

7.1.1. Chemical Fate and Effect

Chemicals can enter the body through the skin, food, or inhalation. They may act immediately upon contact, or they may be absorbed, enter the bloodstream, and travel to other locations to act. Toxic substances are removed from the blood by biological conversion, excretion, or buildup at different locations. Toxicants can also be metabolized by enzymes in the kidneys, lungs, gastrointestinal system, skin, and other tissues in addition to the liver, which is active in this process. Certain toxicants build up in tissues or organs, where they may or may not have harmful effects. While some volatile toxicants can be expelled from the body through the lungs, the majority are removed by the kidneys and liver through the bile or urine. Instead of concentrating on hazardous environmental materials, the majority of research on how aging affects chemical absorption, distribution, metabolism, and elimination has been done on pharmaceuticals. The same pathways that cause drugs to biotransform also transform many toxic chemicals into less toxic, or occasionally even more toxic, substances, so information on drugs is relevant to toxicologic concerns. There are numerous thorough reviews of geriatric pharmacology available for information on drug disposition and aging.

Almost all of the data on toxicants have come from experiments on animals, unlike the data on pharmaceutical agents, which are based on studies involving both humans and animals. Furthermore, many of the animal data and the human data are related to neonatal and young subjects, as documented in a monograph written by Calabrese (1986). The potential impact of aging on carcinogen detoxification, procarcinogen conversion to carcinogen, and carcinogen interaction with putative inducing agents is of particular interest. Age-related variations in the metabolism of carcinogens in both young and old animals, who came to the conclusion that there was a lack of information and conflicting evidence. Studies on metabolism are influenced by strain, species, gender, and substrate. Seldom has research been done on age-related alterations in the monoxygenase components of nonhepatic tissues. Therefore, it would be oversimplified to assume that the increased incidence of cancer with aging is caused by changes in carcinogen metabolism that vary with age. Age-related differences in a given tissue's biotransformation of a given compound may or may not lead to a higher concentration or longer half-life of carcinogenic chemicals or reactive metabolites at susceptible target sites.

Clinical researchers have paid less attention to this issue, despite the fact that many, but not all, animal studies have revealed that aging is not linked to a loss of the ability of oxidative metabolism to respond to inducers—such as barbiturates, polycyclic hydrocarbons, and steroids. Aside from metabolism, age can also affect toxicokinetic measurements like absorption, distribution, renal and biliary excretion, as well as toxicodynamic factors that determine tissue sensitivity. Therefore, a complex interaction of multiple processes that have not been thoroughly studied in humans or animals may lead to an increased sensitivity to carcinogens in older adults. Understanding how aging affects a drug's absorption, distribution, metabolism, and excretion (ADME) can help understand how altered responses to chemicals generally work. Age differences in pharmacokinetics (absorption, distribution, metabolism, and elimination) may also need to be considered in studies of age differences in pharmacodynamics (biochemical and physiologic effects of drugs and their mechanisms of action). For instance, research generally indicates that older people are more susceptible to the analgesic and depressant effects of narcotics (like morphine) and neuroactive medications (like diazepam); in contrast, the age-related decline in the heart's in vivo sensitivity to isoproterenol and its antagonist propranolol appears to occur. Additionally, there is proof that aging modifies the biochemical reactions of cells to specific medications.

7.1.1.1. Absorption

The main mechanism through which toxins pass through bodily membranes is absorption. The gastrointestinal system, lungs, and skin are where toxic agents are primarily absorbed. Numerous toxins have the ability to penetrate the skin and enter the bloodstream. The permeability of the skin can be increased by physical or chemical injury, among other factors. Gases and solid or liquid aerosols are the forms of toxins that are absorbed by the lungs. Because the lungs have a large surface area and a blood supply located close to the inhaled air in the alveoli, absorption can occur quickly and completely. Numerous environmental pollutants pass through the digestive system and into the food chain. The physical and chemical characteristics of the toxicant, gastrointestinal content, and gastrointestinal motility are just a few variables that can affect how well toxicants are absorbed through the gastrointestinal tract.

It is possible that several physiological changes brought on by aging will have an impact on gastrointestinal absorption. These consist of a rise in the pH of the stomach, a fall in intestinal blood flow, a decrease in the quantity of absorbing cells, a reduction in gastrointestinal motility, and a slowing down of the emptying of the stomach. There are few specific data on the range of pH values that can be encountered in the elderly population and the effects of increased pH on bioavailability. An increase in gastric pH may affect the ionization and solubility of some substances. It makes sense that slower stomach emptying and decreased gastrointestinal motility in older adults would slow down absorption. A longer time to peak plasma concentration following oral medication administration has been observed in certain studies. Because there was no difference in the amount of absorption between the elderly and the young subjects, this has very little clinical significance. The majority of research on drug absorption in the elderly, despite the paucity of data, does not show that age has a discernible impact on the rate and extent of absorption.

7.1.1.2. Distribution

A toxin can spread throughout the body as soon as it enters the bloodstream. Only toxicants that are free of plasma protein binding can pass through to other sites. Toxicants bound to those proteins have the potential to be displaced by other chemical agents and, once released, travel to target organs and cause harm there, which is why toxicologists and medical scientists are particularly concerned about this type of binding. Toxicants are distributed according to their affinity for different body parts and their capacity to pass through cell membranes. These two features are highly variable among toxicants. Some are only widely distributed because they are not easily able to pass through cell membranes. Others attach themselves to different parts of the body like bone, fat, liver, or kidneys. A toxicant's primary toxic effect may occur where it binds, but this is not always the case. In actuality, binding sites frequently act as storage facilities whose presence aids in shielding the body from the harmful action.

Many aging-related changes can affect how substances are distributed in terms of volume throughout the body. Among the most significant is body composition. Between the ages of 20 and 80, there is a 10–15% decrease in total body water (both in absolute terms and as a percentage of body weight); lean body mass decreases proportionately to body weight as people age, while body fat increases. It is anticipated that these modifications will result in elevated blood concentrations of compounds primarily found in lean body mass or body water. Changes in body fat can cause highly lipid-soluble substances to accumulate and take longer to act. Furthermore, as people age, their serum albumin levels decline, which allows more drugs that bind to albumin—like the anticonvulsant phenytoin—to diffuse into body tissue. On the other hand, weak bases, like the antidepressant imipramine and the antiarrhythmic medication lidocaine, have less plasma-protein binding in the elderly due to an increase in serum a1-acid glycoprotein. Thus, changed plasma-protein binding may be one factor contributing to altered pharmacokinetics in the elderly, as free-drug concentration is a significant factor in determining drug distribution and elimination. However, the information that is currently available indicates that illness and immobility have a bigger impact on albumin concentration than age does.

7.1.1.3. Metabolism and Elimination

While many chemical agents that enter the body undergo biological transformations due to metabolic processes, some can stay as intact molecules. Simple, reversible chemical or physical interactions that mainly impact transport across membranes and throughout the body can be a part of metabolic processes. In other situations, metabolic processes have the power to significantly change the toxin's chemical makeup, making it either more or less toxic. The body's ability to eliminate waste can be aided by metabolic processes. Thinking of the metabolic processes as two different types has proven helpful. The first involves oxidation, reduction, or hydrolysis procedures that mainly modify or introduce functional (reactive) moieties to the target molecule. In the second, different endogenous chemicals (such as amino acids, sulfate, and glucuronic acid) react chemically with pre-existing or newly formed functional groups on the molecule to form conjugates, or new chemicals. These products' lipid or water solubility and ionization properties frequently change during biosynthesis in ways that facilitate secretion and excretion.

Chemical agents are primarily eliminated from the body through the kidneys and urine, the liver and bile and feces, and the lungs and exhaled air. Minor routes include the body's secretions, which include hair, nails, and desquamated epithelial tissue, as well as bodily fluids like sweat, tears, saliva, mucus, and digestive juices. The above discussion highlights how age and conditions that impair kidney function or hepatic biliary excretion can impact a chemical's potential for toxicity. Filtration in the glomeruli and secretion and reabsorption in the renal tubules are two of the kidney's excretory processes. Therefore, blood flow to the kidneys, molecular volume in relation to glomerular filter pore size, physicochemical properties of the molecule that impact membrane transport, and enzymatic or other systems that may activate or facilitate secretion and reabsorption all play a role in elimination through the kidneys. Chemicals that attach themselves to big molecules, like plasma proteins, may not be removed by filtration and may stay in the body for extended periods of time. Since the liver filters the majority of blood from the gastrointestinal tract before it enters the general circulation, it plays a crucial role in the body's removal of ingested chemicals. With its enzymatic systems, the liver is uniquely positioned to metabolize a substance and secrete the metabolites into the bile. Bile drains into the intestines, where the substance may be excreted in feces or changed and reabsorbed. This method of elimination is frequently hampered by liver injury, which also affects biliary function.

Pharmacokinetic measurements, which are frequently based on the remaining concentration of a chemical or its metabolites in the blood in relation to time, can be used to study the elimination of chemicals from the body. Such data typically yields a reliable approximation of the chemical's toxic action-available concentration. The toxicity of unmeasured, activated intermediate chemical forms or the preservation of the chemical in tissue depots, however, may occasionally be more significant. Age-related changes in metabolism and excretion are possible, although there is only circumstantial evidence of altered drug metabolism in the human liver. According to autopsy studies, liver blood flow and liver mass in relation to body weight both decrease with advancing age after middle age. There is no discernible relationship between age and metabolism for certain drugs, primarily those that undergo liver-based conjugation. The rates at which drugs that are oxidized in the liver are metabolized, however, are not affected by age. Instead, a multitude of genetic and environmental factors are most likely responsible for the large interindividual variation in drug metabolism. Age does not appear to have an impact on the inhibition of drug metabolism, according to the data that are currently available. However, there is conflicting evidence regarding the elderly's susceptibility to the induction of hepatic drug metabolism, with some studies reporting no age differences and others showing a decrease in the extent of induction. More research is needed to determine how aging affects other drug interactions in addition to inducing and inhibiting drug metabolism.

Polycyclic hydrocarbons, found in cigarette smoke, can induce certain isozymes of cytochrome P-450 strongly. Most cross-sectional studies have shown that smoking cigarettes is linked to a lower induction of biotransformation in older adults compared to younger adults. The only way to determine whether this is a natural part of aging or the product of selective mortality would be to conduct longitudinal studies, which have not yet been carried out. However, when prescribing medication for elderly patients, it is important to keep in mind that some may have significantly decreased ability to metabolize and excrete drugs. This can be accomplished by closely monitoring the patients to guarantee that prescribed medications are therapeutically effective and to identify any unwanted drug side effects as soon as possible, or by gradually lowering the dosage of strong drugs with low therapeutic indices. Research conducted on aged laboratory animals has revealed decreased hepatic enzyme activity, which in turn has led to a decreased ability to metabolize drugs and a decreased induction of hepatic enzymes. Since rats and mice have provided the majority of the data, it is possible that the apparent age-related changes are not universal. In rodent studies, species, strain, and sex differences have all been significant variables. Research utilizing nonhuman primates' liver tissue has not demonstrated a discernible decrease in either the amount of cytochrome P-450 or the particular activity of NADPH cytochrome c (P-450) reductase. Similarly, age has no effect on microsomal drug-metabolizing activity, according to limited in vitro studies using human liver tissue. The outcomes disagree with those found in rats and, to a lesser extent, with human in vivo research. (No in vivo research has been done on nonhuman primates. They do, however, stress the challenges of generalizing findings from experimental animals to people and the necessity of clinical research to assess how chemicals and pharmaceuticals are metabolized in people.

Alcohol is a significant chemical that is frequently used as a drug by people of practically all ages. Alcohol is absorbed by all bodily fluids. With aging, its volume of distribution declines in both humans and rodents. The elderly experience higher blood concentrations following equivalent doses due to this decrease compared to the younger population. In a normal liver, acute alcohol exposure inhibits oxidative drug metabolism, while chronic alcohol exposure causes it. The hepatic microsomal enzyme system and cytoplasmic hepatic enzyme alcohol dehydrogenase both contribute to the oxidation of alcohol. Even though older people are more susceptible to the behavioral and cognitive effects of alcohol, research has not shown that human alcohol metabolism varies with age. It has been demonstrated that age affects how rats metabolize alcohol. One significant environmental factor influencing drug toxicity and metabolism is dietary composition. The majority of research has been done using test animals. Research conducted on fit human subjects has demonstrated that eating a high-protein, low-carb diet along with charcoal-broiled beef and dietary brussels sprouts and cabbage boost the metabolism of phenacetin and antipyrine as well as theophylline. Benzo[a]pyrene and other polycyclic hydrocarbons found in charcoal-broiled beef cause the rat liver and placenta to begin metabolizing benzo[a]pyrene more quickly. Spinach, broccoli, cauliflower, cabbage, turnips, Brussels sprouts, and broccoli all cause the rat to produce benzo[a]pyrene hydroxylase. The rat gut is stimulated to metabolize phenacetin, hexobarbital, and 7-ethoxycoumarin by indole compounds found in cabbage and Brussels sprouts.

It is necessary to investigate the potential differences in response to dietary manipulations of cruciferous vegetables, protein, carbohydrates, polycyclic hydrocarbons, and other constituents between older adults and younger adults. Clinical situations involving micronutrient deficiencies have received some attention. In older patients admitted to a geriatric ward, treating ascorbic acid deficiency was linked to an increase in antipyrine plasma clearance; however, there was no difference in basal values between deficient and nondeficient patients, and treating ascorbic acid had no effect on the nondeficient group. In a different study, dietary ascorbic acid variations had no effect on the way older adults metabolized caffeine. The complicated alterations in hepatic drug metabolism that are observed in old age may be caused by poor nutrition and dietary habits, but the data that are currently available are insufficient to support this theory. Unlike hepatic function, decreased renal function in the elderly is common and quantifiable. Research has demonstrated that aging impacts both tubular and glomerular function. Up to 50% can happen to the glomerular filtration rate (GFR) as determined by the clearance of creatinine or inulin. Annually, the flow of renal plasma decreases by roughly 2%. Drugs that are excreted unchanged by the kidney are eliminated at a slower rate when renal function declines. In clinical medicine, it is frequently necessary to lower the maintenance doses of medications such as cardiac glycoside digoxin and aminoglycoside antibiotics to prevent toxicity. Renal function decline is highly variable; some individuals show little to no discernible decline. To attain therapeutic concentrations, it is crucial in clinical practice to measure the plasma concentrations of potentially toxic drugs and modify dosages accordingly.

Not only do elderly patients exhibit different drug elimination rates from normal adults, but so do fetuses, neonates, and children. These differences can be substantial depending on the drug and individual. For instance, children ages 1–6 eliminated antipyrine and phenylbutazone roughly twice as quickly as healthy adults. Two children with both clinical and biochemical signs showed increased plasma antipyrine half-lives. Eight children without clinical symptoms of acute or chronic lead poisoning but with biochemical manifestations had the same rates of antipyrine and phenylbutazone elimination as normal children. Chelation therapy was started, and the children's half-lives went back to normal. Studies with comparable findings have shown that children eliminate phenobarbital, clindamycin, and diazoxide more quickly than adults do. Although human fetuses and neonates, unlike certain rodents, show detectable hepatic microsomal drug-metabolizing activity, human fetuses and newborns have a far lower capacity to eliminate drugs than do children or adults. Certain drug elimination rates seem to be even lower in premature babies than in healthy, full-term babies. For instance, the mean value of plasma indomethacin half-lives was 4/7 h in full-term healthy newborns and 2–3 or 7/02 h in healthy adults, but it was 2 and 24 h in two premature infants. Practically speaking, the significant variations in elimination rates between full-term newborns, adults, children, and premature infants impact determining the right dosages. They also highlight the necessity of looking into the pharmacokinetic and pharmacodynamic mechanisms of many more medications in relation to different age groups. Every feature listed here is significant when researching how environmental chemicals affect aging. People who are exposed to chemicals may not all respond the same way if the effects of those chemicals on aging are similar to other effects on human health. Even among individuals with similar exposures, there will be genetic heterogeneity within the human population, ensuring variations in reactions to environmental chemicals.

7.1.2. Mechanisms of Toxicity at the Molecular, Cellular, and Tissue Level

There is a vast array of mechanisms through which toxic agents operate. These mechanisms differ between agents and between dosages of the same agent. The dose at which the primary toxic effect is induced and the specificity of that effect can be used to describe mechanisms of toxic action. Although the precise mechanism of aging is still unknown, the age-associated functional decline in physiologic systems and the lack of specificity as to cells and tissues have been characterized for elderly people, making this kind of characterization probably most relevant for the consideration of aging.

7.1.2.1. Molecular Action

Toxic agents can act molecularly by producing harmful chemical species that target particular moieties in biological molecules. Given that aging generally affects all tissues, agents with very broad actions should be included in the search for toxic mechanisms shared by aging and specific toxic agents. However, various sorts of mechanisms can lead to varying degrees of breadth of action. Finding substances whose molecular mode of action affected a particular senescent phenotype would also be ideal, as this would enable a more detailed analysis of the underlying mechanisms. A particular molecule may sustain damage, and its changed function may have a wide range of harmful effects. One example is DNA damage which has pleiotropic effects. Agents whose molecular damage results in the emergence of a general damaging species can also have general toxic effects. For instance, free radicals are created either directly or indirectly by ionizing radiation and a variety of chemical substances, as well as by internal metabolic processes. These free radicals have the ability to interact with a wide range of biomolecules to produce different types of damage with varying biological effect potentials, either directly or through a cascade of processes.

Also, different tissues may be susceptible to different levels of exposure, with one tissue being susceptible at one level and others at another. For example, x-rays cause a range of ions and radicals to be produced in tissue that has been exposed to ionizing radiation. High doses (above 100 Gy) of x-rays can cause the CNS to collapse in humans in a matter of minutes or hours. The primary toxic effect at lower doses (10 Gy) is caused by a suppression of the gut crypt stem cell proliferation, which depletes the intestinal mucosa and causes death in a matter of days. X-rays cause cancer in populations exposed to them even at lower doses (1 Gy), in addition to disrupting the hematopoietic system. Ultralow radiation doses (less than 1 Gy) result in both heritable mutation and excess cancer; cancer is thought to pose a higher risk. Investigations on animals as well as epidemiology have shown the reactions to the reduced levels. As was mentioned, in addition to their other harmful effects, x-rays have the potential to shorten life. They therefore give an illustration of an agent that generates a toxic free radical that is nonspecific and targets biomolecules that are vulnerable. On the other hand, the biologic response can be dose-dependent, meaning that it can be unique to different tissues. The above example relates to another principle of toxicology, which is the limitation of toxicity. Should the more severe and immediate effects of radiation not limit them, animals that die from extremely high doses of radiation would also experience other harmful effects. When contemplating the potential impacts of any hazardous substance on the aging process and the elderly, we must perceive this type of induced reaction as one among several harmful behaviors that vary according to the dose, exposure mode, exposure duration, species, and observation period.

Other poisonous substances most likely have more targeted initial and lasting effects. For instance, toxicity is produced when carbon monoxide binds to hemoglobin and lowers its ability to carry oxygen. Whether a particular toxic action can take on more universal forms is a last thought regarding molecular damage that could cause the pleiotropic manifestations seen in aging. It has been suggested that a particular tissue's action can cause different tissues to go through different deteriorative processes. Although changes to the molecules that govern regulatory processes can impact different tissues or present in different ways (e.g., in diabetes), no instance of an induced reaction comparable in scope to the signs of aging has been noted.

7.1.1.2. Cellular Effects

Generally speaking, there are two ways that toxic mechanisms can operate at the cell level: either a single cell experiencing toxic stress can result in some toxic effects (like cancer), heritable mutations, and teratogenesis, or a specific tissue function may fail if sufficient cells of a particular type in that tissue are affected by the exposure. As aging is a phenomenon in which the majority of cells in the majority of tissues can be seen to have changed, it makes sense to think of aging in terms of the first cellular effect described, i.e., as acting through deterioration in the majority of cells in a particular tissue. Based on the findings of certain studies on aging, it has been suggested that the cell is the fundamental building block of aging, with cellular degradation leading to the appearance of symptoms at the tissue, organ, and organism levels. Although the goal of aging research has been to identify the molecular damage or alteration responsible for cellular aging, attempts to identify a molecular etiology have been fruitless. Consequently, comparisons at the cell and tissue levels are appropriate in the hunt for toxic agents that mimic aging.

7.1.1.3. Effects at the Tissue Level

The most common way to characterize toxic action in intact animals is at the tissue level due to the frequent observation of altered tissue structure or function. This specificity could result from toxic stress at the exposure site (e.g., skin, or digestive system), at the location of the metabolic process (e.g., liver, brain, or kidney), or in target cells that are vulnerable. Determining the etiology of the toxic mechanism operating at the cellular and molecular levels is crucial for comprehending the tissue-level mechanism. Referring back to the ionizing radiation example, the inability of the intestinal lining to function as a barrier is directly caused by the inability of stem cells to proliferate, resulting in the sloughing of the intestinal mucosa. The action of free radicals produced by x-rays in the stem cells' chromatin is thought to be the cause of their inability to proliferate through mitotic inhibition. Therefore, determining the sequence of events from molecular changes to their aftereffects at the level of the cell, the tissue, and the organism is the fundamental goal when examining toxic effects linked mechanistically to aging.

7.1.3. Pharmacogenetics

Significant individual differences in response to drugs and in the ability to metabolize and dispose of drugs have been observed during studies of human drug metabolism and disposition. Variations can be attributed to a variety of factors, including genetic, age-dependent (developmental), environmental, and complex interactions between them. Pharmacogenetics is the scientific study of genetic variables that explain individual variations in drug metabolism and response. Pharmacogenetics is important to toxicology because it shows how certain individuals experience toxic effects from exposure to xenobiotics at doses that other people can tolerate due to their genetic makeup. The connection between genetic variations in subjects' rates of metabolism and the production of potentially hazardous biotransformation products from a parent drug or other chemical is particularly intriguing. Because the hepatic drug-metabolizing enzyme system changes lipid-soluble substances that might otherwise stay in the body indefinitely into more polar metabolites that are easily eliminated in urine, it has historically been thought of as a detoxification system. However, it has recently been discovered that this enzyme system can also produce highly reactive, potentially toxic metabolites that can react with DNA and other tissue macromolecules to cause mutations, necrosis, and immunologic reactivity.

The regulation and control of such tissue damage may be influenced by subject-to-subject variations in the drug metabolism pathways and quantitative variations in the activities of the enzymes that catalyze those reactions and pathways. Therefore, genetic variations among participants may cause some to be more sensitive to the toxicity of particular reactive metabolites than others. The effects of aging on the expression of genetic entities often become clear as they are studied in greater detail. Expression of a phenotype, and consequently genetically modified (increased or decreased) susceptibility to chemical agents, may not happen until a person with genes predisposing them to a specific type of environmental chemical is first exposed to it, which may not happen until later in life. Given that older adults receive drug prescriptions more frequently than younger ones, it stands to reason that the prevalence of pharmacogenetically related drug toxicity would rise with age. Furthermore, certain genetically based illnesses, like Huntington's chorea, certain types of neuromuscular disease, and diabetes mellitus, manifest only at a later age.

The wide interindividual differences that define human disposition and xenobiotic response have been thoroughly studied and found to be caused by a variety of factors (Figure 7.1). The variables include age, the condition of the heart, liver, kidneys, and endocrine organs; the time of day or season that drugs are taken; the presence of disease; hormonal and nutritional status; stress; and exposure to activators or inhibitors of the hepatic microsomal drug-metabolizing enzymes (including chronic administration of any of several hundred drugs).

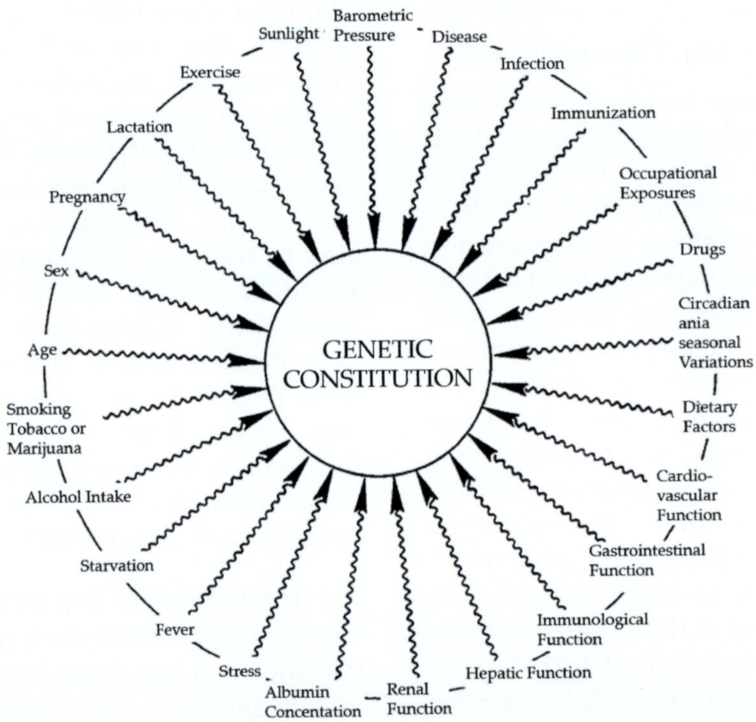

Figure 7.1. *Schematic depiction of established or suspected environmental factors that can alter genetically controlled rates of drug elimination. Lines from each environmental factor to a central circle are wavy, to suggest that modification of genetically controlled rates can occur at different magnitudes. Such environmental effects need not occur directly at the genetic level. In the outer circle, a line joins environmental factors, to suggest that several are associated and interdependent, rather than independent.*

Source: https://www.ncbi.nlm.nih.gov/books/NBK218724/bin/p20004bfeg63001.jpg.

Genetic factors that directly impact human xenobiotic response and disposition have been identified during the last 20 years. There are presently about 60 known factors, and there are undoubtedly many more. Genetic variables may be the primary or even the only reason for these interindividual variations in certain individuals under particular circumstances. For instance, there are significant interindividual differences in how human subjects respond to and dispose of xenobiotics even when factors such as age, sex, diet, and exposure to environmental chemicals that either activate or inhibit the hepatic drug-metabolizing enzyme system remain constant. There is a genetic basis for many of these variations. In US teaching hospitals, 20% of patients are there to treat adverse drug reactions, and between five and 30% of patients have experienced at least one of these reactions (Cluff et al., 1965). Compared to younger patients, elderly patients experience drug adverse reactions more frequently and with greater severity. Although it is only one cause of adverse reactions, including drug toxicity, the typical wide variation in each patient's response to medication plays a significant role in this serious medical issue.

Almost always, there is a toxic reaction as a result of drug buildup brought on by a significant decrease in the parent drug's enzymatic conversion to pharmacologically inactive metabolites. A point mutation in the gene regulating the synthesis of the enzyme causes it to function abnormally. Similar to the majority of other inborn errors of metabolism, the conditions mentioned in Table 7.1 are typically passed down through autosomal recessive traits. As a result, two parents with normal phenotypes each pass on a mutant allele to the affected subjects.

Table 7.1. *Monogenic Metabolic Pharmacogenetic Conditions and Putative Aberrant Enzymes*

Condition[a]	**Aberrant Enzyme and Normal Location**
Acatalasia	Catalase in erythrocytes
Slow inactivation of isoniazid	N-Acetyl transferase in the liver
Suxamethonium sensitivity or atypical pseudocholinesterase	Pseudocholinesterase in plasma
Phenytoin toxicity due to deficient parahydroxylation (autosomal dominant)	Mixed-function oxidase in the liver that parahydroxylates phenytoin b
Bishydroxycoumarin sensitivity (mode of inheritance unknown)	Mixed-function oxidase in the liver that hydroxylates bishydroxycoumarin b
Acetophenetidin-induced methemoglobinemia	Mixed-function oxidase in the liver that de-ethylates acetophenetidin[b]
Polymorphic serum aryl esterase activity	Serum aryl esterase (paraoxonase)
Deficient N-hydroxylation of amobarbital	Mixed-function oxidase in the liver that N-hydroxylates amobarbital[b]
Polymorphic hydroxylation of debrisoquine in man	Mixed-function oxidase in the liver that 4-hydroxylates debrisoquine
Polymorphic hydroxylation of mephenytoin	Mixed-function oxidase in the liver that hydroxylates S-mephenytoin[b]

[a]Autosomal recessive, unless otherwise noted.

[b]Probable but not fully established site of genetic defect.

Source: https://www.ncbi.nlm.nih.gov/books/NBK218724/table/ttt00004/?report=objectonly.

The gene frequencies of various pharmacogenetic conditions vary geographically. Age effects on the acetylase polymorphism have also been found, but further research on the other pharmacogenetic entities in Table 7.1 concerning age is required. The history of the age effect's identification on the acetylation polymorphism gene frequency is especially instructive, as it shows how cautious one must be when looking for these kinds of effects. Age was not taken into consideration as a significant factor in the initial observations. Subsequent research on a limited sample size appeared to support that finding. The slow-acetylator phenotype is more common as people age, and this phenotype is particularly interesting because it is linked to a significantly higher risk of bladder cancer development after long-term industrial exposure to arylamines and hydrazines. There has also been a claim that a pharmacogenetic phenotype and cancer susceptibility are related: patients with bronchogenic carcinoma were found to have a higher prevalence of extensive debrisoquin metabolizers than age- and sex-matched controls (Ayesh et al., 1984).

These variations among healthy individuals suggest, among other things, that a drug given by a given route at a given dose may be toxic in one subject, therapeutic in another, and have no pharmacologic effect in a third. A doctor who must individualize therapy faces a great challenge because of these differences (especially for drugs with low therapeutic indexes). Determining the mechanism responsible for the large interindividual variations in the disposition of many drugs is necessary because of the therapeutic implications. Because of the extreme genetic and environmental heterogeneity of humans, such identification is fraught with challenges. However, heterogeneity can be managed in lab animals like mice and rats. It is possible to manipulate each variable separately, examine each one's quantitative contribution to interindividual differences in drug disposition, and create dose-response curves. These studies have identified numerous factors that can influence drug disposition over the past ten years. Pharmacogenetic conditions in humans can be divided into two categories: pharmacokinetic conditions, which influence how the body responds to drugs, and pharmacodynamic conditions, which affect how drugs react with the body (Vesell, 1973).

Given their rarity and the fact that only a small number of drugs are toxic due to monogenetic (simple, single-gene) conditions, it is likely that these conditions have only a minor impact on the major medical issue of adverse drug reactions. Nonetheless, a recent advancement in the field of pharmacogenetics indicates that genetic variations that impact the disposition of xenobiotics significantly contribute to prevalent types of drug toxicity. When exposed to phenylbutazone, bishydroxycoumarin, antipyrine, halothane, ethanol, phenytoin, nortriptyline, or salicylate, large interindividual variations were not seen in pairs of monozygotic twins, but they were in most, but not all, pairs of dizygotic twins (Vesell, 1973, in press). Nortriptyline had the largest interindividual differences in drug elimination rates among unrelated individuals, with a factor of 30, bishydroxycoumarin having the largest, phenylbutazone and antipyrine having the largest, halothane having the largest, and ethanol having the smallest. It is challenging to assign a portion of the overall interindividual variation to any one environmental factor because of the existence and functioning of numerous environmental factors, each of which has a different capacity to change the basal, genetically controlled rate of drug disposition. The close relationships between seemingly pure environmental factors like diet and smoking and other environmental factors, as well as genetic factors, make it more difficult to divide up the total variation in drug elimination across large heterogeneous populations.

Numerous factors related to the environment, development, nutrition, or endocrine system can impact how quickly a person gets rid of a drug. These factors are connected in Figure 7.1 because, rather than existing independently, they are frequently linked to one another in a particular subject. As a matter of fact, they frequently interact dynamically to alter the basal rates of drug absorption, distribution, metabolism, excretion, or receptor interaction that are typical for a subject. As a result, even within the same subject, the effects of each of these factors on drug response can be complex and vary over time (Vesell, 1980, 1982a,b).

7.1.4. Biologic Markers

An event in a biological system or sample can be indicated by a biochemical, cellular, structural, or functional marker. Biologic markers indicate internal or circulating dose, stored body burden, dose at a target tissue, or the early onset of a pathologic effect, and can be used to assess exposure to or injury caused by a xenobiotic in humans, animals, or other biota. The idea of biological markers originated in the field of cancer research, which aimed to determine whether host factors or exogenous agents were responsible for human cancer. Molecular cancer epidemiology was defined by Perera and Weinstein (1982) as an approach that combines molecular techniques and analytical epidemiology to measure early morphologic, biochemical, or functional responses to carcinogens and identify carcinogens in human tissues, cells, or fluids. Molecular epidemiology was defined by Lower and Kanarek (1982) as the measurement of molecular traits associated with neoplastic disease.

Numerous workshops and symposia have been held to discuss the application of biological markers in disease prevention since those initial publications. Enhancing the predictive relationship between exposure, dose, and response is the ultimate aim of marker research. By accurately determining the level of risk, identifying high-risk individuals or groups, and providing early disease warning, a deeper comprehension of the role of markers will aid in the prevention of disease. The environmental health sciences should benefit greatly from the creation of cellular and molecular markers that span the time span from exposure to the onset of disease. When hazard identification is applied, markers that show the existence of internal or biologically effective doses or of an impending disease can be helpful as the qualitative step that links an environmental agent to a negative outcome. Moreover, markers can be utilized to ascertain dose-response relationships, especially at the low dosages that are pertinent to the majority of environmental chemicals. Clarifying the amount of human exposure in populations, the amount of exposure on an individual basis, and the percentage of high responders or outliers in the human population are some of the main functions of markers (Fowle, 1984).

Many significant ethical questions were brought up by the use of biologic markers (Ashford, 1986). One of these worries is that biologic screening might promote a change in workplace monitoring from environmental to human. There are worries that identifying a susceptibility marker, for instance, might be used to bar someone from employment and that efforts to eliminate hazardous chemicals from the workplace could be replaced by concentrating on identifying susceptible populations and barring them from the workplace. On a time continuum, markers can be identified as indicators of exposure, biologically effective dose (also known as the dose at the receptor site), circulating internal dose, susceptibility, and possible or actual health impairment. Regardless of exposure, markers of susceptibility point to physiological variations in an individual or population that influence how they react to environmental stimulants. These include variances in immunoglobulins, metabolism, receptors, organ reserve capacity, and other factors that affect how the body reacts to environmental stimuli. These factors can include sex, age, physiologic state, and even diet. For example, α-1-antitrypsin enzyme deficiency indicates a higher risk of developing chronic obstructive pulmonary disease.

Biologic events or circumstances that provide details about external exposure, internally absorbed dose, or dose at the receptor site or site of toxic action are known as markers of exposure. Pharmacokinetic features like blood flow, capillary permeability, transport mechanisms, number of receptor sites, material metabolism, and route of administration are examples of markers of internal dose, which show how much of a substance is absorbed into the body. Gibaldi and Perrier (1982) list data on the material's stability and structure, half-life, and peak or cumulative circulating dose as additional factors. Pre-existing susceptibilities, reserve capacity, and rates of metabolic activation and detoxification are examples of target-organ characteristics that serve as indicators of a biologically effective dose. Early biologic responses, like changes in target or nontarget tissue functions soon after exposure, are indicators of possible health impairment. The modified function of the affected tissue, which may be regarded as a preclinical stage of the disease, is one of the markers of health impairment later in response to a toxicant or after the accumulation of high doses.

A biologically effective dose may be absorbed as a result of exposure to environmental contaminants, which may cause either reversible or irreversible harm. It is possible to use various marker types in different ways to assess exposure, dosage, or impairment of health. These types of markers, though, don't always distinguish from one another. Thus, it is frequently challenging to distinguish between markers of exposures and markers of effects. An effect marker may not always be specific to a particular pollutant because the body reacts to injury with a limited number of biochemical or cellular changes.

7.1.5. Toxicity Testing

To evaluate a chemical or physical agent to ascertain its general or particular toxic properties, as well as to screen a large number of agents for the possibility of producing specific toxic effects, are the two main goals of toxicity testing. Decisions regarding the type and scope of testing are influenced by both pragmatic and scientific factors. Every choice is a scientific assessment based on data from numerous chemical tests conducted according to specific protocols, as well as established toxicological mechanisms. The testing of any given agent is constrained by realistic resource and time constraints. Tens of millions of dollars could be spent thoroughly testing an agent across the vast array of standard protocols that are currently in use. In theory or in practice, few agents are significant enough to warrant such costs. There are two types of toxicity-testing protocols: whole-animal testing and screening/auxiliary testing. Auxiliary or screening tests are typically brief assessments intended to determine the possibility of causing particular harmful outcomes. Whole-animal tests can be conducted for a short or long period, and their purpose is to quantitatively assess risk and confirm or refute any potential toxicity.

The usefulness of screening tests is determined by two factors. First, is there a possibility that the biological process being tested for in a test is not the same as the process causing the toxic effect of interest? Regarding the Salmonella typhimurium test, for example, is mutation as observed in the test a necessary and sufficient process in some or all types of carcinogenesis for which the test is used as a screen? The answer to this particular question regarding the Ames assay is probably not, as other processes relevant to the induction of cancer are also not detectable by this test. Still, the Ames assay's predictive value makes it a valuable test due to its second feature. The capacity of a test to forecast the results of additional tests or human behavior is known as predictive value. It is a probabilistic indicator of the degree of correlation between the results of the straightforward test and the "truth" as determined by whole-animal research. Essential biology has no bearing on predictive value. On the other hand, a short-term test is close to ideal if it can accurately predict the response of the entire animal and also replicate important aspects of biology.

In designing screening tests from the toxicologic perspective of detecting agents that accelerate aging, the same criteria apply:

- Does the proposed test mimic the essential biology of aging?
- Does the proposed test detect agents that accelerate aging when tested in whole animals?

These questions accent the problems of designing screening tests for agents that accelerate or interact with aging.

Human response and quantitative risk are best predicted by whole-animal experiments, especially those conducted over extended periods of time. When it comes to displaying comparable toxic responses and simulating human absorption, metabolism, and biodistribution of the chemical agent under test, the tested species should be representative of human populations. Despite the fact that all animals age, some species may not be a suitable substitute for the metabolic response of humans to a given agent. The choice of species for whole-animal, long-term testing on aging must fulfill the requirements of both toxicologists and gerontologists; the toxicologist's choice of species will vary based on the particular agent under test. For practical reasons, only a limited number of animals can be used in laboratory tests. Environmental agent tests are typically conducted at dosages significantly higher than those to which the general public is exposed. Data from these tests must be extrapolated to forecast how people will react to dosages they encounter in the environment. For this extrapolation to work, the dose-response curve's shape must be measured, or at the very least, predicted or assumed. Whether there is a threshold dose (below which no toxic effects will be observed) or whether toxic effects will only be produced in a small percentage of exposed animals at low dosages are two common classifications for toxic effects. Toxic interactions with aging also require consideration of this crucial distinction.

Measuring dose-response relationships for life span reduction is challenging. Life-shortening dose-response curves are complicated and difficult to extrapolate simply to low doses. A test for the theory that radiation exposure causes early aging would be to show that all diseases start at the same time and are influenced by a factor that is proportionate to the degree of life span reduction. The extrapolation from the lab to the real world is another that needs to be considered. The majority of laboratory experiments have been conducted using protocols that evaluate the toxic effects of a single agent; nevertheless, the human environment is made up of numerous agents that may interact. Furthermore, there isn't much proof that interactions happen between substances at the low concentrations that are frequently present in the environment, but it's still vital to take them into account. The toxic effects of combining different agents are currently being investigated, and the findings may direct similar research into the effects of aging.

7.2. Toxicology of Drug Therapy in Older Adults

Age significantly raises the prevalence of prescription drug use. According to survey data collected between 2010 and 2011, nearly 90% of older adults regularly take one prescription medication, nearly 80% regularly take two prescription medications, and 36% regularly take five prescription medications (Qato, Wilder, Schumm et al., 2005). Including dietary supplements and OTC medications significantly raises these prevalence rates. Patients in hospitals, assisted living facilities, and fragile older adults are the groups most likely to use drugs.

Providing safe, effective drug therapy for older adults is challenging for many reasons:

- They use more drugs than any other age group, increasing the risk of adverse effects and drug interactions and making adherence more difficult,
- They are more likely to have chronic disorders that may be worsened by the drug or affect drug response,
- Their physiologic reserves are generally reduced and can be further reduced by acute and chronic disorders,
- Aging can alter the pharmacodynamics and pharmacokinetics of drugs,
- They may be less able to obtain or afford drugs.

There are 2 main approaches to optimizing drug therapy in older adults:

- Using appropriate drugs as indicated and to maximize cost-effectiveness,
- Avoiding adverse drug effects by ensuring drugs are dosed correctly, discontinuing unnecessary drugs, and avoiding drug-drug and drug-disease interactions.

Because the risk of adverse drug effects is higher, overprescribing (polypharmacy) has been targeted as a major problem for older adults. However, underprescribing appropriate and therapeutically beneficial drugs must also be avoided.

7.2.1. Pharmacokinetics in Older Adults

The study of pharmacokinetics in older adults examines how aging influences a drug's ADME. Numerous physiological changes that come with aging can have a substantial effect on these pharmacokinetic processes. First, modifications in gastrointestinal function, such as decreased splanchnic blood flow, delayed gastric emptying, and decreased gastric acid secretion, can affect absorption. The speed and degree of medication absorption may be impacted by these modifications. Second, age-related changes in body composition—such as an increase in body fat and a decrease in lean body mass and total body water—impact how drugs are distributed throughout the body. Hydrophilic drugs may have a lower volume of distribution and higher plasma concentrations because of these modifications, whereas lipophilic drugs may have higher concentrations in fat tissues and longer durations of action. Aging has an impact on metabolism, which is a crucial pharmacokinetic process that mostly occurs in the liver. Reduced liver size, decreased hepatic blood flow, and decreased liver enzyme activity can all have a negative impact on hepatic metabolism. This decrease in metabolic capacity may result in longer half-lives for drugs as well as a higher chance of toxicity and drug accumulation. Drug metabolism is further complicated by the fact that cytochrome P450 enzymes, essential for the metabolism of many medications, may become less active as people age.

As people age, their excretion also varies, mostly through the kidneys. Age-related reductions in renal blood flow, GFR, and tubular function usually cause a decline in renal function. Drugs and their metabolites may accumulate as a result of this decrease in renal clearance, raising the possibility of toxicity, particularly for medications that are mainly eliminated unaltered by the kidneys. Furthermore, the pharmacokinetic profile of drugs can be further affected by complex drug interactions and polypharmacy, which is the use of multiple medications in addition to the presence of multiple comorbidities. For example, some drugs can cause or inhibit the enzymes that carry out drug metabolism, changing how co-administered drugs behave pharmacokinetically.

Clinical practice will be significantly impacted by these pharmacokinetic changes in older adults. It might be necessary to modify dosage schedules for older adults to prevent under- or overdosing. These schedules are safe and effective for younger populations. When prescribing drugs, medical professionals need to take these modifications into account. They should start with lower dosages and titrate gradually, keeping a careful eye out for both beneficial effects and side effects. Drug dosing optimization can be aided by pharmacokinetic modeling and simulations specifically designed for the elderly population.

Pharmacokinetics is best defined as what the body does to the drug; it includes

- Absorption
- Distribution across body compartments
- Metabolism
- Excretion

All these domains undergo changes with age, with certain changes having greater clinical significance. Certain medications must have their dosages lowered because of the decreased metabolism and excretion of numerous medications. Because the concentrations of drugs used chronically increase for five to six half-lives before reaching a steady state, toxicity may develop slowly. For instance, the active metabolites of some benzodiazepines, such as flurazepam, chlordiazepoxide, and diazepam, can have half-lives of up to 96 h in elderly patients; symptoms of toxicity might not manifest for days or weeks after the start of therapy.

7.2.1.1. Absorption

Changes in drug absorption tend to be clinically insignificant for most drugs despite age-related decreases in small-bowel surface area, slowed gastric emptying, and increased gastric pH. Calcium carbonate is one exception that is clinically significant because it needs an acidic environment to be absorbed as well as possible. Thus, elevations in stomach pH can reduce calcium absorption and raise the risk of constipation. These elevations can be caused by drugs (like proton pump inhibitors) or age (like atrophic gastritis). Therefore, older adults ought to use a calcium salt that dissolves more readily in less acidic environments, like calcium citrate. The early release of enteric-coated dosage forms (such as enteric-coated aspirin and enteric-coated erythromycin), which raises the possibility of gastrointestinal side effects, is another illustration of altered absorption with elevated stomach pH. Drugs may take longer to pass from the stomach into the small intestine if they are taken with anticholinergic medications or if their gastrointestinal motility slows down with age. Slowing gastrointestinal motility can delay the absorption and onset of action of drugs absorbed in the upper small intestine, like acetaminophen, as well as lower peak drug concentrations and pharmacologic effects.

7.2.1.2. Distribution

Body fat tends to rise with age, while total body water tends to decrease. When fat content rises, the volume of distribution of highly lipophilic medications (e.g., chlordiazepoxide, and benzodiazepines) and could significantly lengthen their elimination half-lives. As people age, their serum albumin levels fall and their alpha 1-acid glycoprotein levels rise; however, the clinical impact of these changes on serum drug binding varies depending on the medication. Serum concentrations of the unbound (free) drug may rise in patients with acute disorders or malnourishment, so that drug effects can be amplified by quickly reducing serum albumin. Medications that are highly protein-bound, such as warfarin and phenytoin, are more likely to have toxic side effects when serum albumin levels drop.

7.2.1.3. Hepatic Metabolism

As people age, their liver's ability to metabolize various drugs via the cytochrome P-450 enzyme system declines. The clearance of medications with reduced hepatic metabolism usually drops by 30 to 40%. Theoretically, this percentage should be subtracted from maintenance drug doses; however, since each person's rate of drug metabolism differs significantly, dose adjustments should be customized. In older adults, the hepatic clearance of drugs metabolized through phase I reactions is more likely to be prolonged. Drugs that are metabolized by conjugation and glucuronidation (phase II reactions) are typically not significantly affected by age. Age has an impact on first-pass metabolism as well; this type of metabolism, which is usually hepatic and happens before a drug enters the systemic circulation, declines by roughly 1% annually after the age of 40. Therefore, older adults may have higher circulating drug concentrations for a given oral dose. Propranolol, phenobarbital, nifedipine, nitrates, and age-related decreases in first-pass metabolism are significant examples of medications that have an increased risk of toxic effects. The hepatic metabolism of drugs can also be impacted by smoking, heart failure patients' reduced hepatic blood flow, and the use of medications that induce or inhibit the cytochrome P-450 metabolic enzymes.

7.2.1.4. Renal Elimination

A major pharmacokinetic alteration linked to aging is a reduction in the amount of medication removed by the kidneys. GFR declines by 8 mL/min/1.73 m^2/decade (0.1 mL/sec/m^2/ decade) on average after age 40; however, the age-related decline differs significantly between individuals. Because older adults often have less muscle mass and are less physically active than younger adults, they produce less creatinine, which is why serum creatinine levels frequently stay within normal limits even when GFR decreases. Clinicians may be misled into believing that normal serum creatinine levels indicate normal kidney function if those levels are maintained. Similar to declines in glomerular function, tubular function also decreases with age. Many drugs' renal elimination is lowered by these modifications (see Table 7.2). The therapeutic index of the medication (the ratio of maximum tolerated dose to minimum effective dose) and the degree to which renal elimination contributes to overall systemic elimination will determine the clinical consequences. For the majority of medications excreted by the kidneys, dosage is determined by creatinine clearance. Medication that is primarily removed by the kidneys should have a lower daily dose and/or a lower dosage frequency. Due to the dynamic nature of renal function, patients may require adjustments to their medication maintenance doses when they become ill, become dehydrated, or have recovered from dehydration.

Table 7.2. *Effect of Aging on Metabolism* and Elimination of Some Drugs*

Class or Category	Decreased Hepatic Metabolism	Decreased Renal Elimination
Analgesics and anti-inflammatory drugs	Diclofenac Ibuprofen Meperidine Morphine Naproxen	Meperidine Morphine Oxycodone
Antidiabetic drugs	—	Alogliptin Canagliflozin Chlorpropamide Dapagliflozin Empagliflozin Ertugliflozin Exenatide Glimepiride Glyburide Lixisenatide Metformin Saxagliptin Sitagliptin
Antimicrobial agents	—	Amikacin Ciprofloxacin Gentamicin Levofloxacin Nitrofurantoin Streptomycin Tobramycin Trimethoprim

Cardiovascular drugs	Amlodipine Diltiazem Lidocaine† Nifedipine Propranolol Quinidine Verapamil Warfarin	*N*-Acetylprocainamide Apixaban Captopril Dabigatran Digoxin Dofetilide Edoxaban Enalapril Enoxaparin Heparin Lisinopril Procainamide Quinapril Rivaroxaban
Diuretics	—	Amiloride Furosemide Hydrochlorothiazide Spironolactone Triamterene
Psychoactive drugs	Alprazolam† Chlordiazepoxide Desipramine† Diazepam Imipramine Nortriptyline Trazodone Triazolam†	Brexpiprazole Lurasidone Paliperidone Risperidone

Others‡	Cimetidine Levodopa Theophylline	Allopurinol Amantadine Cimetidine Famotidine Gabapentin Lithium Metoclopramide Oseltamivir Ranitidine
** When aging's effect on hepatic metabolism of a drug is controversial, effects reported in the majority of studies are listed.*		
† The effect occurs in men but not in women.		
‡ The drugs listed are examples only and not an exhaustive list.		

Source: https://www.msdmanuals.com/professional/geriatrics/drug-therapy-in-older-adults/pharmacokinetics-in-older-adults.

7.2.2. Pharmacodynamics in Older Adults

Pharmacodynamic effects, as opposed to pharmacokinetic ones, are characterized by the actions of the drug on the body or the body's reaction to it; these effects are influenced by chemical interactions, postreceptor effects, and receptor binding. Similar drug concentrations at the site of action (sensitivity) may have different effects in older adults than in younger adults. Variations may result from altered drug-receptor interactions, post-receptor events, or adaptive homeostatic reactions. In patients who are frail, pathologic organ alterations are frequently the cause of these variations. It can be challenging to distinguish between pharmacodynamic and pharmacokinetic effects in clinical settings. The effects of anticholinergic medications can particularly affect older adults. Anticholinergic effects are present in many medications, such as tricyclic antidepressants, sedating antihistamines, urinary antimuscarinic agents, some antipsychotics, antiparkinsonian medications with atropine-like activity, and a lot of OTC hypnotics and cold remedies. The adverse effects of these drugs on the central nervous system (CNS) can make older adults, especially those with cognitive impairment, more susceptible to confusion and drowsiness. In addition, anticholinergic medications frequently result in dry mouth, blurred vision, orthostatic hypotension, constipation, and urinary retention (particularly in elderly men with benign prostatic hyperplasia). These medications can raise the risk of heatstroke even at low doses by preventing diaphoresis. In general, anticholinergic medications should be avoided by older adults whenever feasible (Table 7.3).

Table 7.3. *Effect of Aging on Drug Response*

Class	Drug	Action	Effect of Aging
Analgesics	Morphine	Acute analgesic effect	↑
	Pentazocine	Analgesic effect	↑
Anticoagulants	Heparin	PTT (partial thromboplastin time)	↔
	Warfarin	PT/INR (prothrombin time/ international normalized ratio)	↑
Bronchodilators	Albuterol	Bronchodilation	↓
	Ipratropium	Bronchodilation	↔
Cardiovascular drugs	Angiotensin II receptor blockers	Decreased blood pressure	↑
	Diltiazem	Acute antihypertensive effect	↑
	Enalapril	Acute antihypertensive effect	↑
	Felodipine	Antihypertensive effect	↑
	Isoproterenol	Increased heart rate	↓
		Increased ejection fraction	↓
		Venodilation	↓
	Nitroglycerin	Venodilation	↔
	Norepinephrine	Acute vasoconstriction	↔
	Phenylephrine	Acute venoconstriction	↔
		Acute hypertensive effect	↔
	Prazosin	Acute antihypertensive effect	↔
	Propranolol (and other beta-blockers)	Decreased heart rate	↓
	Verapamil	Acute antihypertensive effect, cardiac conduction effects	↑
Diuretics	Bumetanide	Increased urine flow and sodium excretion	↓
	Furosemide	Latency and size of peak diuretic response	↓
Oral hypoglycemics	Glyburide*	Chronic hypoglycemic effect	↑
Psychoactive drugs	Diazepam	Sedation	↑
	Diphenhydramine	Psychomotor dysfunction	↑
	Haloperidol	Acute sedation	↑
	Midazolam	Electroencephalogram (EEG) activity	↑
		Sedation	↑

	Temazepam	Postural sway	↑
		Psychomotor effect	↑
		Sedation	↑
	Thiopental	Anesthesia	↔
	Triazolam	Sedation	↑
Others	Atropine	Impaired gastric emptying	↔
	Levodopa	Adverse effects	↑
	Metoclopramide	Sedation	↔
□ = unchanged; □ = increased; □ = decreased. ** Older adults are particularly susceptible to the hypoglycemic action of glucose-lowering drugs. Hypoglycemia may be difficult to recognize in older adults.*			

Source: https://www.msdmanuals.com/professional/geriatrics/drug-therapy-in-older-adults/pharmacodynamics-in-older-adults.

7.2.3. Drug-Related Problems in Older Adults

Drug-related issues frequently affect older adults, including ineffective medication, unwanted side effects, incorrect dosage, insufficient monitoring, noncompliance, and interactions with other drugs. Inadequate dosing may occur due to concerns about adverse effects, while poor adherence can result from financial or cognitive limitations. Adverse effects can be uncomfortable or dangerous, such as oversedation, confusion, falls, and bleeding. Older adults experience adverse drug effects at a significantly higher rate than younger adults, with hospitalization rates four times higher. The majority of these hospitalizations are due to just four medications or drug classes—warfarin, insulin, oral antiplatelet drugs, and oral hypoglycemic drugs.

7.2.4. Reasons for Drug-Related Problems

Any patient can experience adverse drug effects, but older adults are particularly vulnerable due to specific characteristics. For instance, age-related changes in pharmacodynamics and pharmacokinetics, as well as the frequent use of multiple medications by older adults, all raise the possibility of side effects. When medications are prescribed and taken as directed, side effects can happen to anyone at any age. For example, allergic reactions that develop suddenly are unpredictable and unpreventable. However, in at least 25% of cases involving older adults, adverse effects are believed to be avoidable. Antipsychotics, warfarin, antiplatelet agents, hypoglycemic medications, insulin, antidepressants, and sedative-hypnotics are among the drug classes that are frequently involved. Many common reasons for ineffectiveness, side effects, or both in older adults can be avoided. Inadequate communication between medical professionals and patients is a major contributing factor (especially during healthcare transitions). If medication reconciliation were given more consideration during hospital admissions, discharges, and other care transitions (such as moving from a skilled nursing facility to a nursing home or from a nursing home to a hospital), many drug-related issues could be avoided.

7.2.4.1. Drug-Disease Interactions

Regardless of the patient's age, a medication prescribed to treat one illness may worsen another, but these interactions are especially dangerous for older adults. It can be challenging to distinguish the effects of a disease from the often-subtle adverse drug effects, which could result in a cascade of prescriptions. When a new medication is prescribed to treat an adverse drug effect that is mistakenly interpreted as a symptom or indication of a new disorder, this is known as a prescribing cascade. The novel, superfluous medication might have more negative effects, which could be misdiagnosed as yet another illness and treated needlessly, and so on (Table 7.4).

Table 7.4. *Preventable Causes of Drug-Related Problems*

Category	Definition
Drug interactions	Use of a drug results in a drug-drug, drug-food, drug-supplement, or drug-disease interaction, leading to adverse effects or decreased efficacy.
Inadequate monitoring	A medical problem is being treated with the correct drug, but the patient is not adequately monitored for complications, effectiveness, or both.
Inappropriate drug selection	A medical problem that requires drug therapy is being treated with a less-than-optimal drug or is generally ineffective for treating the medical problem.
Inappropriate treatment	A patient is taking a drug for no medically valid reason, or the treatment risks outweigh the potential benefits of the drug.
Lack of patient adherence	The correct drug for a medical problem is prescribed, but the patient is not taking it as directed.
Overdosage	A medical problem is being treated with too much of the correct drug.
Poor communication	Drugs are inappropriately dosed, duplicated, continued, or stopped when care is poorly transitioned between providers and/or facilities.
Underprescribing	A medical problem is being treated with too little of the correct drug.
Untreated medical problem	A medical problem requires drug therapy, but no drug is being used to treat that problem.

Source: https://www.msdmanuals.com/professional/geriatrics/drug-therapy-in-older-adults/drug-related-problems-in-older-adults#Reasons-for-Drug-Related-Problems_v1133524.

Many drugs have adverse effects that resemble symptoms of disorders common in older adults or changes due to aging. The following are examples:

- Parkinson's disease-like symptoms may be brought on by antipsychotics. These symptoms in older adults may be misdiagnosed as Parkinson disease and treated with dopaminergic medications, which may cause side effects from the anti-Parkinson's medications (e.g., delirium, nausea, hallucinations, orthostatic hypotension, and so on).
- Patients with dementia may be prescribed cholinesterase inhibitors such as donepezil, rivastigmine, and galantamine. These medications can potentially lead to side effects like diarrhea or urinary issues. In some cases, patients may be prescribed an anticholinergic drug like oxybutynin to manage these new symptoms. However, adding another medication unnecessarily can increase the risk of harmful drug effects and interactions. A more effective approach would be to lower the dosage of the cholinesterase inhibitor or explore alternative dementia treatments like memantine, which works through a different mechanism.
- In patients with hypertension, calcium channel blockers (such as amlodipine, nifedipine, and felodipine) may be prescribed. These medications may effectively treat hypertension, but they also run the risk of causing peripheral edema. Following the prescription of diuretic medication (such as furosemide), patients may experience hypokalemia, which calls for the use of potassium supplements. Reducing the dosage or stopping the calcium channel blocker in favor of other antihypertensive medications, like angiotensin receptor blockers or angiotensin converting enzyme inhibitors, is a better course of action.

In older patients, prescribers should always consider the possibility that a new symptom or sign is due to existing drug therapy (Table 7.5).

Table 7.5. *Drug-Disease Interactions of Concern in Older Adults*

Disease	Drugs	Reason to Avoid
Cardiovascular		
Heart failure	Avoid: Cilostazol Avoid only in heart failure patients with reduced ejection fraction: nondihydropyridine calcium channel blockers (diltiazem, verapamil) Use with caution in heart failure patients who are asymptomatic and avoid in patients with symptomatic heart failure: NSAIDs, COX-2 inhibitors, thiazolidinediones (pioglitazone, rosiglitazone), dronedarone	May promote fluid retention and/or exacerbate heart failure (NSAIDs, COX-2 inhibitors, nondihydropyridine calcium channel blockers, and thiazolidinediones) May increase mortality in older adults with heart failure (cilostazol and dronedarone)
Syncope	Acetylcholinesterase inhibitors, peripheral alpha-1 blockers (e.g., doxazosin, prazosin, terazosin), tertiary TCAs, antipsychotics (chlorpromazine, thioridazine, and olanzapine)	Increased risk of orthostatic hypotension or bradycardia

Central Nervous System		
Delirium	Anticholinergics, antipsychotics, benzodiazepines, corticosteroids*, H2 receptor blockers (cimetidine, famotidine, nizatidine, ranitidine), meperidine, sedative hypnotics (eszopiclone, zaleplon, zolpidem)	Worsened delirium in older adults with or at high risk of delirium Antipsychotics increase the risk of stroke and mortality in patients with dementia and should be avoided for behavioral problems of delirium unless nonpharmacologic options (e.g., behavioral interventions) have failed or are not possible and the patient is threatening substantial harm to self or others
Dementia and cognitive impairment	Anticholinergics, antipsychotics (chronic and as-needed use), benzodiazepines, sedative hypnotics (eszopiclone, zolpidem, zaleplon)	Adverse CNS effects Antipsychotics increase the risk of stroke and mortality in patients with dementia and should be avoided for behavioral problems of dementia unless nonpharmacologic options (e.g., behavioral interventions) have failed or are not possible and the patient is threatening substantial harm to self or others
History of falls or fractures	Antiseizure drugs, antipsychotics, benzodiazepines, sedative hypnotics (eszopiclone, zaleplon, zolpidem), opioids, antidepressants (TCAs, SSRIs, SNRIs)	Ataxia, impaired psychomotor function, syncope, and additional falls Shorter-acting benzodiazepines are not safer than long-acting ones If one of the drugs must be used, reduce the use of other CNS-active drugs that increase risk of falls and fractures and implement other fall risk reduction strategies; data for antidepressants are mixed but no compelling evidence indicates that certain antidepressants confer less fall risk than others Avoid antiseizure drugs except for seizure and mood disorders Avoid opioids except for pain management in the setting of severe acute pain, such as pain due to recent fractures or joint replacement
Parkinson's disease	Antiemetics (metoclopramide, prochlorperazine, promethazine), antipsychotics (except for quetiapine, clozapine, and pimavanserin)	Dopamine receptor antagonists with potential to worsen parkinsonian symptoms (less likely with pimavanserin and clozapine)
Gastrointestinal		

History of gastric or duodenal ulcers	Aspirin (> 325 mg/day), non–COX-2 selective NSAIDs	Exacerbate existing ulcers or cause new ulcers Avoid unless other alternatives are not effective and patients can take a gastroprotective drug (e.g., a proton pump inhibitor or misoprostol)
Kidney and Urinary Tract		
Chronic kidney disease (stage IV or higher: creatinine clearance < 30 mL/min [0.5 mL/sec])	NSAIDs (non-COX and COX-selective, oral, and parenteral, nonacetylated salicylates)	May increase the risk of acute kidney injury and further decline of renal function
Urinary incontinence (all types) in women	Estrogen, oral and transdermal (excludes intravaginal estrogen), peripheral alpha-1 blockers (doxazosin, prazosin, terazosin)	Lack of efficacy (oral estrogen) Worsened incontinence (alpha-1-blockers)
Lower urinary tract symptoms, benign prostatic hyperplasia	Drugs that have strong anticholinergic effects (except antimuscarinics for urinary incontinence)	May decrease urinary flow and cause urinary retention in men
** Excludes inhaled and topical forms. Oral and parenteral corticosteroids may be required for conditions such as exacerbations of COPD (chronic obstructive pulmonary disease), but should be prescribed in the lowest effective dose and for the shortest possible duration.*		
CNS = central nervous system; COX-2 = cyclooxygenase-2; NSAIDs = nonsteroidal anti-inflammatory drugs; SNRIs = serotonin-norepinephrine reuptake inhibitors; SSRIs = selective serotonin reuptake inhibitors; TCAs = tricyclic antidepressants.		

Source: https://www.msdmanuals.com/professional/geriatrics/drug-therapy-in-older-adults/drug-related-problems-in-older-adults#Reasons-for-Drug-Related-Problems_v1133524.

7.2.4.2. Drug-Drug Interactions

Older adults are especially susceptible to drug-drug interactions because they frequently use multiple drugs. Additionally, older adults often use dietary supplements and medicinal herbs, but they might not disclose this to their healthcare providers. Medicinal herbs and prescription medications may interact negatively and cause side effects. For instance, taking warfarin along with ginkgo biloba extract may raise the risk of bleeding, and St. Combining St. John's wort with an SSRI may raise your chance of developing serotonin syndrome. As a result, doctors ought to question patients directly about dietary supplements, such as vitamin and herbal blends. There is little difference between drug-drug interactions in the general population and those in older adults. Still, some drugs (e.g., rifampin, carbamazepine, phenytoin) may be reduced in older adults; consequently, the shift (increase) in drug metabolism may be less noticeable in this population. Numerous other medications block CYP450 metabolism, which raises the possibility of toxicity for medications that rely on that pathway for excretion. Due to their increased drug usage, older adults are more likely to experience numerous, unpredictable CYP450 interactions. Additionally, using more than one medication at the same time that has similar side effects can make side effects more likely or severe.

7.2.4.3. Inadequate Monitoring

Monitoring drug use involves

- Documenting the indication for a new drug
- Keeping a current list of drugs used by the patient in medical records
- Monitoring for achievement of therapeutic goals and other responses to new drugs
- Monitoring necessary laboratory tests for efficacy or adverse effects
- Periodically reviewing drugs for continued need

For elderly patients in particular, these precautions are crucial. Inadequate supervision raises the risk of polypharmacy, side effects, and inefficiency, particularly after new medications are prescribed. As part of the drug utilization review criteria, an expert consensus panel from the Health Care Financing Administration developed criteria to help with monitoring. The criteria center on therapy duplication, potential drug-drug interactions, and improper dosage or duration of treatment.

7.2.4.4. Inappropriate Drug Selection

A drug is inappropriate if its potential for harm exceeds its potential for benefit. Inappropriate use of a drug may involve

- Choice of an unsuitable drug, dose, frequency of dosing, or duration of therapy
- Duplication of therapy
- Failure to consider drug interactions and appropriate indications for a drug
- Appropriate drugs that are mistakenly continued once an acute condition resolves (as may happen when patients move from one health care setting to another and the indication is not reevaluated)

Certain drug classes pose particular risks for older adults. Certain drugs are so harmful that older adults should never take them, while others should only be taken under specific circumstances and can be used with greater caution. Other comparable lists are available (4). The American Geriatrics Society Beers Criteria is a list of drugs that may be inappropriate for older adults based on drug class. There is also a list of some drug-therapy substitutes along with citations (5). Potential advantages and risks of therapy to each patient must be considered by clinicians. When a patient is nearing the end of their life, different criteria apply for drug therapy decisions. Inappropriate medications are still prescribed for older adults despite their awareness of the American Geriatrics Society Beers Criteria® and other criteria. Approximately 20% of older adults who live in the community receive at least one inappropriate medication. Adverse effect risk is elevated in these patients. Inappropriate use also raises the risk of hospitalization and death in residents of nursing homes. In a study involving hospitalized patients, 27.5% were given the wrong medication.

A few improper medications (e.g., diphenhydramine, and oral nonsteroidal anti-inflammatory drugs [NSAIDs]) are available OTC; as a result, healthcare professionals should ask patients directly if they use OTC medications and address any possible side effects. Proton pump inhibitors, hypnotics, and analgesics are the most common medications prescribed to older adults for minor symptoms (including side effects from other medications) that may be better managed with nonpharmacologic therapies (e.g., physical therapy, massage, dietary modifications, cognitive-behavioral therapy) or by reducing the dosage of the medication that is having negative side effects. It is frequently inappropriate to start taking new medications because they may have little benefit, increase costs, or cause more toxicity. It takes more than just staying away from a short list of drugs and identifying drug categories of concern to address the issue of inappropriate drug use in older adults. A patient's complete medication regimen should also be routinely evaluated to ascertain whether the drug is still necessary and whether there may be more benefit than harm.

7.2.4.5. Lack of Patient Adherence

Drug effectiveness is often compromised by a lack of patient adherence among the ambulatory older adults. Adherence is affected by many factors, including language barriers, but not by age per se. Up to half of older adults do not take drugs as directed, usually taking less than prescribed (underadherence). Causes are similar to those for younger adults. In addition, the following contribute:

- Financial and physical constraints, which may make purchasing drugs difficult
- Cognitive problems, which may make taking drugs as instructed difficult
- Use of multiple drugs (polypharmacy)
- Use of drugs that must be taken several times a day or in a specific manner
- Lack of understanding about what a drug is intended to do (benefits) or how to recognize and manage adverse effects (harms)

Patients may find it difficult to adhere to a regimen that calls for either too frequent or too infrequent dosing, multiple medications, or both. Physicians should evaluate their patients' health literacy and medication adherence skills (e.g., dexterity, hand strength, vision, and intellect) and make an effort to work around their limitations by setting up or suggesting large print drug labels and instructions, alarm-equipped containers filled according to daily drug requirements, phone reminders, or medication assistance. Every time they see an elderly patient, pharmacists and nurses can support them by educating them and going over prescription instructions. By observing if patients get refills on time or if a prescription seems strange or incorrect, pharmacists may be able to spot an issue. If prescriptions are not being filled at the proper intervals, many pharmacies can track refill trends and get in touch with patients, prescribers, or both.

7.2.4.6. Overdosage

If the prescriber does not take into account age-related changes that affect pharmacokinetics and pharmacodynamics, older adults may be prescribed an excessive dose of a medication that is appropriate. Drugs that are cleared by the kidneys, for instance, have different dosages, for example, digoxin, gabapentin, and a few antibiotics) should be modified in patients with renal impairment. Generally speaking, medications should be started at the lowest dose in older adults, even though individual dose requirements vary greatly. When a drug has a narrow therapeutic index, when it may exacerbate another condition, and especially in patients who are frail, starting doses of roughly one-third to one-half the usual adult dose are recommended. Once the desired effect is achieved, the dose is titrated upward as tolerated. Whenever possible, drug levels should be tracked and patients should be assessed for side effects before receiving a higher dose. In addition, drug interactions that increase the quantity of a drug available or therapeutic duplication—the practice of one practitioner prescribing a medication without the knowledge of another practitioner—can also result in overdosage.

7.2.4.7. Poor Communication

Up to 50% of medication errors and up to 20% of adverse drug effects in hospitals are the result of inadequate medical information transferred between healthcare settings during transitions. When hospitalized patients are released from care, medication regimens that were initiated and required exclusively while in the hospital (e.g., laxatives, proton pump inhibitors, and sedative hypnotics) may be continued unnecessarily by the discharging prescriber. This may be the result of negligence, a lack of time, or an inability to get in touch with the primary care physician. On the other hand, poor communication upon admission to a medical facility may cause an inadvertent omission of a critical maintenance medication. Drug reconciliation is a formal process that helps eliminate mistakes and omissions by going over all prescribed medications at each change in care.

7.2.4.8. Underprescribing

It's possible to under prescribe appropriate medications—i.e., not employed to get the most benefit. Underprescribing has the potential to lower quality of life and raise morbidity and death. Physicians should administer appropriate dosages of medications and multidrug regimens when necessary. Anticoagulants, beta-blockers, heart failure, depression, Alzheimer's disease, atrial fibrillation, and hypertension are among the medications that are frequently under prescribed to older adults. Additionally, vaccinations aren't always administered the recommended way.

- **Beta-blockers:** In patients with a history of myocardial infarction and/or heart failure, even in older patients at high risk of complications (e.g., those with pulmonary disorders or diabetes), these drugs reduce mortality rates and hospitalizations.
- **Antihypertensives:** Guidelines for treating hypertension in older adults are available, and treatment appears to be beneficial (reducing the risk of stroke and major cardiovascular events) even in frail older adults. Nonetheless, studies indicate that hypertension is often not optimally controlled in older patients.
- **Drugs for Alzheimer's disease:** Acetylcholinesterase inhibitors and NMDA (N-methyl-d-aspartate) antagonists have been shown to benefit patients with Alzheimer's disease. The amount of benefit is modest and variable, but patients and family members should be given the opportunity to make an informed decision about their use.
- **Anticoagulants:** Anticoagulants (both warfarin and the newer direct oral anticoagulant drugs) reduce risk of stroke in patients with atrial fibrillation. Although there is an increased risk of bleeding with anticoagulation in general, some older adults who might benefit from anticoagulation are not receiving it.
- **Immunizations:** Older adults are at greater risk of morbidity and mortality resulting from influenza, pneumococcal infection, and herpes zoster. Vaccination rates among older adults can still be improved.

Acute or unrelated disorders may go untreated in older patients with chronic illnesses (e.g., an untreated case of hypercholesterolemia in individuals with chronic obstructive pulmonary disease. Clinicians are worried about lengthening the time it takes for a patient with a lower life expectancy to benefit from treatment or raising the risk of side effects, therefore, they may decide not to administer these treatments. Physicians may believe that treating the main issue is all that patients are capable of or desire, or that they are unable to pay for the additional medications. For clinicians to comprehend patients' priorities and concerns, it is important that patients and caregivers actively participate in decision-making regarding drug treatment.

7.2.5. Drug Categories of Concern in Older Adults

The Beers Criteria categorize potentially inappropriate drugs into three groups:

- Potentially inappropriate for all older adults: To be avoided if possible
- Potentially inappropriate due to drug-disease and drug-syndrome interactions: To be avoided in older adults with certain diseases or syndromes
- Benefit may offset risk in some patients: To be used with caution

A few drug classes (e.g., analgesics, anticoagulants, antihypertensives, diuretics, hypoglycemic medications, antiparkinsonian medications, and psychoactive medications) present unique risks for elderly patients. Certain drugs are safe enough for younger adults to use, but they pose such a risk that older adults shouldn't use them. For identifying such inappropriate drugs, the American Geriatric Society Beers Criteria® are most frequently utilized.

7.2.5.1. Analgesics

Oral nonsteroidal anti-inflammatory drugs (NSAIDs) are used by > 30% of people aged 65 to 89, and half of all NSAID prescriptions are for people > 60. Several NSAIDs are available without prescription.

Older adults may be prone to adverse effects of these drugs, and adverse effects may be more severe because of the following:

- NSAIDs are highly lipid-soluble, and because adipose tissue usually increases with age, distribution of the drugs is more extensive.
- Plasma protein is often decreased, resulting in higher levels of unbound drugs, and exaggerated pharmacologic effects for drugs that are highly protein-bound.
- Renal function is reduced in many older adults, resulting in decreased renal clearance and higher drug levels.

Peptic ulceration and upper gastrointestinal (GI) bleeding are serious side effects that can occur; the risk increases with the initiation of an NSAID and with increasing the dosage. Aspirin, warfarin, direct oral anticoagulants, corticosteroids, and other antiplatelet medications increase the risk of upper gastrointestinal bleeding when NSAIDs are taken together e.g., clopidogrel). NSAIDs have the potential to raise cardiovascular event risk, induce fluid retention, and occasionally cause nephropathy. NSAIDs have the additional potential to raise blood pressure; this effect may go unnoticed and result in a prescribing cascade whereby antihypertensive medication is increased. Clinicians should therefore be aware of this effect when older adults' blood pressure rises and inquire about their use of NSAIDs, especially OTC NSAIDs.

Compared to other NSAIDs, selective COX-2 (cyclooxygenase-2) inhibitors, or coxibs, cause less GI discomfort and platelet inhibition. However, patients taking warfarin or aspirin (even at a low dose) or who have experienced GI events are more susceptible to bleeding during coxib use. Although the risk may differ between drugs, coxibs as a class seem to increase the risk of cardiovascular events; therefore, they should be used with caution. The effects of coxibs on the kidneys are similar to those of other NSAIDs. Alternatives with less risk (e.g., when feasible, use acetaminophen, topical diclofenac gel. The lowest effective dose and regular reviews of continued need are recommended when using NSAIDs in older adults. Serum creatinine and blood pressure should be regularly monitored when using NSAIDs for an extended period, particularly in patients who have additional risk factors (e.g., heart failure, kidney impairment, volume depletion, cirrhosis with ascites, diuretic use), and a gastroprotective medication (e.g., Misoprostol or a proton-pump inhibitor) should be taken into consideration for concurrent use.

7.2.5.2. Anticoagulants

Growing older may make one more susceptible to warfarin's anticoagulant effects. When older adults take warfarin, their increased risk of bleeding can be largely mitigated by careful dosing and regular monitoring. Additionally, because warfarin and other drugs frequently interact, patients who take multiple medications should consult computerized drug interaction programs before starting new ones or stopping old ones. Additionally, patients should be watched for interactions between warfarin and alcohol, food, OTC medications, and supplements. In comparison to warfarin, the newer anticoagulants dabigatran, rivaroxaban, apixaban, and edoxaban may be simpler to dose and have fewer drug-drug and food-drug interactions. In patients with atrial fibrillation, the newer anticoagulants are as effective as or more effective than warfarin in lowering the risk of stroke and intracranial hemorrhage; however, they still raise the risk of bleeding in older adults, especially those with impaired renal function.

7.2.5.3. Antidepressants

Even though tricyclic antidepressants (TCAs) are useful, older adults should not often take them. Although they are less toxic and just as effective as TCAs, mixed reuptake inhibitors like serotonin-norepinephrine reuptake inhibitors (SNRIs) and selective serotonin reuptake inhibitors (SSRIs) raise certain concerns. Furthermore, in older adults, the use of any SSRI, SNRI, or TCA may raise the risk of falls and hyponatremia.

- In addition to having anticholinergic effects and being more sedating than other SSRIs, paroxetine can also inhibit the activity of the hepatic cytochrome P-450 2D6 enzyme, which may affect the metabolism of several medications, including tamoxifen, some antipsychotics, antiarrhythmics, and TCAs.
- Citalopram and escitalopram: Doses in older adults should be limited to a maximum of 20 mg/day and 10 mg/day, respectively, because QT prolongation is a concern.
- Venlafaxine and duloxetine: These drugs may increase blood pressure.
- Mirtazapine: This drug can be sedating and may stimulate appetite/weight gain.
- Sertraline: This drug confers the highest risk of diarrhea.

7.2.5.4. Antihyperglycemics

Patients with diabetes mellitus should have their antihyperglycemic medication doses carefully titrated. The age-related risk of hypoglycemia from sulfonylureas may rise. Chlorpropamide is not advised for use in older adults due to the increased risk of hypoglycemia and hyponatremia caused by the syndrome of inappropriate antidiuretic hormone secretion, as detailed in the table, "potentially inappropriate drugs in older adults". Because renal clearance is decreased in older adults taking glyburide and glimepiride, the risk of hypoglycemia is also higher than with other oral antihyperglycemics. Given alone or in combination with sulfonylureas, metformin, a biguanide excreted by the kidneys, increases peripheral tissue sensitivity to insulin. The degree of renal impairment and patient age are associated with an increased risk of lactic acidosis, an uncommon but serious complication. A contraindication is heart failure with symptoms. Among patients with impaired renal function, sodium-glucose cotransporter-2 (SGLT2) inhibitors (canagliflozin, dapagliflozin, and empagliflozin) should be avoided due to the increased risk of fungal infections, hypovolemia with orthostatic hypotension, and urinary tract infections.

7.2.5.5. Antihypertensives

For the majority of older adults with hypertension, standard doses and multidrug therapy are required to achieve blood pressure goals; however, in many cases, lower starting doses of antihypertensives may be required to minimize risk of side effects. Depending on comorbidities, the initial treatment of hypertension in older adults usually consists of a dihydropyridine calcium channel blocker, angiotensin-converting enzyme (ACE) inhibitor, thiazide-type diuretic, or angiotensin II receptor blocker. Beta-blockers ought to be kept for people with heart conditions or to regulate the rate of atrial fibrillation. The use of short-acting nifedipine as it may raise the risk of mortality is not recommended. Blood pressure should be checked while sitting and standing, especially if using multiple antihypertensives, to look for orthostatic hypotension, which raises the risk of fractures and falls. Because many older adults experience white-coat syndrome, which is an increase in blood pressure while at a doctor's office, or masked hypertension, which is a decrease in blood pressure while at a doctor's office, ambulatory or home blood pressure monitoring may also be more accurate in older adults than in-clinic blood pressure readings. Physicians need to strike a balance between the objectives of blood pressure targets and the possibility of unfavorable outcomes in older adults (like causing orthostatic hypotension or raising the risk of falls).

7.2.5.6. Antiparkinsonian Drugs

Older adults have lower levodopa clearance and are more vulnerable to side effects, especially orthostatic hypotension and confusion. As a result, levodopa should be started at a lower dosage for older adults and their effects should be closely monitored. Not only may patients who experience confusion while on levodopa be unable to tolerate dopamine agonists (e.g., ropinirole, pramipexole). Due to the possibility of concurrent cognitive symptoms in older adults with Parkinsonism, medications with anticholinergic effects (e.g., trihexyphenidyl, diphenydramine) ought to be steered clear of.

7.2.5.7. Antipsychotics

Antipsychotics ought to be reserved for cases of psychosis. Antipsychotics have serious side effects and only slightly better symptom control than a placebo in agitated, nonpsychotic patients. The FDA releases a "black box" warning regarding their use in these patients. In general, behavioral issues associated with dementia (e.g., straying, shouting, and disobedience) do not react well to antipsychotics. Antipsychotics should not be administered only in response to a behavioral issue (e.g., shouting, or repeating words) irritates people besides the patient. When using an antipsychotic, the initial dosage ought to be roughly 25% of the typical adult starting dose. It should then be progressively increased while being closely monitored for side effects and response. If possible, the dose should be titrated down to the lowest effective dose once the patient responds. If the medication is not working, it has to be stopped. There is a dearth of clinical trial information on the dosage, safety, and effectiveness of these medications in older persons.

Antipsychotics may make confusion worse while also lessening paranoia. The frequently irreversible condition known as tardive dyskinesia is more common in older adults, particularly in women. Up to 20% of older adults taking antipsychotics may experience akathisia, or subjective motor restlessness, sedation, orthostatic hypotension, anticholinergic effects, and akathisia; additionally, drug-induced Parkinsonism may last for up to 6 to 9 months after the medication is stopped. Although second-generation antipsychotics (e.g., risperidone, olanzapine, quetiapine, and others) are used, particularly in larger dosages. The patient or the person in charge of the patient's care should be informed of the advantages and disadvantages of using an antipsychotic. Antipsychotics ought to be taken into consideration for behavioral issues only in cases where nonpharmacologic treatments have proven ineffective and the patient's actions endanger others or themselves.

7.2.5.8. Anxiolytics and Hypnotics

Prior to using hypnotics, treatable causes of insomnia should be identified and addressed. Nonpharmacologic strategies like cognitive-behavioral therapy and good sleeping habits (e.g., cutting back on naps during the day, changing bedtime) should be attempted initially. If not successful, nonbenzodiazepine hypnotics (e.g., eszopiclone, zolpidem, and zaleplon) are available for short-term usage. These medications lessen sleep disturbances than benzodiazepines because they primarily bind to a subtype of benzodiazepine receptor. Although lower doses are recommended for older adults, they have a quicker onset, fewer rebound effects, fewer next-day effects, and less potential for dependence. When treating insomnia in older adults, nonbenzodiazepine hypnotics and short-, intermediate-, and long-acting benzodiazepines should be avoided due to their increased risk of cognitive impairment, delirium, falls, fractures, and motor vehicle crashes. For older adults experiencing anxiety or panic attacks, benzodiazepines may be helpful. If possible, the length of hypnotic or anxiolytic therapy should be kept to a minimum because withdrawal symptoms like insomnia or rebound anxiety can result from tolerance and dependence. The antihistamines (e.g., since they have anticholinergic effects and tolerance to the sedative effects sets in quickly, they are not advised for use as hypnotics or anxiolytics. For general anxiety disorder, buspirone, a partial serotonin agonist, can be helpful; dosages up to 30 mg/day are well tolerated by older adults. In emergency situations, the anxiolytic effect's delayed (up to two or three week) onset may be detrimental.

7.2.5.9. Digoxin

Digoxin is a cardiac glycoside that is used to treat supraventricular arrhythmias and strengthen myocardial contractions. In older adults, though, it needs to be used carefully. A higher risk of death is linked to serum digoxin levels > 0.8 ng/mL (1.0 nmol/L) in men with heart failure and a left ventricular ejection fraction of ≤ 45%. Its limited therapeutic index usually relates to adverse effects. Digoxin was found to be helpful in women when their serum levels were between 0 and 9 ng/mL (0 and 6 nmol/L), but it may be hazardous if the levels were greater than 1 ng/mL (1 nmol/L). There are several factors that make older adults more susceptible to digoxin toxicity. Digoxin renal clearance can be lowered by renal impairment, transient dehydration, and the use of nonsteroidal anti-inflammatory drugs (NSAIDs), all of which are prevalent in older adults. Furthermore, digoxin clearance falls by an average of 50% in older adults with normal serum creatinine levels. Additionally, digoxin's volume of distribution decreases with a decrease in lean body mass, which can happen as people age. For this reason, starting doses ought to be modest (0.125 mg/day), and they ought to be modified in accordance with response and serum digoxin levels (which typically range from 0.08 to 2.0 ng/mL [1.0 to 2.6 nmol/L]). Serum digoxin levels, however, do not always indicate a higher risk of toxicity. Additionally, for the first line of treatment of heart failure and atrial fibrillation, the American Geriatric Society Beers Criteria® recommend avoiding doses greater than 0 to 125 mg/day and avoiding digoxin.

7.2.5.10. Diuretics

Compared to other diuretics, lower dosages of thiazide diuretics, such as hydrochlorothiazide or chlorthalidone 12 ppm to 25 mg, have a lower risk of hypokalemia and hyperglycemia and can effectively control hypertension in many older adults. Potassium supplements might therefore be needed less frequently. When administering potassium-sparing diuretics to older adults, care should be taken to monitor the patient's potassium level. This is especially important if the patient has impaired kidney function or is taking ACE inhibitor or angiotensin II receptor blocker along with the diuretics.

A Closer Look

Polypharmacy and Drug-Drug Interaction

Polypharmacy refers to the concurrent use of multiple medications by an individual, typically involving the use of four or more medications simultaneously. While polypharmacy can be necessary for managing multiple chronic conditions, it also presents significant challenges and risks, particularly in older adults. The prevalence of polypharmacy has increased in recent years due to aging populations, the rising burden of chronic diseases, and advances in medical treatments. While each medication may be prescribed with good intentions to address specific health concerns, the cumulative effects of multiple drugs can lead to adverse outcomes, including drug interactions, increased risk of side effects, medication non-adherence, and reduced quality of life.

One of the primary concerns associated with polypharmacy is the increased risk of drug-drug interactions (DDIs). A drug-drug interaction occurs when the effects of one medication are altered by the presence of another medication, leading to changes in pharmacokinetics or pharmacodynamics that may result in therapeutic failure or toxicity. DDIs can occur through various mechanisms, including interference with drug metabolism, competition for binding sites, and additive or synergistic effects. For example, concomitant use of warfarin (an anticoagulant) and nonsteroidal anti-inflammatory drugs (NSAIDs) can increase the risk of bleeding due to their combined effect on platelet function and blood clotting. Polypharmacy and drug-drug interactions are particularly concerning in older adults due to age-related changes in pharmacokinetics and pharmacodynamics, as well as the higher prevalence of comorbidities and frailty. Aging is associated with alterations in liver and kidney function, which can affect drug metabolism and excretion, leading to prolonged drug half-lives and increased drug concentrations in the bloodstream. Additionally, older adults may have reduced physiological reserves and a higher susceptibility to adverse drug effects, making them more vulnerable to the consequences of polypharmacy and drug interactions.

Managing polypharmacy and preventing drug-drug interactions require a comprehensive and individualized approach that involves healthcare providers, patients, and caregivers. Healthcare providers play a crucial role in conducting medication reviews, assessing the appropriateness of drug regimens, and identifying potential interactions. This may involve using tools such as Beers Criteria and STOPP/START criteria, which provide guidance on potentially inappropriate medications in older adults and appropriate alternatives. Pharmacists also play a vital role in medication management by providing medication reconciliation, counseling patients on drug interactions and side effects, and collaborating with prescribers to optimize therapy. Patient education and engagement are essential components of managing polypharmacy and reducing the risk of drug interactions. Patients should be encouraged to actively participate in their care by keeping an up-to-date list of medications, including OTC drugs and supplements, and discussing any concerns or questions with their healthcare providers. Patients should also be informed about the importance of medication adherence, proper dosing, and potential side effects, as well as the risks associated with self-medication and non-prescription drug use.

Summary

- Geriatric toxicology is a specialized field of toxicology that focuses on the study of adverse effects of substances on the elderly population. This branch of toxicology is particularly important due to the unique physiological and pharmacokinetic changes that occur with aging, which can alter the way drugs and other toxic substances are metabolized and excreted.
- The science of toxicology has a dual nature. It is the study of mechanisms by which environmental agents exert their toxic effects, and it is the empirical definition of the magnitude of toxicity of such agents and the risk they present to exposed human populations.*
- Nutrition underscores the usefulness of considering aging as a toxic end point. For example, both deficiency and excess of vitamin B6 can lead to neurologic damage (and these changes superficially resemble those accompanying aging).
- The absence of universal mimicry of aging by toxic agents, even in a given tissue, is an important observation that must not be overinterpreted. A toxic agent might produce molecular lesions similar to aging-induced lesions.
- Neurotoxicology and immunotoxicology should also be emphasized. Most environmental agents have not been screened for neurotoxic and immunotoxic effects, and some neurologic and immunologic deficits of unknown etiology are observed in a large proportion of the aged.
- Absorption is the major process by which toxicants are transported across body membranes. The main sites of absorption of toxic agents are the skin, lungs, and gastrointestinal tract. Many toxicants can be absorbed through the skin and enter the bloodstream. Chemical or physical injury and other circumstances can increase the skin's permeability.
- Some chemical agents that enter the body can remain as intact molecules, but many are biologically transformed by metabolic processes. Metabolic processes might involve simple and reversible chemical or physical interactions that primarily affect transport throughout the body and across membranes.
- The mechanisms by which toxic agents exert their actions are extremely diverse. Such mechanisms vary between specific agents and between doses of a given agent.
- The molecular action of toxic agents can result from the creation of damaging chemical species that attack specific moieties of biologic molecules. The search for toxic mechanisms that are shared by aging and by specific toxic agents should include agents whose action is very broad, because aging broadly affects all tissues. Breadth of action can result from different types of mechanisms, however.
- Toxic mechanisms can act at the level of the cell in two general ways: specific tissue functions can fail if enough cells of a specific type in that tissue are altered by the exposure, and toxic stress of a single cell can produce some toxic effects (as in cancer), heritable mutation, and teratogenesis.

References

1. Ashford, N. A. (1986). Policy considerations for human monitoring in the workplace. *Journal of Occupational Medicine, 28*(8), 563–568.
2. Ayesh, R., Idle, J. R., Ritchie, J. C., Crothers, M. J., & Hetzel, M. R. (1984). Metabolic oxidation phenotypes as markers for susceptibility to lung cancer. *Nature, 312*(5991), 169–170.
3. Calabrese, E. J. (1986). *Age and Susceptibility to Toxic Substances.* New York: John Wiley & Sons.
4. Campbell, T. C., & Hayes, J. R. (1974). Role of nutrition in the drug-metabolizing enzyme system. *Pharmacological Reviews, 26*(2), 171–197.
5. Cluff, L. E., Thornton, G. L., & Smith, J. (1965). Epidemiological study of adverse drug reactions. *Transactions of the Association of American Physicians, 78*, 255–268.
6. Forster, A. J., Clark, H. D., Menard, A., et al. (2004). Adverse events among medical patients after discharge from hospital. *CMAJ, 170*(3), 345–349. https://doi.org/10.1503/cmaj.1030250.
7. Fowle, J. R., III. (1984). *Workshop Proceedings: Approaches to Improving the Assessment of Human Genetic Risk—Human Biomonitoring* (Report No. EPA-600/9–84–016). Washington, D.C.: U.S. Environmental Protection Agency, Office of Health and Environmental Assessment. Available from National Technical Information Service, Springfield, VA, as PB85–103018.
8. Hanlon, J. T., Semla, T. P., Schmader, K. E., et al. (2015). Alternative medications for medications in the use of high-risk medications in the elderly and potentially harmful drug-disease interactions in the elderly quality measures. *Journal of the American Geriatrics Society, 63*(12), e8–e18. https://doi.org/10.1111/jgs.13807.
9. Hayes, A. W. (1982). *Principles and Methods of Toxicology*. New York: Raven Press.
10. Lower, G. M., Jr., & Kanarek, M. S. (1982). Risk, susceptibility and the epidemiology of proliferative neoplastic disease: Descriptive vs. mechanistic approaches. *Medical Hypotheses, 9*(1), 33–49.
11. Perera, F. P., & Weinstein, I. B. (1982). Molecular epidemiology and carcinogen-DNA adduct detection: New approaches to studies of human cancer causation. *Journal of Chronic Diseases, 35*(8), 581–600.
12. Qato, D. M., Wilder, J., Schumm, L. P., et al. (2016). Changes in prescription and over-the-counter medication and dietary supplement use among older adults in the United States, 2005 vs 2011. *JAMA Internal Medicine, 176*(4), 473–482. https://doi.org/10.1001/jamainternmed.2015.8581.
13. Tam, V. C., Knowles, S. R., Cornish, P. L., et al. (2005). Frequency, type and clinical importance of medication history errors at admission to hospital: A systematic review. *CMAJ, 173*(5), 510–515. https://doi.org/10.1503/cmaj.045311.
14. The American Geriatrics Society 2019 Beers Criteria Update Expert Panel. (2019). American Geriatrics Society updated Beers Criteria® for potentially inappropriate medication use in older adults. *Journal of the American Geriatrics Society, 67*(4), 674–694. https://doi.org/10.1111/jgs.15767.
15. Vesell, E. S. (1982). Dynamically interacting genetic and environmental factors that affect the response of developing individuals to toxicants. In V. R. Hunt, M. K. Smith, & D. Worth (Eds.), *Environmental Factors in Human Growth and Development* (Banbury Report 11, pp. 107–124). Cold Spring Harbor Laboratory.

16. Vesell, E. S. (1982). On the significance of host factors that affect drug disposition. *Clinical Pharmacology and Therapeutics, 31*(1), 1–7.

17. Wong, J. D., Bajcar, J. M., Wong, G. G., et al. (2008). Medication reconciliation at hospital discharge: Evaluating discrepancies. *Annals of Pharmacotherapy, 42*(10), 1373–1379. https://doi.org/10.1345/aph.1L190.

16. Vesell, E.S. (1982). On the significance of host factors that affect drug disposition. *Clinical Pharmacology and Therapeutics*, 32(1), 1–2[illegible].

17. Wong, J. D., Bajcar, J. M., Wong, G. G., et al. (2008). Medication reconciliation at hospital [illegible] *Annals of Pharmacotherapy*, 42(10), 1373–1379. https://doi.org/10.1345/aph.1L190

Chapter

8

PEDIATRIC TOXICOLOGY

Contents

Introduction

A specialty area of medicine called pediatric toxicology is devoted to the investigation, diagnosis, and management of poisonings and toxic exposures in children. It covers a broad spectrum of substances that may be harmful to children, such as drugs, household goods, chemicals, plants, and poisonous animals. Recognizing children's particular vulnerabilities owing to things like their smaller stature, developing organ systems, and behaviors that could raise their risk of exposure is essential to understanding pediatric toxicology. To treat children who have been poisoned, this field integrates concepts from pharmacology, toxicology, pediatrics, emergency medicine, and environmental health. Poison prevention (Walton WW. 1982), toxic exposure identification, toxicity severity assessment, and the application of suitable management techniques are important facets of pediatric toxicology. The goal of poison prevention initiatives is to inform parents, kids, and caregivers about potential risks found in the house, how to store medications and household chemicals, and how to handle them safely. Pediatric toxicologists employ a methodical approach to evaluate the child's clinical state, obtain pertinent medical history, and pinpoint the toxin in question following toxic exposures. This frequently entails carrying out a comprehensive physical examination, obtaining test results from laboratories, and carrying out diagnostic imaging studies as required.

Making treatment decisions requires having a clear understanding of the degree of toxicity. Pediatric toxicologists assess several variables, such as the child's age and weight, the substance's toxic qualities, the amount and duration of exposure, and the existence of any underlying medical conditions. For mild exposures, treatment options might include straightforward observation and supportive care; for more serious poisonings, treatment options might include more aggressive measures like antidote administration, decontamination techniques, and advanced life support. Pediatric toxicologists are essential in treating chronic exposures and environmental pollutants that can have long-term effects on children's health in addition to acute poisonings. This could entail evaluating the long-term health impacts, counseling families on lowering environmental exposures, and pushing for public health initiatives to shield kids from potentially harmful substances in their environment. In the field of pediatric toxicology, cooperation between emergency physicians, intensivists, clinical pharmacists, and poison control centers is crucial for the prompt and efficient management of children who have been poisoned. Furthermore, to improve treatment outcomes, advance our knowledge of toxicology principles, and create preventive measures to protect children's health and wellbeing, it is imperative that research and education continue.

Orientation and Directional Terms

Term	Definition	Illustration
Pharmacology	Pharmacology is the science of drugs and medications, including a substance's origin, composition, pharmacokinetics, pharmacodynamics, therapeutic use, and toxicology.	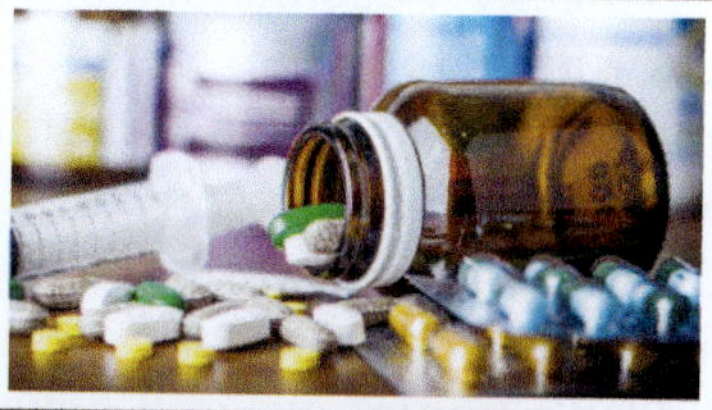
Liquid medications	Most commonly used by patients who have difficulties swallowing tablets and capsules such as children and the elderly.	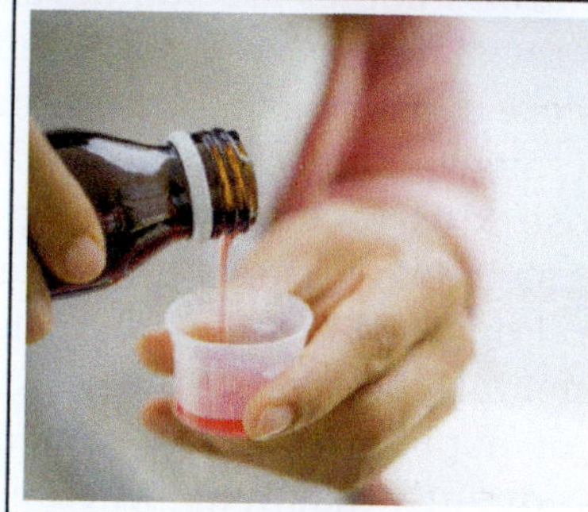
Chlorpyrifos	Chlorpyrifos is an organophosphate insecticide, acaricide and miticide used primarily to control foliage and soil-borne insect pests.	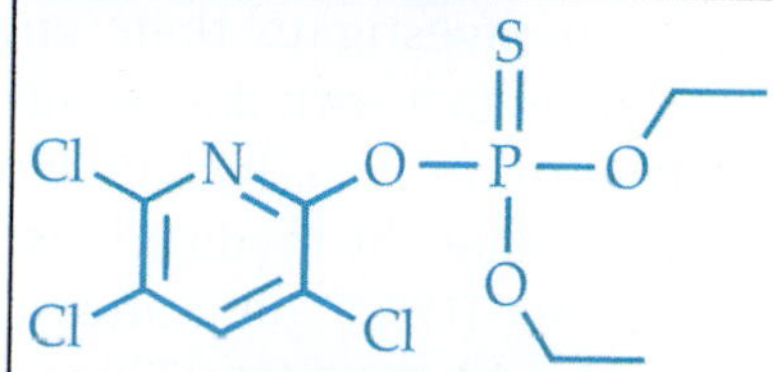 Chlorpyrifos
Hand sanitizers	Hand sanitizer, agent applied to the hands for the purpose of removing common pathogens (disease-causing organisms).	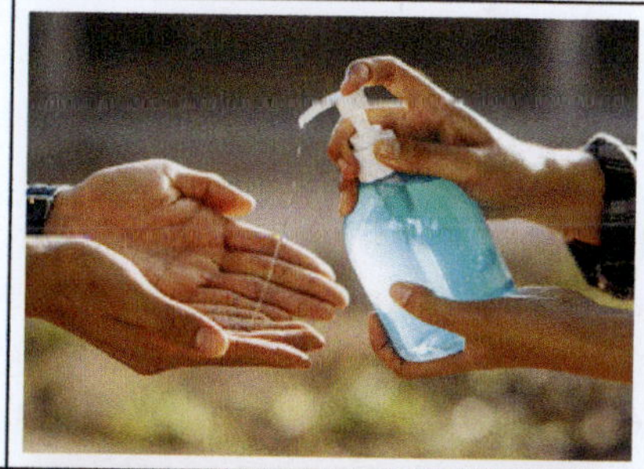
Nicotine	Nicotine is a naturally produced alkaloid in the nightshade family of plants and is widely used recreationally as a stimulant and anxiolytic. As a pharmaceutical drug, it is used for smoking cessation to relieve withdrawal symptoms.	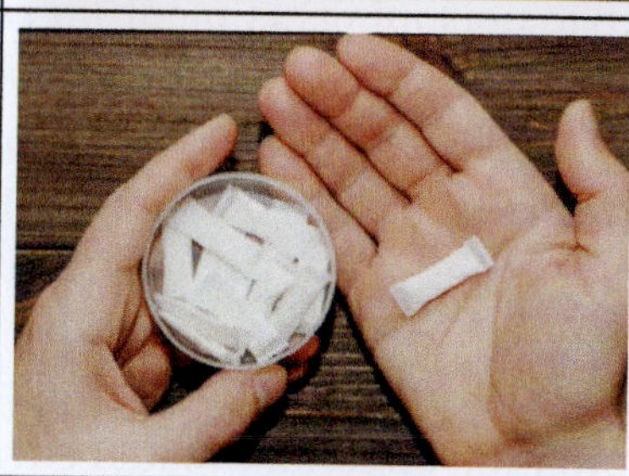

8.1. Common Pediatric Poisonings

Children typically become poisoned at home when they inhale, touch, or come into contact with a toxic substance. Usually unintentional, the poisoning affects children younger than five. Children's poisoning is frequently caused by medications, household cleaners, and alcohol. Since children's bodies are still developing and have less resistance to the poison's effects than adults', these substances may be toxic to them. include a range of materials and situations that can expose kids to toxins. Among the main causes of pediatric poisonings are medications, common household chemicals, plants, and environmental pollutants. The most frequent method of exposure is accidental ingestion, which frequently happens when inquisitive young children investigate their environment and come into contact with dangerous materials that are left within reach. Pediatric poisonings are frequently caused by medications, especially over-the-counter (OTC) painkillers, vitamins, and cough and cold remedies. This is especially true when the medications are not stored properly or are mistaken for candy.

Children are at serious risk from household chemicals like pesticides, cleaning products, and laundry detergents because they could accidentally swallow or inhale these substances while playing in areas or opening cabinets where they are kept. Another frequent cause of pediatric poisonings is plant ingestion, both indoors and outdoors. This is because kids may be drawn to vibrant berries or foliage without realizing how toxic it could be. Furthermore, children may be at risk from environmental toxins like lead, carbon monoxide, and mold, especially in older homes or buildings with poor ventilation or contaminated environments. Because lead is found in paint, soil, and water sources, lead poisoning in particular is still a serious concern. Reducing the risk of pediatric poisonings requires the implementation of preventive measures like childproofing homes, locking cabinets, or keeping toxic materials out of reach, using child-resistant packaging, and teaching caregivers about potential dangers. If a poisoning does occur, it is imperative to recognize the symptoms as soon as possible and seek medical attention right away because prompt treatment can lessen the effects of toxicity and avoid major complications.

8.1.1. Medicine Poisoning

The most frequent cause of poisoning in children is medications. A number of the medications you or a family member take may be harmful to young people. Not only are opioids and barbiturates known to be dangerous, but medications for diabetes, mental illness, and elevated blood pressure can also be harmful. For a small child, a single tablet can be lethal. Many of the medications your child is prescribed may be dangerous in larger dosages. Your child's pediatrician will weigh them and recommend a dosage that is both safe and efficient. To make sure you are administering the dose correctly, always read the label before giving it. Never take liquid medications with a regular spoon. Use the designated measuring cup, dropper, or other dosing tool that came with the medication. Keep your kids' medications in a safe place. Since liquid medications are frequently sweet, a child who manages to get their hands on a bottle could drink a lot of them. To prevent double dosing, effective communication is crucial if multiple adults are administering medication to your child (Deeths & Breeden, 1971).

These guidelines from the American Academy of Pediatrics will keep children safe:

- Keep all medicines in their original containers, which usually have child safety caps. Nothing is childproof.
- Store medicines high up, where children cannot reach or see. For

dangerous medicines, consider locks on the cabinet.

- Children who crawl, eat anything they find on the floor. If you drop a pill, do not stop looking until you find it.
- Get rid of unused medicines, using safe disposal methods.
- Know basic first aid and have the poison control center number available.
- If medication is dropped or spilled, sweep and/or vacuum the area to be sure no medicine was left out.

8.1.1.1. Storing Medicines Safely

Medications left in places where kids can access them can frequently result in poisoning. Medication must be kept high and secure in a locked cabinet. The cabinet ought to have child-resistant locks and be at least 1.5 meters high, if at all feasible. Additionally, after using a medication, put it back in the cabinet right away. Never put medications in reach of minors.

Here are more tips for storing medicines safely:

- Leave all medicines in their original containers.
- Ask your pharmacist to put child-resistant caps on your medicines if they are not already on the bottle. But remember that child-resistant caps are not child proof. You still need to store these medicines up high in a locked cupboard.
- Make sure you always put caps back on the bottles correctly and immediately after use.
- Clean out your medicine cupboard regularly. Return unwanted and out-of-date medicines to your local pharmacist for safe disposal.
- Keep any measuring cups and droppers used for medicine separate and safe.
- Rinse empty medicine containers with water before you discard or recycle them.

8.1.1.2. Preventing Medicine Poisoning

These safety precautions can help you keep your child safe from medicine poisoning:

- If your child needs to take medicine, read the label, dosage, and instructions carefully. Double-check everything before you give your child the medicine.
- If someone else regularly gives your child medicine, set up a 'checking system' to avoid giving your child double doses of medicine. Write down the time and dose each time you give your child their medicine. Keep this information with the medicine.
- When you're giving medicine to your child, take care that other children can't reach the medicine.
- If you're not sure about how much medicine to give or for how long, ask your doctor or pharmacist.
- Avoid distractions when giving your child medicines. If possible, have a routine for giving or taking medicines. And always supervise while your child is taking medicine.
- Refer to medicines by their proper names. This is better than calling them 'special lollies,' which can confuse your child and tempt your child to try them.

- Keep bags away from your child's reach and ask visitors to do the same, because bags can contain medicine.
- Take care when visiting older people. They might not be used to having children around and might leave medicine within easy reach. Check to make sure your child canot get to their medicines.

8.1.2. Pesticide Poisoning

A wide range of chemicals are categorized as pesticides and are used to eradicate or manage insects, unwanted plants, molds, and animals (e.g., rodents). Although the term "pesticide" refers to a broad range of products, it is frequently and incorrectly used to exclusively refer to insecticides. A thorough analysis of every active ingredient in the vast array of pesticide types and products is outside the purview of this report. Based on past experience and/or new research, this review concentrates on particular insecticides, herbicides, and rodenticides, as well as particular chemical classes within these categories, that have the highest acute and long-term toxicity for children (Table 8.1).

Table 8.1. *Major Pesticide Classes and Selected Examples*

Pesticide Class	Examples	Toxicity	Comment, Uses
Organochlorines	DDT, endrin, aldrin, chlordane, lindane	☐ High toxicity	☐ Many organochlorines now banned in the United States ☐ Lindane has been banned in California, elsewhere used for control of lice and scabies ☐ DDT and other organochlorines have long metabolic disposition and are stored in fatty tissues and can persist in the environment
Organophosphates	Parathion, chlorpyrifos, dichlorvos, acephate, methyl-parathion, malathion, phorate	☐ Most OPs are highly toxic ☐ Malathion is considered relatively less toxic than other OPs	☐ Parathion is banned for use in the United States ☐ Chlorpyrifos is no longer approved for residential use ☐ Most others are used for insect control in both agricultural and home settings ☐ Malathion is an approved treatment of head lice

N-Methyl carbamates	Aldicarb, carbaryl, carbofuran, pirimicarb, propoxur	☐ Aldicarb and carbaryl are both highly toxic ☐ Other carbamates have a relatively moderate toxicity	☐ Insect control in agricultural and home settings
Pyrethrins and pyrethroids	Permethrin, cyano-pyrethroids: deltamethrin, cypermethrin, fenvalerate	☐ Permethrin has relatively low toxicity ☐ Other pyrethroids have moderate toxicity	☐ Permethrin is a common pediculicide ☐ Most other pyrethroids are commonly used to control insects, often used in home and garden
Neonicotinoids	Imidacloprid	☐ Relatively newer class of insecticides ☐ Have relatively lower toxicity than OPs and carbamates	☐ Selective affinity toward insect nicotinic acetylcholine receptors compared with mammalian nicotinic acetylcholine receptors ☐ Often used as spot-on flea control for domestic animals
N-Phenylpyrazole insecticides	Fipronil	☐ Relatively newer class of insecticides	☐ Often used as spot-on flea control for domestic animals ☐ Yard treatments for insect control
Phosphonate herbicides	Glyphosate	☐ Because of primary mechanism of action, has relatively low toxicity from active ingredient. ☐ Toxicity often due to the accompanying organic solvent	☐ Acts on plant cell wall ☐ Commercially available in many products
Chlorophenoxy herbicides	2,4-D, 2,4,5-T	☐ Moderate toxicity	☐ Weed control
Dipyridyl herbicides	Paraquat, diquat	☐ Highly toxic	☐ Infrequently used ☐ Paraquat toxicity often requires a lung transplant
Long-acting anticoagulants	Brodifacoum (superwarfarins)		☐ Rodenticides ☐ Longer-acting than warfarin ☐ Recently eliminated packaging as loose pellets

2,4,5-T, 2,4,5-trichlorophenoxy acetic acid.

Source: https://www.ncbi.nlm.nih.gov/pmc/articles/PMC5813803/.

This report does not address a number of pesticide types. Despite their potential for toxicity, fumigants and fungicides are generally not associated with acute childhood exposure or poisoning, so they are left out. This report does not include wood preservatives that contain arsenic. Since January 2004, the particular compound that contained arsenic, copper chromium arsenate, has been taken off the market. Homes, playgrounds, and yards still contain older wood structures that were treated with copper chromium arsenate. These structures should be sealed annually with a waterproof material. Insect repellents, such as picaridin and N, N-diethyl-meta-toluamide, differ from most pesticides in that they are applied to human skin on purpose to ward off insect bites and are not actually insecticides. These substances are distinct and have just undergone evaluation.

This technical report focuses on exposures that are most pertinent to children living in the United States, even though the severity of pesticide exposures and toxicity may be higher in developing nations with less regulatory oversight and information. Commonly used insecticides are covered, along with the relatively new class of neonicotinoids. These include the carbamate, pyrethroid, and organophosphate (OP) classes. The phosphonate herbicides (such as glyphosate), chlorophenoxy herbicides, and long-acting anticoagulants (rodenticides) are additional pesticides that will be covered in some detail. See other sources for a more thorough analysis of the acute toxicity resulting from the variety of pesticide active ingredients and products.

8.1.2.1. Children's Unique Vulnerabilities

Due to dietary, physiological, and developmental factors, children are especially susceptible to the absorption of pesticides and their negative effects. Exposure can happen through skin contact, inhalation, or ingestion. Children may inadvertently consume food or liquids at a significantly higher dose than adults due to their higher food or fluid intake per pound of body weight. When compared to adults, frequent hand-to-mouth behavior of a child is a significant source of increased exposure.

8.1.2.2. Residential Factors

Fortunately, children in the US rarely experience acute toxicity linked to pesticide poisoning, so a general practice pediatrician may not come across such an occurrence. Subacute and chronic low-level exposure is typical, though. The use of herbicides and fungicides on lawns, as well as insecticides and rodenticides inside the house, are residential factors that affect chronic exposure. Broadcast applications such as foggers, "flea bombs," and sprays can leave behind persistent residues in carpet, toys, and household dust when used indoors. Playing on the floor and crawling across it are examples of typical exploratory behavior that raises the risk of skin, respiratory, and oral exposure to residues as they settle on surfaces or in the air. Incidental exposure that happens again and again can also accumulate. In addition to being measurable in indoor air samples, pesticides can be carried home from the office and are also present in dust vacuumed from carpeted areas, upholstered furniture, and children's toys like stuffed animals. Over time, residues from herbicides used on the lawn or garden can find their way inside the house. Diazinon applications to lawns have been shown to be carried indoors by pet dogs' paws. Geographically, residential pesticide residue levels also differ based on the particular pesticide requirements in the area. Because there are a lot of termites, fleas, and crawling insects in Los Angeles, high concentrations of chlorpyrifos and other insecticides have been found there. In contrast, weed-control applications in Iowa resulted in high concentrations of the herbicides

2,4-dichlorophenoxyacetic acid (2,4-D) and dicamba. Residentially related sources might be pertinent in other places where kids hang out, like daycare centers, schools, relatives' houses, etc., based on patterns of indoor and outdoor pesticide use and proximity to pesticide use. All indoor air and dust samples from 142 urban homes and preschools in North Carolina showed evidence of chlorpyrifos.

8.1.2.3. Biomonitoring Data for Exposure Assessment

In connection with the NHANES, the Centers for Disease Control and Prevention (CDC) runs a population-based biomonitoring program. Biomarker data for numerous herbicides, pyrethroid insecticides, carbamate, OP, and organochlorine insecticides, as well as some other pesticides, are included in the most recent report. Out of 44 pesticide metabolites tested, 29 could be found in the majority of samples analyzed (ages 6–59). The most common pesticides in the US, according to reports, are OP and organochlorine insecticides. While the health effects of these "snapshot" sampling data are not well understood, they do offer a point of reference for the distribution of pesticide metabolites. Evaluations of exposure trends at the population level are also made possible by periodic reassessment. As was previously mentioned, children are frequently more likely than adults to absorb higher doses from contaminated environments due to their distinct behaviors and metabolic rates. One example that stands out from the biomonitoring data is the non-persistent OP insecticide chlorpyrifos. Despite being outlawed in 2000 for domestic use, it is still utilized in agriculture to grow crops like apples and pears and other staple foods for kids. According to the biomonitoring data of CDC, the youngest age group evaluated (6–11 years) had the highest levels of urine metabolites specific to chlorpyrifos when compared to older children and adults. Conversely, the youngest age group under observation (12–19 years) had lower concentrations of the organochlorine insecticides and their metabolites, such as DDT, dieldrin, and chlordane, which were all outlawed in the United States in the 1970s and 1980s, according to biomonitoring of serum markers of these substances. Even at comparatively lower concentrations, the continuous detection and rising levels as one ages probably indicate the lifetime accumulation of these persistent, fat-soluble compounds.

8.1.2.4. Exposures from the Food Supply

The main way that the general public is exposed to OPs and organochlorines is through their food. Food residues and household pesticides are significant sources of pyrethroids. By establishing "tolerances," or the highest concentration of pesticides that are permitted to be used in or on food and animal feed, the US Environmental Protection Agency (USEPA) controls the exposure of consumers to pesticides in food. Enforcing these tolerances is the responsibility of the US Food and Drug Administration. As part of its modest monitoring program, 7234 samples were examined in total in 2003. Of the domestically produced samples, there were detectable but legally permissible pesticide residues in 49% of the fruit, 29% of the vegetables, 26% of grain products, 24% of fish and shellfish, and 0% of milk and dairy products. The only food items with residues above the permitted limits were fruits and vegetables (about 2% each). Overall, fewer residues were found in the samples of imported fruits and vegetables that were tested; however, there were more exceedances of legal tolerances (5–7% of the imported fruits and vegetables that were sampled). A study where children were fed an organic diet for five days straight showed that eating organic food may reduce exposure to pesticides. During the organic diet phase, a noticeable and swift decrease was noted in the metabolites of chlorpyrifos and malathion OP insecticides excreted in their urine.

8.1.2.5. Agriculturally Related Exposures

Some children may also be exposed to pesticide contamination in their home environment if they live close to agricultural areas that have been treated with pesticides or if household members use pesticides. Pesticide levels in carpet dust and pesticide metabolites in urine of residents increased with self-reported proximity of homes to orchard fields and during the pesticide application season, according to a Washington State study of children of agricultural workers and non-agricultural workers in an agricultural setting. Similar results were found in a California agriculture center where house dust samples from nearby homes and urine samples from the residents showed a significant correlation with pesticide residues of three chemicals that had recently been used on crops. The results were observed in farmworkers as well as non-farm workers. Pesticide levels are also raised in homes occupied by agricultural workers due to "take-home" exposures. The levels of pesticide metabolites in the urine were higher in kids who lived on farms than in kids who did not. Youngsters may engage in agricultural labor involving the application of pesticides or come into contact with foliage that has been treated with them.

8.1.2.6. Exposures from Drinking Water

Another way that some children's residential environments could become contaminated is if they live close to agricultural areas that have been treated with pesticides or if any household members work with pesticides. In a Washington State study involving children of agricultural workers and non-agricultural workers in an agricultural setting, residents' self-reported proximity to orchard fields and the time of year when pesticides are applied led to an increase in pesticide levels in carpet dust and pesticide metabolites in urine. Similarly, in a California agriculture center, there was a significant correlation found between house dust samples from nearby homes and urine samples from the residents and pesticide residues of three chemicals that had recently been used on crops. Both farmworkers and non-farm workers were subject to the findings. Due to "take-home" exposures, having an agricultural worker in the house also raises pesticide levels. Compared to children who did not live on a farm, those who lived on one had higher urine levels of pesticide metabolites. Youngsters themselves may engage in pesticide-treated foliage contact or agricultural labor involving the use of pesticides.

8.1.3. Cleaning Product Poisoning

Caustic agents are chemicals found in most cleaning products that can burn people's skin, eyes, throats, mouths, and lungs. Even in small doses, poisoning with these potent bases can harm your child's digestive system and result in other severe injuries. Benzalkonium or sodium hypochlorite, which can be extremely toxic if inhaled, are ingredients in a lot of hand sanitizers. When kids are not around, use them and then store them in a locked cabinet.

8.1.4. Alcohol Poisoning

Youngsters might discover alcoholic beverages and take a sip. Alcohol is also present in mouthwash, colognes, sanitizers, and OTC cold medications. Drinking alcohol when young can result in coma, seizures, and low blood sugar.

8.1.5. Carbon Monoxide Poisoning

The gas carbon monoxide has no color and no smell. Burning hydrocarbons in a closed space without enough ventilation can result in poisoning. Generators, heating systems, charcoal grills, engine-driven tools, camp stoves and lanterns, gas ovens and ranges, and gas water heaters are common items that can result in carbon monoxide poisoning. Children (and adults) who are exposed to carbon monoxide poisoning experience nausea, dizziness, and sleepiness before going into a coma. If carbon monoxide poisoning is not treated quickly, death could result. Every carbon monoxide-producing device needs to be placed outdoors or in an area with adequate ventilation. Install and routinely test carbon dioxide detectors in your home. Never leave an automobile running in a garage that is connected to a home.

8.1.6. Plants Poisonous to Kids

While some garden plants are beautiful additions to your house and yard, others are harmful due to their toxins, which can harm the skin, stomach, liver, and heart, among other body parts. If consumed, they could make your child ill. Daffodils, dumb cane, hydrangea, foxglove, lilies, oleanders, rhododendrons, and wisteria are a few of them. For instance, oleanders contain glycosides that can be deadly if ingested and cause heart damage. The names of every plant in your garden should be known to you. Remove those that are known to be dangerous, if possible.

8.1.7. Hydrocarbon Poisoning

Gasoline (petrol), kerosene, lamp oil, lighter fluid, motor oil, and paint thinners and removers are hydrocarbons. Exposure by ingestion or inhaling can affect the brain and respiratory and central nervous systems.

8.1.8. Liquid Nicotine Poisoning

Liquid nicotine, which is used in e-cigarettes, is a highly concentrated and harmful chemical. A small amount spilled on a young child's skin or consumed can be fatal. Cigars, chewing tobacco, nicotine gum, patches, and cigarettes are additional dangerous products containing nicotine. Should your child consume them, they may be toxic.

8.1.9. Child Poisoning Treatment

If a child has swallowed something extremely toxic and fast-acting, you may need to do first aid right away and call for emergency medical help. Then follow these steps:

- **Swallowed poison.** Take the substance from the child, and get them to spit out any in their mouth. Do not force them to vomit without medical advice.
  - Touched poison. If poison touches the skin, immediately wash the area with soap and warm water for 10–30 min. If there is blistering, take the victim to the emergency room right away.
- **Inhaled poison.** Take your child out in the open air, away from the poisonous place. You may need to give cardiopulmonary resuscitation (CPR) until help arrives.

Other treatments for poison exposure include:

- If a toxic substance gets in the eyes, flush eyes continuously with warm water for 10 min.
- If the victim has stopped breathing or does not have a heartbeat, perform CPR and call 911 right away.
- If the victim is unconscious or breathing is difficult or labored, call 911.

Note: The American Academy of Pediatrics now recommends against using syrup of ipecac to cause vomiting when children swallow a poisonous substance.

8.1.10. Child Poisoning Prevention

For the majority of substances, the general population's use of drugs for abuse has not changed over the past ten years. In Spain, cocaine is currently the most commonly used illegal stimulant and the drug that people between the ages of 15 and 64 consume the most frequently, after cannabis. Over the past ten years, there has been a rise in the use of cannabis and cocaine in Spain, reaching up to 7.1% and 8.8%, respectively. While the prevalence of cocaine use in Europe has been declining since peaking at 3% in 2007. In a prior study, our team of researchers discovered that 10% of prenatals were exposed to drugs of abuse overall. Another study using hair as an alternative matrix on patients who came to our hospital's pediatric emergency room revealed that 23.3% of children ages 1–4 and 13.5% of children ages 10–14 are chronically exposed to drugs of abuse in their immediate surroundings.

The cases that have been documented show that acute intoxication with drugs of abuse in children is frequently the initial clinical sign of repeated, chronic exposure. Babies, toddlers, and young children may be passively exposed to these substances through hand-to-mouth behaviors that result in the ingestion of drug residue from an active user's home or by breathing in the smoke produced by their consumption. Additionally, they could be administered purposefully by the adult, as well as passively through the placenta, breastfeeding, the user's saliva, or sweat. On the other hand, there is a paucity of published research regarding persistent exposure to drugs of abuse following the neonatal stage. Many published clinical cases have already documented this possibility.

8.1.11. Purposes

Toxicology screening in pediatrics serves several important purposes, each with its own set of causes and motivations:

- **Identification of Acute Poisonings:** Finding children who have suffered acute poisoning is one of the main goals of toxicology screening in pediatrics. Accidental ingestion of prescription drugs, common household chemicals, plants, or other toxic substances can result in these poisonings. Typical situations include kids discovering unsupervised medication, pesticides or household cleansers getting into their mouths, or kids inadvertently eating plants or mushrooms from the surrounding area. Healthcare professionals can promptly determine the precise toxin in question, evaluate how it might affect the child's health, and start the necessary treatment with the aid of toxicology screening.
- **Evaluation of Suspected Drug Overdoses:** A toxicology screening may be carried out to determine whether drugs or other harmful substances are present in a child's system if their symptoms point to a drug overdose. Adolescents may unintentionally overdose on drugs when they take too much of a prescription drug or have access to illegal drugs at home. In addition, deliberate drug overdoses can happen in teenagers who abuse substances or who self-harm. In addition to helping determine the kinds and amounts of drugs used, toxicology screening also helps with treatment planning and addresses any underlying psychosocial problems that may have contributed to the overdose (Schille et al., 2009).

- **Assessment of Environmental Exposures:** Children's distinct behaviors, developmental stages, and physiological makeup make them especially susceptible to environmental exposures to toxic substances. When children are exposed to environmental toxins like lead, pesticides, industrial chemicals, or pollutants in air or water sources, toxicology screening may be necessary. These exposures can have short-term or long-term health effects and can happen through a variety of channels, such as ingestion, inhalation, or skin contact. Screening aids in determining the level of exposure, evaluating any possible health risks, and directing the right interventions to prevent more harm.
- **Evaluation of Suspected Child Abuse:** Toxicology screening may be used as a part of the diagnostic process when child abuse or neglect is suspected to look for signs of drug exposure or poisoning. Victimized children might be exposed to drugs in utero because of maternal substance abuse during pregnancy, or they might be purposefully exposed to harmful substances by caregivers. By enabling the right interventions and preventative measures, toxicology screening can support forensic investigations, offer objective proof of exposure, and contribute to the child's safety and welfare.
- **Monitoring of Therapeutic Drug Levels:** In some medical situations, toxicology screening may be done to keep track of the levels of therapeutic drugs in children who are taking medications with a limited safe range or a known risk of toxicity. This is particularly important for drugs like antiepileptics, immunosuppressants, and psychotropic medications, where maintaining the right drug levels is crucial for their effectiveness and safety. Checking drug levels helps in finding the best dosing schedules, avoiding harmful reactions, and ensuring that the drugs work as intended while reducing the chances of toxicity.

Toxicology screening in pediatrics is primarily motivated by the need to monitor therapeutic drug levels, detect evidence of child abuse, evaluate environmental hazards, identify, and manage toxic exposures, and determine the extent of poisoning or drug overdose. To ensure prompt and accurate screening, result interpretation, and implementation of appropriate interventions catered to the specific needs of pediatric patients, collaboration amongst healthcare providers, toxicologists, clinical laboratories, and poison control centers is imperative (Bronstein and Spyker, 2010, 2011, 2012).

8.1.12. Diagnosis

Acute intoxications can result in a wide range of clinical symptoms, many of which are neurological in nature. When several substances are taken at once, even doses that are generally safe for adults can cause serious health problems in kids. Conversely, long-term intoxications brought on by persistent drug abuse exposure seldom manifest particular symptoms; instead, they are typically identified through toxicological examination of biological materials. The only method of identifying exposure that has been employed historically, outside of emergency room visits due to acute intoxications, has been asking the child's or parents' medical history. Although there is evidence that using questionnaires to diagnose drug intake is unreliable and has a low diagnostic yield due to underreporting or nonexistent drug use, questionnaires remain the most widely used tool for identifying prenatal and postnatal exposure to drugs of abuse. There is no standardized toxicology screen that can be agreed upon and used in pediatric emergency rooms. Every laboratory has access to a selection of commercial rapid detection tests, each with its own set of limitations regarding the substances it can identify and the thresholds for positive results. The most popular techniques use urine as the biological matrix and entail enzyme immunoassay for semiquantitative detection. Hospital testing typically identifies the presence of amphetamines, methadone, benzodiazepines, barbiturates, cocaine, cannabis, opioids, and tricyclic antidepressants. Urine tests will only identify substances that have been actively or passively consumed in the hours or days prior to sample collection, with very few exceptions (e.g., long half-life benzodiazepines, or cannabis used regularly).

Recent advancements in analytical techniques have significantly enhanced the objective detection of parent drugs and their metabolites, known as biomarkers, across various biological matrices. This progress has facilitated definitive diagnoses, establishing a foundation for appropriate treatment and monitoring of infants and children who have been passively exposed to substances of abuse. Different biological matrices offer distinct time windows for detecting drug exposure, with acute detection possible in urine, blood, or saliva, and chronic detection achievable through hair or meconium analysis. Historically, blood and urine have been the primary biological matrices utilized for toxicology screening due to their ability to indicate recent drug consumption.

- Blood tests for drugs have a very narrow detection window, which is between 0 and 1 h after consumption or exposure, though it can go up to 24 h for some substances. The main drawback is the invasive nature of the sample collection process.
- The detection window for drugs of abuse in urine is somewhat longer, ranging from 30 min to 5 h from intake or exposure, although it can extend to 24–48 h for cannabis, or even 1 week.
- When compared to traditional matrices, alternative or nonconventional biological matrices (hair, meconium, sweat, and saliva) have the following advantages: the collection process is typically noninvasive, and some have very broad retrospective detection windows, such as the past two trimesters in the case of meconium, while each centimeter of hair, starting at the scalp, is equivalent to one month in the past.
    - When a child presents with acute intoxication or lives in a high-risk environment, hair is thought to be the best matrix to rule out chronic exposure to drugs of abuse. The Society of Hair Testing has set standards for reference values for the identification and measurement of different substances in hair, as well as guidelines for the processing and cleaning of samples to prevent contamination from outside sources and the clinical interpretation of the results. Another method for identifying prenatal

passive exposure brought on by substance use during pregnancy is maternal hair testing.

- Meconium allows assessment of prenatal exposure to substances of abuse in the second and third trimesters of gestation, including fetal production of metabolites starting on weeks 12–16.

In pharmacotoxicology, the identification of drugs of abuse in hair represents a novel analytical technique since it enables the verification of past drug use or passive exposure over several months. Apart from its widely recognized use in forensic toxicology, the identification of drugs of abuse in hair can also be employed in epidemiological investigations to impartially evaluate passive exposure in high-risk groups, including expectant mothers, new babies, and kids raised in drug-using households. Previous cohort studies conducted in Spain have shown that children are exposed to drugs of abuse, and there is a high likelihood that parents will also test positive for the same drugs. According to the scientific literature, there is a significant chance that either passive or active exposure will have detrimental effects. Urine tests for drugs of abuse are used to confirm acute exposure to these substances when intoxication is suspected. To rule out chronic exposure, a positive result should be followed by confirmation using conventional biological matrices (urine) and testing alternative matrices (hair) using extremely sensitive and specific techniques (liquid or gas chromatography and mass spectrometry). A urine sample must be saved for a confirmatory test and a hair sample must be taken whenever a clinical presentation suggests drug abuse. The hair sample should be a lock from the nuchal region, 2–3 cm in diameter, cut as close to the scalp as possible, fixed at the proximal end to a sheet of paper with a paperclip, and stored in an envelope at room temperature. This is especially true if the suspicion is confirmed by rapid urine testing. When a child's exposure to the drug of abuse is confirmed, samples from adults and other children living in the home of the intoxicated child should be taken, and the relevant social services department should be notified. The confirmatory urine test can be carried out in hospital reference laboratories, but hair analysis needs to go through exceptional channels through clinical research or legal medicine specialty centers.

8.1.13. Indications for Toxicology Screening

Drug abuse can affect newborns, kids, and teenagers in different ways, and the exposure can be either acute (resulting in acute intoxication) or chronic. The scenarios that can occur are as follows: (1) inadvertent active intake; (2) passive exposure to smoke resulting from substance consumption; (3) purposeful recreational use (adolescents); (4) purposeful self-administration during an attempted suicide; and (5) purposeful forced exposure (child abuse, Munchausen syndrome by proxy, attempted murder, drug-facilitated crime, etc.). (6) maternal use during pregnancy resulting in prenatal exposure; (7) exposure through perspiration or breast milk. Thus, in the context of pediatric practice, the following scenarios would be considered indications for toxicology screening (rapid urine test with confirmation in reference laboratory for cases of acute intoxication, and hair testing in reference laboratory for cases of chronic exposure): (1) suspected acute intoxication or chronic exposure (both based on history taking or clinical manifestations); (2) all cases of acute intoxication; (3) known accidental exposure; (4) reported intake; and (5) suspected prenatal exposure (based on history of maternal use or clinical manifestations) or postnatal exposure.

We cannot suggest that hair testing be used for broad screening because it is still an expensive method with restricted availability for detecting drugs of abuse.

Consequently, we suggest that it be indicated for paediatric patients that seek care in the primary care or hospital systems in any of the following scenarios:

- Geographical area with a high prevalence of substance use and of low socioeconomic status.
- Clinical suspicion of acute intoxication with any drug of abuse.
- Clinical suspicion of chronic intoxication with any drug of abuse.
- Suspicion, evidence or report of substance use by the adult accompanying the child.
- Evidence of a high-risk environment for the child.
- Newborn at risk of or with suspected prenatal exposure.

In emergency situations, routine medical care must include the evaluation of children who have been exposed to drugs of abuse both acutely and chronically. The public health system and social services must implement interventions to raise public awareness of the risks to child health and the need to abstain from substance use during pregnancy and in places where children spend time with adults in order to prevent drug exposure and intake in newborns, children, and adolescents. In addition, guidelines for clinical practice need to be created and put into effect for social workers and medical professionals who deal with drug abuse exposure in newborns, kids, and teenagers.

8.1.14. Physical Examination

Sometimes, in an emergency room, vital treatments must begin before a thorough examination can be finished. In these situations, initial stabilization and essential therapy will be followed by a thorough examination. In order to assess the efficacy of treatment, monitor the course of the illness, and ultimately decide on the patient's course of action, repeated examinations are frequently required. When a child has been poisoned, a focused physical examination involves checking vital signs, mental state, and neurological function in addition to looking for specific toxidromes in the eyes, mucous membranes, skin, bowel, and bladder.

8.1.14.1. Vital Signs

The vital signs are often very useful in identifying the toxidrome that is involved. Furthermore, keeping the child's vital signs within reasonable bounds is essential to providing supportive care for the poisoned child. The abnormal vital signs associated with specific poison types are summarized in Table 8.2. When using this information, keep in mind that extreme stress and decompensation can cause vital signs that aren't usually linked to the poison in question. For instance, exposure to cocaine or other sympathomimetic substances is usually linked to tachycardia and/or hypertension; however, decompensation can lead to bradycardia and hypotension. It is useful to remember that the expected results in the table may not appear when in extremis.

Table 8.2. *Vital Sign Abnormalities Typical with Certain Types of Poisons*

Vital Sign Abnormality	Poison
Tachycardia	Amphetamine Albuterol Antihistamines Caffeine Cocaine Pseudoephedrine Salicylate Theophylline Tricyclic antidepressant
Bradycardia	Beta blocker Calcium channel blocker Clonidine Digoxin Opioid Sedative-hypnotic
Tachypnea	Caffeine Cyanide Ethylene glycol Methanol Salicylate Theophylline
Bradypnea	Barbiturate Clonidine Ethanol Opioid Sedative-hypnotics
Hypertension	Amphetamine Cocaine Pseudoephedrine
Hypotension	Albuterol Beta blocker Caffeine Calcium Channel Blocker Clonidine Imidazolines Nicotine Opioids Theophylline Tricyclic antidepressants
Hyperthermia	Amphetamine Caffeine Cocaine MAO inhibitor Malignant hyperthermia Neuroleptic malignant syndrome Phencyclidine (PCP) Salicylate Serotonin syndrome Theophylline
Hypothermia	Depressed consciousness in setting which may result in heat loss to environment Hypoglycemic agents
Hypoxia	Barbiturates Ethanol Opioids
False pulse oximetry measurement	Carboxyhemoglobin Methemoglobin Methylene Blue Sulfhemoglobin

Agents, such as propoxyphone, may result in tachycardia and mydriasis, atypical in opiod exposure.

Source: https://www.ebmedicine.net/media_library/aboutUs/Table%207.%20Vital%20Sign%20Abnormalities.JPG.

8.1.14.2. Mental Status and Neurologic Exam

The doctor needs to record if there is a change in mental status. First and foremost, a bedside measurement of the serum glucose level should be performed as soon as possible in response to any change in sensorium or neurologic status that may be indicative of hypoglycemia. Certain findings during the physical examination may include weakness, hyperreflexia, altered muscle tone, tremors, fasciculations, twitching, dystonic posturing, hallucinations, formications, altered muscle tone, cranial nerve deficit, or other neurologic abnormality. Evaluation for intracranial hemorrhage or lesion should be prompted by focal neurologic findings or decerebrate or decorticate posturing. Distinguishing between neurologic and behavioral changes or psychiatric findings is crucial. While psychiatric side effects are typically managed by providing a safe environment for the patient to stay in while the drug's effects wear off, neurologic findings are much more concerning for CNS injury or lesion and may warrant intensive imaging and management techniques that require ICU level care.

The topic of substance withdrawal is not covered in this article, but it is important to remember that withdrawal from barbiturates, benzodiazepines, and other sedative-hypnotic substances frequently results in changes in mental status. These withdrawal symptoms have the potential to be fatal. The age group most likely to exhibit signs of substance withdrawal is newborns. Withdrawal from a variety of substances, such as amphetamines, barbiturates, cocaine, caffeine, opioids, and selective serotonin reuptake inhibitors, can cause significant behavioral changes in a newborn. The Glasgow Coma Scale (GCS) or AVPU (alert / verbal / painful / unresponsive) scale has been recommended for use in poisoning cases in recent publications. Such a practice cannot be justified by the available data regarding the usefulness of GCS in the prognosis or treatment of poisoned patients.

8.1.14.3. Pupils, Extra Ocular Motions, and Nystagmus

Though constricted pupils indicate exposure to opiates, cholinergic agents, imidazolines, and clonidine, dilated pupils may indicate a sympathomimetic or anticholinergic toxidrome. Theoretically, anticholinergic drugs should cause a dilated nonreactive or sluggish pupil and sympathomimetic stimulants a dilated reactive pupil; however, we find that pupil reactivity does not always indicate the presence of anticholinergic toxicity. Although toxicity from other drugs may also cause this effect, rotatory as well as horizontal nystagmus is commonly linked to phenytoin and carbamazepine toxicity, as well as related drugs such as ketamine, dextromethorphan, and phencyclidine (PCP). Although the presence of nystagmus aids in raising the index of suspicion for the aforementioned agents, the absence of the finding does reliably exclude toxicity from them.

Luoroscein stain should be used to check for corneal abrasions in the eyes if there is a possibility of caustic exposure, following thorough irrigation and pH evaluation. Assuring that all the caustic material has been removed requires rechecking the pH 20 min after irrigation is finished. This is crucial for alkali exposures because alkali penetrate more quickly and are less easily neutralized by eye surface proteins than acids. The best course of action is to use a Morgan lens for irrigation; gravity-dependent IV tubing drips of fluid into the eye, but this is not a sufficient substitute.

8.1.14.4. Skin and Mucus Membranes

The patient should be undressed and carefully examined, noting the skin color, hydration status, and temperature. Table 8.3 summarizes findings that may provide a key to a final diagnosis.

Table 8.3. *Poison-Associated Dermatologic Findings and their Causes*

Skin Finding	Cause
Cyanosis	Hypoxia Methemoglobinemia
Diaphoresis	Amphetamines/cocaine/ sympathomimetics Caffeine Cholinergic agents Nicotine Salicylates Theophylline
Dry skin	Anticholinergic drugs
Flushed skin	Anticholinergic drugs- flushed skin Boric acid- erythroderma or boiled-lobster red skin Carbon monoxide- pink skin Cyanide- pink skin Niacin- brightly flushed skin Scombroid- brightly flushed skin
Jaundice	Carotenemia (excess carrot intake) Hemolysis Hepatic failure Hepatotoxins Lycopenia (excess tomato intake)

Source: https://www.ebmedicine.net/spaw/uploads/aboutUs/Table%208.%20Poison-Associated%20Dermatologic.JPG.

8.1.15. Diagnostic Testing

8.1.15.1. Bedside Glucose Monitoring

A dextrose assessment is useful when tending to the poisoned patient. Of all the harmful effects of poisoning, hypoglycemia is the easiest to identify and treat. A bedside blood glucose measurement should be performed on any patient who has experienced a change in mental state or has been exposed to a poison that could result in hypoglycemia.

8.1.15.2. Electrocardiogram (ECG)

The mnemonic for initial stabilization of patients with poison exposure is "A,B,C,D,E," with "E" signifying ECG. Any patient who has changed mental status, irregular blood pressure or heart rate, or who has been exposed to a poison that can cause cardiac dysrhythmia should have an ECG. Novel or atypical antipsychotics, phenothiazines, tricyclic antidepressants, digitalis, beta-blockers, calcium channel blockers, clonidine, opioids, antidysrhythmics, alpha-blockers, theophylline, cocaine and other sympathomimetics, and sodium-channel blockers are among the substances that may cause cardiac abnormalities. In adults, exposure to tricyclic antidepressants is confirmed by finding R' in the terminal 40 ms in lead AVR (Augmented vector right), S' in AVL, and I.48 In cases when these terminal 40 ms changes and tachycardia are present, lengthening of the QRS (represents the depolarization of ventricles) interval beyond 100 ms is indicative of TCA (Tricyclic Antidepressant) toxicity. Since there is significant right axis deviation in children, it is unsafe to presume that terminal 40 ms changes have the same prognostic value in children as in adults.

It is dangerous to assume that terminal 40 ms changes in children have the same prognostic value as in adults because there is significant right axis deviation in children. TCAs, antidysrhythmics, phenothiazines, cocaine, diphenhydramine, propoxyphene, ethanol, and quinine are additional substances that can result in widened QRS. Bradycardia may indicate the use of sedative-hypnotic medications, lithium, beta-blockers, calcium channel blockers, opioids, clonidine, or digoxin.

8.1.15.3. Qualitative Urine Toxicology Screen

A discussion of the management of poisoned patients would be incomplete without addressing the issue of "toxicology screening." Discussing toxicology screening (TS) is difficult because there is no standard definition of what constitutes TS. Generally, a "tox screen" involves qualitative detection of specific drugs or metabolites in urine or serum. The term is most frequently used to denote assay detection of commonly abused drugs, most frequently amphetamines, cocaine, marijuana, opioids, and phencyclidine (PCP), though many other abused drugs are detectable as well. The drugs of abuse mostly widely available in multiple substance assays are commonly called the "NIDA 5," an abbreviation indicating the National Institute of Drug Abuse 5-panel drug screen; these five drugs are amphetamines, cannabinoids (marijuana), cocaine, opioids, and phencyclidine. Benzodiazepines and sometimes barbiturates may be included in drug of abuse screening assays as well.

The screening process for drug abuse has several limitations. Ample instances of how the conventional five-drug panel is insufficient for modern applications include the amphetamine screening assay. When the drug screening panel was created, amphetamines—typically pharmaceutical amphetamines—were heavily abused. Nevertheless, modern amphetamines that are most commonly used, like MDMA (ecstacy), methamphetamine, or methylphenidate, cannot be consistently detected by amphetamine screening. A healthcare facility screening for drug abuse will be screening for a relatively uncommon amphetamine rather than the most commonly abused ones unless they have made an effort to update their drug of abuse screening assay.

Most importantly, it has been repeatedly shown that using drug abuse screening assays to manage poisoned patients is not thoughtful. A review of 463 pediatric TS cases was conducted in a retrospective study. In this study, 50% of patients were younger than eleven years old, and 16% were younger than five. Seven (3%) of the 234 positive screening results from a TS assay that tested for over 550 toxins were positive without a clinical suspicion of exposure. The patients' medical care was unaffected by any positive test results, and the tests themselves cost $88,433. Treating physicians recorded whether TS had an impact on how they handled suspected pediatric drug ingestions in another prospective study. This study found that while quantitative assays for some medications, like salicylates, acetaminophen, and anticonvulsants, may help with patient management, qualitative screening of more than 500 other toxins has not shown a comparable benefit. Similar findings were obtained from a second retrospective review of TS in pediatric emergency department patients. Tox screens are expensive, but they don't change the way care is given to patients or improve patient outcomes. Despite multiple studies assessing TS in the emergency department setting, there is no proof that toxicology screening will help in the diagnosis and medical management of poisoned patients, despite intuition to the contrary.

The use of urine toxicology screening for forensic purposes is a crucial disclaimer to this. Screening for illicit drugs is necessary in any situation where it is thought that a child has unintentionally been exposed to them. This is different from using these screens for medical management, but it could be important for the patient's outcome and the steps taken by child welfare authorities. A second assay using a different methodology must confirm a positive result to be used in forensic testing. This verification is typically accomplished using gas chromatography mass spectroscopy. The results of forensic testing are typically useless in deciding how to dispose of ED patients because this confirmation is not easily obtained and can take several days.

8.1.15.4. Quantitative Drug Assays

There are some toxins for which quantitative assays can help guide clinical management, see Table 8.4.

Table 8.4. *Drug for Which Quantitative Serum Levels may be Clinically Useful*

• Acetaminophen	• Lead
• Anticonvulsants (carbamazepine, phenytoin, valproate)	• Iron
	• Lithium
• Barbiturates	• Methanol
• Caffeine	• Methotrexate
• Digoxin	• Salicylate
• Ethanol	• Theophylline
• Ethylene glycol	

Source: https://www.ebmedicine.net/media_library/aboutUs/Table%209.%20Drugs%20For%20Which%20Quantitative%20Serum.JPG.

These tests, apart from acetaminophen levels, ought to be ordered sparingly when specific drug exposures are suspected rather than on a regular basis. Acetaminophen is a common co-ingestant that may not cause symptoms to appear right away after ingestion, so it is wise to measure it on a regular basis in all patients who have been exposed to it or in any patient who has consumed any substance with the intention of harming themselves.

8.1.15.5. Urine Analysis

Urine testing has limited utility in the assessment of pediatric patients who have experienced toxic exposure. Testing for ferric chloride has the potential to verify if salicylate is present in urine. The test is considered successful when ferric chloride and urine combine to form a purple color. A quantitative serum salicylate level is recommended; however, no information regarding toxicity is provided by this test. Sometimes exposure to ethylene glycol is confirmed by urine microscopy. Calcium oxalate crystals are precipitated by ethylene glycol in the kidney and can be observed under a standard microscope. But if appropriate therapy is started, this finding might not be seen at all or it might be absent soon after ingestion. Urinary fluorescence testing has been recommended as a screening technique for ethylene glycol exposure; however, it is not a reliable indicator of ethylene glycol exposure in children. The clinician should be alerted to suspect hemolysis or myoglobinuria from rhabdomyolysis if the urine is heme-positive and shows no visible erythrocytes.

8.1.15.6. Serum Electrolytes and Osmolarity

These should be obtained whenever the clinician suspects a toxic exposure that can produce an anion gap metabolic acidosis. Evaluation of the anion gap can help to rapidly narrow down the diagnosis. Anion gap is calculated easily from serum electrolytes.

- Anion Gap=Na-(Cl+HCO3).
- Normal gap: 8 to 12

Elevated unmeasured anions are present when the value is greater than 12. Increased gap can be caused by uremia, lactate, toxins, and ketones, among other things. Regular testing can easily rule out the first three categories at this point, and the presence of an unexplained anion gap should alert the clinician to the possibility of toxins. It is necessary to compute the osmol gap in these patients. Measurement of the osmolal gap should be done to look into toxic alcohol exposure if a specific diagnosis is not made.

- Osmol gap=measured osmolality calculated osmolarity
- Calculated osmolarity=(2Na+ + Glucose/18+BUN/2.8 + ETOH/4.6)
- Normal osmolar gap=-2+/-6 mOsm
- Osmol gap=N/Molecular Weight (4.6 for ethanol, 3.2 for methanol,
- 6.2 for ethylene glycol, and 6.0 for isopropanol)

Methanol, ethylene glycol, or isopropanol are examples of unmeasured osmoles present when the osmol gap is > 10. Using the formula, the physician can determine the serum concentration of these substances. An osmol gap of less than 10 does not rule out the presence of these substances, even though an increased gap is helpful. This is because different individuals have different baseline variations, and depending on when the substance is presented, the parent compound may have been largely metabolized and left with little in the serum.

8.1.15.7. Radiological Studies

Depending on the specific clinical situation and suspected toxin, radiological studies may or may not be ordered. A standard radiograph will not show the majority of ingested agents because they are radiolucent. The acronym COINS serves as a helpful reminder of some notable exceptions to this rule: calcium, chloral hydrate, iron and other metals, opioid (or other drug) packets, neuroleptic agents, and enteric and sustained-release coated preparations. Radiographs can also be used to diagnose ingested or spilt foreign bodies that are radio-opaque. When identifying severe side effects of toxic exposures, like chemical or aspiration pneumonitis, radiological studies may be useful.

8.1.16. Treatment

Treatment entails a methodical assessment of the child's clinical status, determination of the particular toxin implicated, determination of the degree of toxicity, and application of suitable management techniques customized for each patient. Principles from emergency medicine, pediatrics, toxicology, pharmacology, and critical care serve as the foundation for this multimodal strategy. The first thing to do when a child who has been poisoned is discovered is to evaluate their breathing, circulation, and airway in order to guarantee rapid stabilization. Interventions like airway management, supplemental oxygen administration, or assisted ventilation may be required to maintain appropriate oxygenation and ventilation for children whose airways have been compromised or who have breathing difficulties as a result of exposure to toxins. Similarly, to maximize hemodynamic stability, children exhibiting signs of cardiovascular instability, such as hypotension or arrhythmias, may need to undergo fluid resuscitation, vasopressor support, or other cardiac interventions.

Once the patient is stabilized, the next stage of treatment is to pinpoint the particular toxin that caused the poisoning. This frequently necessitates getting a thorough history from caregivers or witnesses about the specifics of the exposure, such as the kind and quantity of substance consumed, when it was consumed, and any concurrent medications or preexisting medical conditions. Diagnostic tests can also be carried out to evaluate the child's organ function and general clinical status, or to confirm the presence of specific toxins. Examples of these tests include imaging studies, laboratory studies, and toxicology screening tests. The degree of toxicity is evaluated after the toxin has been identified to inform treatment choices. The amount and length of exposure, the child's age and weight, the substance's toxic qualities, and the existence of any underlying medical conditions are all factors that can affect how toxic a substance is. Supportive care measures including observation, vital sign monitoring, and symptomatic management, may be necessary for mild to moderate poisonings in order to reduce symptoms and avoid complications. This can entail giving antidotes or reversal agents for particular toxins, offering supportive therapies like intravenous fluids, electrolyte replacement, or antiemetics, and putting in place strategies to improve toxin removal, like the administration of activated charcoal or increased diuresis.

More aggressive interventions might be required in cases of severe poisoning or potentially fatal toxicity in order to stabilize the child and stop additional harm. To preserve critical organ function, this may entail the use of advanced life support techniques like mechanical ventilation, endotracheal intubation, and hemodynamic support. Extracorporeal treatments like hemoperfusion, plasmapheresis, or hemodialysis may be used in certain cases to reduce systemic effects and eliminate toxins from the bloodstream. Depending on the ingestion time and route of exposure, decontamination procedures might also be necessary. Gastric decontamination techniques, such as the administration of activated charcoal or gastric lavage, may be taken into consideration for ingestions involving toxic substances to stop the toxin from further being absorbed from the gastrointestinal tract. However, the specific toxin involved, the amount of time since ingestion, and the child's clinical condition all affect the efficacy and safety of these interventions, so their use should be carefully weighed against potential risks. To ensure the best possible outcomes and guide ongoing management decisions, it is crucial to closely monitor the child's clinical status, vital signs, laboratory parameters, and response to therapy throughout the course of treatment. In order to address any emotional or psychological distress connected to the poisoning incident and promote recovery, psychosocial support and counseling may also be provided to the child and their family. To coordinate care, share expertise, and maximize treatment outcomes for children poisoned, collaboration with multidisciplinary healthcare teams—including pediatricians, toxicologists, emergency physicians, intensivists, clinical pharmacists, and poison control centers—is essential. Furthermore, lowering the frequency and consequences of poisonings in pediatric populations requires education and prevention initiatives that support safe handling and storage procedures, prompt recognition of toxic exposures, and poison awareness.

8.2. Specialized Approach to the Poisoned Child

A child is seen ingesting a household product or medication, prompting worried parents to rush their child to the emergency department (ED). Even though this situation occurs almost 90,000 times a year in the US, it still holds a special fascination for all parties involved, including the patient, family, and medical personnel. In the most extreme of situations, the child's survival hinges on the emergency department personnel's quick identification of the poisoning, prompt initiation of life support, and provision of effective initial care. After a brief period of benign observation and maybe a few lab tests or a dose of charcoal, the family leaves for home in a few hours for the majority of these visits. It may even be suggested to parents that the next time, a quick call to the local poison control center (PCC) would have prevented the ED visit altogether. Nonetheless, it is likely that the patient's and family's ED experience will remain with them in some capacity in every instance. Young children are uncomfortable with even the thought of the smallest medical procedures and fear strangers, especially doctors. Although parents are their children's natural caregivers and comforters when they are ill, they frequently feel under pressure to act in a quasiprofessional capacity in the emergency department. When it comes to childhood poisoning, they might also experience a great deal of worry about what will happen to their child and guilt for letting the incident happen.

They are essentially patients as well. It is understandable that emergency practitioners (EPs) would prefer not to take blood samples, put in IV lines, or insert nasogastric tubes (NG tubes) into wailing children. If these interventions weren't medically necessary, they would gladly forgo them. EPs also appreciate having the knowledge and assurance to start potentially life-saving treatment in the uncommon situation of a severely ill poisoned child. This chapter focuses on specific toxins that have been shown to be especially dangerous for young children as well as exploratory ingestions to help EPs navigate the wide range of pediatric exposures to potentially toxic substances. In addition, specific pediatric topics receive some attention. These topics include poisons that can be fatal in small doses, pediatric medication errors, child abuse through poisoning, how to approach a seemingly healthy child who may have ingested a toxic substance, and newly discovered (or resurrected) toxic household products and medication formulations.

8.2.1. Cause, Epidemiology, and Prevention

Poisoning in children can occur through various routes, such as ingestion, inhalation, skin contact, envenomation, and exposure during pregnancy. This article focuses on ingestion, which is the most prevalent of these mechanisms. A young child ingesting a nonfood, potentially toxic substance usually results from the complex interaction of environmental, substance-related, and child-related factors. These frequent occurrences were once referred to as "accidental ingestion," but that term has since become obsolete. Instead, inadvertent, unintentional, or perhaps most appropriately, exploratory ingestion is now used to describe these common occurrences. This use highlights the contemporary injury model, which, as explained by Haddon in 1980, sees injuries as predictable events based on a number of crucial variables. This model is similar to the infectious disease model in that it involves a victim (or host), an agent (or microbe), and a favorable environment. The majority of poisoning victims are between the ages of 1 and 5, when they are still too young to understand what is dangerous but are at a developmental stage that permits mobility and the expression of typical exploratory behavior. They frequently exhibit greater impulsivity, hyperactivity, and pica propensity. Certain agents have a higher likelihood of being consumed due to their accessibility or appeal to young children.

Traditionally, pregnant or postpartum women—who frequently have an older toddler in the home—were prescribed adult-intended iron tablets, which looked like candy, were small, easily ingested by toddlers, smooth-coated, and available over-the-counter. Acute iron poisoning consequently ranked among the most common causes of poisoning deaths in children up until 1997, when the US Food and Drug Administration (FDA) mandated that the majority of iron preparations be blister packaged (the regulation was later suspended, but many manufacturers have voluntarily continued this practice, and pediatric iron-related morbidity has since remained low). Laundry detergent pods are a recent example of a new product that has proven to be both harmful and alluring to kids. A new baby, relocating to a new house or apartment, parental illness, or disability, and visiting or caring for elderly parents are among the stressful or environmental changes that can lead to poisoning. Perhaps even more likely to occur is exploratory ingestion when two or three of these factors are congruent. (Beuhler MC, Gala PK, Wolfe HA, et al., 2013)

Many doctors and parents fervently assert that their children will consume anything due to their inclination for exploratory eating. The quantity of ingestions by children is striking, and a wide range of medications and non-pharmaceutical substances can cause poisoning in children. Between 2009 and 2011, the three most recent years for which tabulated data were available, the American Association of Poison Control Centers (AAPCC) National Poison Data System (NPDS) data show an average of more than 1.2 million exposures per year in children younger than 6 years. Typically, these figures account for over 50% of all calls to the country's PCCs related to poisoning. The most often consumed agents recorded in 2011 are listed in Table 8.5.

Table 8.5. *Major Substances most Often Involved in Exposures to Young Children*

Substance Category	Percent of Total Substances[a]
Cosmetics and personal care products	14
Analgesics	10
Cleaning products	9
Foreign bodies, toys, and so forth	7
Topical preparations	7
Vitamins	4
Antihistamines	4
Pesticides	3
Cold and cough medications	3
Antimicrobials	3
Gastrointestinal medications	3
Plants	3

Source: https://renaissance.stonybrookmedicine.edu/sites/default/files/Approach_to_the_Poisoned_Child.pdf.

These agents include noncorrosive cleaners, plants, and cosmetics and personal hygiene products; none of them are likely to have a major negative impact. Published in 1992, it was a great attempt to categorize the long list of pediatric exposures (McFee RB, 2006) into those that had a genuine potential for toxicologic hazards. This was done by looking at the hazard factor, which considers the agent's intrinsic toxicity and frequency of occurrence. The most dangerous pharmaceuticals (Yin S. 2010) at the time were salicylates, antidepressants, iron supplements, and cardiovascular drugs (of which, iron in particular, has become less of a threat due to decreased accessibility, as previously mentioned). Opioids, anticonvulsants, diphenoxylate/atropine, chloroquine, isoniazid, theophylline, and oral hypoglycemics were among the other dangerous medications. Hydrocarbons, pesticides, alcohols/glycols, drain and oven cleansers, and gun bluing agents containing selenium acid were the most dangerous non-pharmaceutical household products; a number of these substances are still very dangerous today. Now, button batteries would also be among the most dangerous non-pharmaceutical substances.

Out of the 3.6 million childhood exposures that were reported to the US authorities between 2009 and 2011, over 2500 of them resulted in a serious illness and 109 of them were fatal due to exposure-related causes. However, compared to fifty years ago, when 300 500 pediatric poisoning deaths annually were common, these summary data show a significant improvement in morbidity and mortality. With good reason, pediatricians, public health officials, and consumer advocates celebrate this development, which they attribute primarily to the adoption of child-resistant packaging for many prescription drugs and dangerous household items following the enactment of the Poison Prevention Packaging Act in 1970. Significant progress has been made in poison prevention efforts since the 1950s, when accidental poisoning was conceptualized within the framework of the modern injury model. This has mainly involved attacking the toxic agent through reduced accessibility through regulations requiring child-resistant packaging and reformulating household products into less toxic forms. The development of emergency and hospital-based care for poisoned patients, as well as the poison center movement, have surely contributed to additional reductions in childhood morbidity.

Notwithstanding these significant advances, new data point to a concerning pattern that has been present since 2000: a rise in pediatric ingestions, and specifically, associated ED visits and hospital admissions. AAPCC data from 2001 to 2008 was analyzed, and it was found that there was a significant increase in pharmaceutical exposures and related ED visits, along with increases in hospital admissions and injuries. Prescription drugs, in particular oral hypoglycemics, opioid analgesics, sedative/hypnotics, and cardiovascular medications, were the agents most frequently implicated in serious exposures. The general rise in the use of such powerful medications, and consequently their presence in the surroundings of young children, was hypothesized as the most plausible explanation for this unsettling trend. Researchers tested this hypothesis by comparing data from the National Ambulatory Medical Care Surveys for adult-intended prescriptions written between 2000 and 2009 with data from the AAPCC for pediatric exposures. Significant correlations between these factors were discovered, especially for kids aged 0 to 5, as well as for opioid analgesics, oral hypoglycemics, and cardiovascular drugs. Therefore, there are still obstacles to overcome to reduce pediatric toxic exposures even more. New initiatives are being made in this regard, such as the use of blister packets inside of conventional child-resistant containers for pill-form medications or "next-generation safety packaging," which restricts the flow rate of liquid medications.

Two etiologic factors warrant particular attention: pediatric medication errors and intentional poisoning of young children. Poisoning as a means of abusing children is rare; only 0.077 to 0.02% of pediatric poisonings reported to the AAPCC involve this practice. When hospital-based cases are examined, the frequency might be higher. According to one investigation, 4% of pediatric poisonings that occurred in hospitals were reported to the regional child protective services agency, and 13% of pediatric poisonings that occurred in emergency departments and inpatients resulted in consultation with the hospital's child abuse team (though many of these were for concerns of inadequate supervision, neglect, or exposure to illicit substances, rather than truly malicious intent). Cases like these could be particularly suspected in poisoned infants under a year old, or in children roughly between the ages of five and eleven (e.g., preadolescent), as well as in cases where the history is erratic or causes the clinician unease in any other way. A history of poisoning in the past or siblings who have experienced poisoning are additional risk factors. Massive overdoses, ingesting multiple agents (unless the child was discovered with an open pill minder or something similar), exposure to illicit drugs, unusual poisonings from common household items like salt, pepper, and even water, and evidence of past child abuse or neglect are also risk factors. These cases typically have a higher morbidity rate, and if child abuse is suspected, these patients need to be reported to child protective services as soon as possible. The clinical and laboratory results must also be precisely documented, and chain-of-custody protocols pertaining to the handling of toxicology specimens must be closely followed.

Medication errors made by parents or other iatrogenic factors can also result in drug toxicity in young children. Youngsters may be more likely to make these mistakes for several reasons, such as the inescapable need to determine dosage based on weight or age and their inability to speak for themselves when it comes to allergy history or early warning signs of a side effect. Furthermore, children in hospital settings who have complex medical needs may be more vulnerable. A 10-fold overdose brought on by an mg/kg dosage calculation error is a frequent occurrence. On the other hand, errors may occur during compounding or when administering different concentrations of medications that do not have a standardized pediatric formulation. Moreover, there are several pediatric oral suspension concentrations of potentially toxic drugs like verapamil, atenolol, carvedilol, labetalol, propranolol, and tacrolimus. The incidence and severity of medication errors in children are significant. They are responsible for 12% of poisoning deaths in young children and up to 6% of all exposures in this age group. Computerized order entry systems, clinical pharmacists stationed on units, and increased communication efforts among health care team members are examples of preventive tactics.

8.2.2. Pediatric Pathophysiologic Considerations

For reasons beyond simply being smaller than adults, pediatric patients react to poisoning in different ways than adult patients do. The child's anatomy and physiology vary greatly, which influences their susceptibility to toxic exposures. Additionally, certain drugs become exceptionally toxic to very young children due to changes in drug disposition and effect that occur with development. Children exhibit a higher body surface area/weight ratio, increased skin perfusion, and increased skin hydration, all of which are indicators of increased dermal absorption. Dermal exposures carry a higher risk of toxicity and increase the risk of dehydration and insensible losses. Another pediatric vulnerability is inhalation absorption; young children's minute ventilation and elevated respiratory rate allow many airborne toxins to reach their body faster and in greater doses. The most prevalent of these poisons is carbon monoxide, which causes a range of exposed individuals to experience symptoms, the most severe of which are frequently observed in the youngest child.

Children are more susceptible to hypoxia and respiratory failure due to a higher metabolic rate and decreased reserve. The abdominal breathing that is frequently observed in young children experiencing respiratory distress is caused by an increased dependence on the diaphragm and a restricted ability of other accessory muscles. This can also lead to a higher risk of fatigue and respiratory failure. A child's capacity to adjust for acid-base disruptions and their resistance to a direct respiratory toxin (like aspirated hydrocarbon) may both be impacted by this circumstance As a result, children may be more acidemic at initial presentation with salicylism and may have more severe acidemia with other clinical scenarios, such as toxic alcohol poisoning. A relative lack of glycogen stores is another metabolic vulnerability that raises the risk of fasting hypoglycemia from ethanol, b-receptor antagonists, and other substances that change glucose homeostasis.

When under stress, children's cardiovascular reserve is more constrained. Heart rate has a major influence on cardiac output, and it cannot be increased by much. Up until the advanced stages of shock, however, normal blood pressure can be maintained due to elevated adrenergic tone. As a result, a child who is about to experience circulatory failure may seem stable at first, showing only tachycardia as the only abnormal vital sign and normal blood pressure. A sharp fall in health may occur if a drug is consumed that disturbs this delicate equilibrium. For instance, very small doses of medications that cause bradycardia, such as calcium channel antagonists or organophosphorus pesticides, can cause circulatory arrest. It is becoming more and more obvious that the way a particular drug is absorbed, distributed, metabolized, and excreted varies significantly throughout childhood, even though a thorough discussion of pediatric pharmacokinetics and pharmacodynamics is outside the purview of this review. During this time, a variety of ion channels and neurotransmitter receptors mature. The phenomenon of agents causing specific toxicity only in young children has been observed for a while; this could be explained by the developmental changes in drug distribution and response. Several opioid receptor agonists, such as codeine, buprenorphine, diphenoxylate antidiarrheals, clonidine, and dextromethorphan cough syrups, cause enhanced central nervous system (CNS) and respiratory depression in children. Infants under the age of one are more likely to experience paradoxical reactions to benzodiazepines and to experience QTc prolongation from sotalol and other prodysrhythmic medications.

8.2.3. Emergency Management Overview

Some become very sick, even though the majority of common pediatric exploratory ingestions result in relatively low rates of serious clinical toxicity (see previous note). Thus, it is still the responsibility of EPs to identify and care for children who have been poisoned. There are great overviews of the general treatment of a poisoned patient in easily accessible recent literature. To expand these overviews to the pediatric context, not much work is required. We make a number of observations that share our understanding of this approach and our experience with it, especially when it comes to the child who is seriously ill or at risk of a rapid decline. The senior author's prior attempt in this area, which was made twenty years ago, is improved upon by the planned method. If a small child has severe poisoning, it can be treated similarly to the multiple trauma model of today. The degree of (chemical) injury at each site can vary greatly, potentially causing multiple organ systems to be affected in a previously healthy child. For emergency physicians and paramedics, there is frequently a small window of time during which they can perform dramatic, life-saving interventions. A more thorough secondary assessment and detoxification phase are made possible by timely and comprehensive evaluation of life-threatening conditions followed by sequential immediate intervention (primary survey). In Table 8.6, this strategy is outlined. The comments are mostly annotated here because EPs are well-versed in this paradigm.

Table 8.6. *Emergency Management of the Poisoned Child*

Phase	Actions and Considerations
Initial Life Support Phase ($ABCD_3EF$)	
Airway	Emphasis on protection in obtunded child Possible compromise in caustic exposures
Breathing	Adequate oxygenation and ventilation
Circulation	Close monitoring of vital signs, capillary perfusion Early IV access
Disability	Level of consciousness Pupillary size, reactivity
Drugs	Dextrose (± rapid bedside testing) Oxygen Naloxone Other ACLS medications as needed
Decontamination	Ocular: copious saline lavage Skin: remove contaminated clothes, copious water, then soap and water GI: consider options (often none)
Electrocardiogram	Rate and rhythm QRS width, QTc length Terminal R wave in lead AVR
Fever	Core temperature check for hyperthermia Emergent cooling as needed
Evaluation, Decontamination, and Supportive Care Phase	
History	Brief, focused Known toxin Estimate amount, elapsed time, early symptoms, home treatment, PMH? Suspected but unknown toxin, consider if Acute onset of illness; age 1–5 y PMH of pica, ingestions Current household stressors Multiorgan system dysfunction Puzzling clinical picture New medication access Suspicious HPI, PMH, or FH for child abuse Institute hospital protocols Consider expanded laboratory testing with chain-of-custody procedures
Physical Examination	Vital signs, pulse oximetry (with core temperature) Level of consciousness, neuromuscular status Eyes: pupillary size and reactivity, extraocular movements, nystagmus Mouth: corrosive lesions, odors on breath, hydration of mucous membranes Cardiovascular: rate, rhythm, capillary perfusion Respiratory: rate, chest excursion, air entry, auscultatory signs GI: tenderness, bowel sounds Skin: color, bullae, burns, autonomic signs (eg, diaphoretic, flushed, dry) Odors: breath, clothing, vomitus
Laboratory (individualize)	CBC, co-oximetry ABG or VBG, ± serum osmolarity Chest radiograph, abdominal radiograph Electrolytes, BUN, creatinine, glucose, calcium, magnesium, liver function tests Rapid overdose toxicology screen Quantitative toxicology tests (especially acetaminophen, salicylate, ethanol) Comprehensive toxicology testing at reference laboratory
Assessment of severity and diagnosis	Clinical findings (see Table 3 toxidromes) Laboratory and ECG abnormalities
Specific detoxification and continued supportive care	Reassess $ABCD_3EF$ (always) Consider GI decontamination options Antidotal therapy, as indicated Enhance elimination, as indicated Supportive care (in every case!)

(*continued on next page*)

Source: https://renaissance.stonybrookmedicine.edu/sites/default/files/Approach_to_the_Poisoned_Child.pdf.

8.2.3.1. Life Support

The initial step in managing poisoned children involves focusing on the traditional ABCs (airway, breathing, circulation) as well as toxicologic aspects expanded to ABCD3EF. This includes assessing disability, starting empirical drug therapy, and conducting initial decontamination, with special attention given to ocular and dermal decontamination. An electrocardiogram evaluation and checking core temperature are also important. Children who are seriously poisoned can quickly deteriorate, potentially leading to coma and respiratory failure. Due to the risk of airway obstruction, it is crucial to be prepared to intubate if needed. Clinical judgment should guide decisions, and endotracheal intubation should be considered early to protect the airway and ensure adequate ventilation. This approach allows for a more organized response and reduces the risk of a sudden cardiac arrest.

In a similar vein, any child who exhibits symptoms of poisoning should receive prompt access to an IV, as well as early evaluation of blood pressure, capillary perfusion, cardiac rate and rhythm (including a 12-lead ECG). When a child is poisoned and experiencing cardiac arrest or severe hemodynamic compromise, the American Heart Association's guidelines for pediatric advanced life support should be followed. There are rare exceptions to this rule, such as when advanced cyclic antidepressant (or other sodium channel blocking agent) toxicity is treated with sodium bicarbonate early on. Other cases include additional specific antidotal therapy for other cardiotoxic drugs, like glucagon for b-adrenergic blocker (BB) toxicity, digitalis antibodies for severe digoxin overdose, and calcium and insulin/glucose therapy for severe calcium channel blocker (CCB) toxicity. Initial management for a child in shock who has not yet arrested usually involves IV crystalloid fluids (e.g., 20 mL/kg bolus, repeated and titrated to clinical effect), once more, and, if necessary, with particular antidotes. For chronic shock, cautious inotrope use is necessary after circulatory filling is accomplished. Such severe cases should prompt a call to the PCC or the need for emergent toxicology advice from an internal consultant.

With the exception of the regular use of thiamine, empirical drug therapy for obtunded young children who are poisoned, or possibly so, is similar to that used in adults. While pediatricians and emergency physicians typically consider and administer dextrose promptly, there are times when they neglect to administer a toddler naloxone trial. Toddlers can, however, get access to a lot of opioids through prescription analgesics (which have become more common in the last ten years, as previously mentioned), OTC cough medications, antidiarrheal medications, illicit drugs, and the partially naloxone-responsive antihypertensive drug clonidine. 61 Every child who has been blinded by poisoning should have a naloxone trial. Deeply obtunded or apneic toddlers can be treated right away with relatively high doses (by adult standards) without much concern about starting withdrawal symptoms; we usually start therapy with 0–1 mg/kg (or 1–2 mg) IV. If opioid toxicity is strongly suspected, this therapy may need to be repeated, particularly for agents like methadone, fentanyl, buprenorphine, and clonidine.

As was previously indicated, the administration of dextrose is a potentially crucial intervention that ought to be taken into consideration at an early stage of caring for a comatose or seizing child. If the blood glucose reading is unquestionably within the normal range, a quick bedside test might be helpful, but one should be cautious when depending solely on a borderline result. Patients with hypoglycemia may present with atypical neuropsychiatric symptoms, such as aphasia, slurred speech, and focal neurologic signs, in addition to coma or seizures. In toddlers (as opposed to adults), hypoglycemia is commonly observed following ethanol ingestions, oral hypoglycemic drug ingestions, and on rare occasions, b-blocker and salicylate intoxication. To minimize osmotic shifts from the typical 50% adult solution, the initial dose of dextrose is 0.5 g/kg. It is given as a 25% solution (2 mL/kg) for toddlers or as a 10% solution (5 mL/kg) for infants. Anticonvulsants and additional advanced life support drugs are administered as needed. Poisoning-related dysrhythmias are frequently due to blockages in the potassium or sodium channels, and conventional antiarrhythmic medications may exacerbate these conditions. Sodium bicarbonate is a common and effective treatment for the former, while magnesium infusion or override pacing is used for the latter. Titrated to effect, benzodiazepine therapy is generally the most effective treatment for seizures caused by toxins. A barbiturate is frequently a second-choice medication. For the most part, phenytoin is ineffective in treating seizures caused by toxins. In all patients who are seizing, blood glucose should be measured. One particular remedy for isoniazid-induced seizures is pyridoxine. When toxin-induced dysrhythmias or seizures occur, particularly when they are not responding to first-line treatment, it is important to consider the possibility of seeking an urgent toxicology consultation or contacting the local PCC.

Extreme hyperthermia in a young poisoned child is an uncommon symptom. This complication may arise from drug overdose in a number of drug classes, such as anticholinergics, salicylates, sympathomimetics, and other uncouplers of oxidative phosphorylation. It may also arise in the context of certain drug-induced hyperthermic syndromes, such as serotonin syndrome, neuroleptic malignant syndrome, and malignant hyperthermia. 64 A toddler presenting to the ED is not likely to be experiencing alcohol or sedative/hypnotic withdrawal, which is another possible cause of hyperthermia. The majority of these cases are treated with high-dose benzodiazepines (along with ventilatory support if needed) and fast external cooling while taking neuromuscular paralysis into account. Particular remedies (e.g., cyproheptadine for serotonin syndrome; bromocriptine for neuroleptic malignant syndrome) may be beneficial and ought to be taken into consideration following a toxicology consultation. The poisoned child should be carefully assessed using the ABCD3EF approach within a few minutes of presentation, and life-support interventions should be started as necessary. Individuals exhibiting markedly altered mental status ought to be evaluated for airway intubation, receive IV access, and participate in appropriate rapid bedside testing for oxygen, naloxone, and glucose empirical trials. extra advanced life support drugs, such as antiarrhythmics or anticonvulsants, as well as cooling techniques for individuals who are overheated.

8.2.3.2. Evaluation, Decontamination, and Supportive Care

- **History.** After the life-support phase is over, a focused and succinct history should be obtained. The standard inquiries about what, when, and how much was consumed are made of the child who has been exposed, whether it was known or suspected. However, young children who have been poisoned frequently arrive at the emergency department (ED) with an acute illness of dubious origin rather than a clear history of toxin exposure. In such cases, patient-related factors such as age (1 to 5 years), history of pica-prone behavior, acute onset, multiple organ system dysfunction, altered sensorium, and any perplexing clinical picture are highly suggestive of occult poisoning. Social and familial history variables might also be beneficial. Have any environmental stressors occurred, as noted earlier? Was the child visiting a grandparent's home, or vice versa, allowing the introduction of new medications into the household in a context that might be less childproofed? Are siblings or parents ill or taking newly prescribed medications, such as the pregnant or postpartum mother with the nearly universal prescription of iron supplementation? Holiday gatherings, with numerous relatives of all ages visiting and a general lessening of parental availability to supervise toddlers, are also high-risk occasions, as are recent moves in residence with boxes full of medications and household products often temporarily on the floor. As previously indicated, an uneven past medical history or a troubling family history could point to intentional poisoning.

- **Physical examination.** It is important to look for the typical physical characteristics of any poisoned patient when examining a small child. It is necessary to carefully reevaluate the capillary perfusion and vital signs, taking the core temperature as well. Examination findings related to the autonomic and central nervous systems, pupil size and reactivity, and any evident abnormalities of the skin, mucous membranes, cardiorespiratory or gastrointestinal tracts should be the main focus. It is important to look for distinctive scents in clothing or breath. The traditional groups of clinical observations, or toxidromes, observed in numerous poisoning categories (e.g., opioids, sympathomimetics, cholinergics, and anticholinergics) are characteristic of both adults and young children when age-corrected vital signs and baseline developmental status are taken into account. Table 8.7 lists several of the more prevalent toxidromes. As previously mentioned, test results that point to possible child abuse or neglect may increase the risk of intentional poisoning.
- **Laboratory and ECG evaluation.** Toddlers are subject to the same issues regarding quantitative drug levels and rapid overdose toxicology panels as adults or adolescents, and these issues are not discussed in detail. When it comes to treating most poisoned patients in an emergency, toxicology screens are not very useful. This observation holds especially true for the toddler whose ingestion of a single agent was observed. The toxicology screen may be useful in the patient with an unknown ingestion (particularly for forensic purposes if child abuse is suspected). However, routine chemistries, blood gas analysis (co-oximetry), and serum osmolarity (to assess anion, osmolal gaps, and pH disturbances) are more beneficial in case management. For the teenager who intentionally overdoses, a quantitative acetaminophen level is frequently recommended because this could be an undetected or unreported coingestant. In small children, routine screening for unreported acetaminophen ingestion is typically not recommended.

Table 8.7. *Major Pediatric Toxidromes*

Toxidrome	Examples	Significant Clinical Findings
Anticholinergic	Atropine Antihistamines Cyclic antidepressants	VS: ↑T, ↑HR, ↑BP (↓BP, dysrhythmias with CAs) CNS: delirium, coma, seizures Eyes: mydriasis (sluggishly reactive), blurred vision Skin: flushed, hot, dry Misc.: ileus, urinary retention
Cholinergic	Organophosphorus and carbamate pesticides Military nerve agents	VS: ↑ or ↓HR, ↑RR (with pulmonary effects) CNS: confusion/drowsiness to coma, seizures Eyes: miosis, blurry vision, lacrimation Skin: diaphoresis Misc.: SLUDGE; bronchorrhea, bronchospasm, pulmonary edema; muscle fasciculations, weakness to paralysis
Sympathomimetic	ADHD medications Amphetamines Cathinones Cocaine	VS: ↑T, ↑HR, ↑BP CNS: agitation, delirium, psychosis Eyes: mydriasis (normally reactive) Skin: diaphoresis Misc.: tremor, myoclonus
Opioid	Prescription analgesics Antitussives Antidiarrheals Antihypertensives (clonidine) ADHD medication	VS: ↓T, ↓HR, ↓BP, ↓ RR CNS: euphoria to coma Eyes: miosis (pinpoint pupils) Skin: normal Misc.: hyporeflexia

Source: https://renaissance.stonybrookmedicine.edu/sites/default/files/Approach_to_the_Poisoned_Child.pdf.

Clonidine, digoxin, CCBs, BBs, iron, and other clinically significant medications are frequently consumed by toddlers and have the potential to cause coma or disrupted cardiovascular function. Typically, a toxicology screen for these drugs comes out negative. All of these, however, have distinct patterns of clinical, ECG, or routine laboratory abnormalities. Clonidine mimics an opioid overdose in that it causes hypotension and bradycardia that appear out of proportion, and it responds differently to naloxone. Digoxin more commonly manifests as sinus bradycardia with typical ECG findings, and in severe cases, hyperkalemia and ventricular dysrhythmias. Iron toxicity can cause marked vomiting, diarrhea, and hypotension, along with an anion gap metabolic acidosis, hyperglycemia, and leukocytosis. CCBs and BBs frequently present with a history of drug availability from family members, especially grandparents, with combined bradycardia and hypotension. This evaluation and supportive care phase calls for a closer look at the ECG. Subtle ECG abnormalities can be brought on by a variety of medications and poisons. These abnormalities represent pathophysiologic changes that can lead to hemodynamic instability and dysrhythmia potential. 65 Specifically, many drug classes cause potassium efflux channel blockade, which can lead to potential torsades de pointes, or sodium channel blockade, which can cause hypotension and a tendency toward ventricular tachycardia or fibrillation. The longer QRS and QTc durations, respectively, are indicative of these conditions. In the final 40 milliseconds of the QRS complex, sodium channel blocking agents may also result in a significant rightward axis deviation. This is especially noticeable when lead AVR exhibits a significant terminal upright R wave, which is not usually seen in healthy children past the neonatal stage. Sodium channel blockers include diphenhydramine, class Ia and Ic antiarrhythmics, carbamazepine, hydroxychloroquine, and cyclic antidepressants. Some nonsedating antihistamines, phenothiazines and butyrophenones, other antipsychotics, some serotonin-selective antidepressants (citalopram and escitalopram), some macrolide and quinolone antibiotics, and once more, class Ic antiarrhythmmics are on a similar list of potassium channel blocking agents.

- **Assessment.** An assessment of the potential severity of the intoxication for the child with a known exposure can be made by the emergency physician through a thorough clinical evaluation, sometimes with additional laboratory data and ECG interpretation. The same method should enable a reasonable estimation of the likely agent or class of agents in charge of the child's illness in the case of an occult poisoning. In either scenario, the practitioner may now take into account additional advice from the PCC or a nearby toxicology consultant to help with the care of children who have been exposed to more unusual substances or who are more seriously ill.
- **Specific detoxification issues.** Rapid topical decontamination is necessary for children with significant ocular or dermal contamination, as is appropriate for any aged patient based on substance and clinical criteria. Over the past ten years, guidelines for intestinal decontamination have changed significantly and are now applicable to both adults and children. Without gastrointestinal decontamination, the majority of poisoned patients are treated in the emergency department (ED) in a safe and efficient manner. It is no longer advised to use ipecac syrup for gastric emptying in hospitals or

at home. Except in cases of high-lethality ingestions in patients who present within 30 to 60 minutes, gastric lavage is rarely indicated. It is also more technically challenging and prone to complications when performed on small children. Similar to this, single-dose AC administration is no longer a standard ED intervention; however, it might be taken into consideration for patients who arrive shortly after ingesting agents that bind to AC, for whom antidotal therapy or supportive care might not be adequate to avoid serious toxicity. When hydrocarbons or caustics are consumed, AC should not be used because the risk of pulmonary aspiration or direct mucosal damage is more serious than systemic toxicity. The pediatric dose, if chosen, is usually 1 g/kg, or 10 to 15 g on average for toddlers. When combined with a fruit-flavored beverage and given by mouth, a lot of kids swallow this much, or nearly so, especially if they can use a straw and a cup with a plastic top to hide the unsightly appearance. About 20% of children who receive AC administration—especially through an NG tube—vomit, so it is generally not recommended for obtunded patients who have not previously had airway protection. Furthermore, the use of NG tubes increases the risk of a potentially fatal consequence in the event that a struggling child unintentionally inserts their trachea. Seldom do we employ an. NG tube for the administration of AC to toddlers, with the exception of the most extremely fatal overdoses; in these instances, it is imperative to confirm the gastric placement prior to using the tube and to give careful thought to a prior endotracheal intubation for comparatively better airway protection. Iron is the only one of the several substances that are not well adsorbed to AC and whose consumption may be lessened by gastrointestinal decontamination in young children. After a large iron exposure, the majority of children throw up a lot, but abdominal radiography can still be helpful in checking for any leftover iron pills, fragments, or concretions. Consideration should be given to whole bowel irrigation (WBI) if it is present, using an electrolyte solution balanced with polyethylene glycol. When WBI is given to toddlers, an NG tube must usually be placed. The dosage is 250–500 mL/h until the rectal effluent is clear, which usually happens in 3 to 4 h. The child who ingests illicit drug packets or vials, the young patient found to have large amounts of lead paint chips in the gastrointestinal tract, the large overdoses of significantly toxic medications, especially if in extended-release formulation (such a scenario is uncommon in toddlers; exceptions include several CCBs and b-blockers), and the uncommon ingestion of various medications in patch formulations can all be treated with WBI.

- **Antidotal therapy.** While supportive care alone is usually sufficient to manage most poisonings, in certain instances, targeted antidotal therapy is necessary. With a few extra considerations, the indications for and selection of antidotes for children are comparable to those for adults. Pediatric experience is frequently limited, and the pediatric indication is off label, similar to many other newer or limited-use therapies. Because these are rarely administered medications that need weight-based dosing and diluent volume, there is a high risk of medication errors. Certain medications, like ethanol infusions and calcium salts, need to be administered continuously through large-bore IV access, which can be challenging to get for a small child. However, a number of crucial antidotes have demonstrated a broad safety margin, and it is not appropriate to withhold antidotal therapy in circumstances where it may be life-saving. A number of the antidotes in Table 8.8 are particularly noteworthy and have a vital but infrequent role in the management of pediatric toxicology.

Table 8.8. *Major Antidotes in Pediatric Poisonings*

Drug or Toxin	Antidote
Acetaminophen	*N*-acetylcysteine
Benzodiazepines	Flumazenil
β-Adrenergic antagonists (β-blockers)	Glucagon[a]
CCBs	Calcium[a] High-dose insulin euglycemia (insulin and glucose)[a] IV lipid emulsion[a]
Coumadin (and similar rodenticides)	Vitamin K_1
Cyanide	Hydroxocobalamin (preferred) Sodium nitrite and sodium thiosulfate
Digoxin	Digoxin immune Fab
Ethylene glycol	Fomepizole (preferred) Ethanol[a]
Iron	Deferoxamine
Isoniazid	Pyridoxine
Lead	British anti-Lewisite $CaNa_2EDTA$ (versenate) Succimer (dimercaptosuccinic acid)
Methanol	Fomepizole (preferred) Ethanol[a]
Methemoglobinemia	Methylene blue
Opioids	Naloxone
Organophosphorus insecticides and nerve agents	Atropine Pralidoxime
Sulfonylureas	Dextrose Octreotide[a]
Rattlesnake (and other crotalid) envenomations	Crotalidae polyvalent immune Fab
Tricyclic antidepressants	Sodium bicarbonate IV lipid emulsion[a]

[a]Without specific FDA approval for this indication

Source: https://renaissance.stonybrookmedicine.edu/sites/default/files/Approach_to_the_Poisoned_Child.pdf.

When it comes to organophosphorus pesticide or nerve agent poisoning, prompt atropine administration can be life-saving, and in more serious cases, pralidoxime may be a necessary adjunct. Because of this, emergency medical services teams frequently carry adult-dose autoinjectors, which provide larger dosages than those advised for small children. It may be possible to find pediatric atropine autoinjectors with lower dosages, and modifying adult dose kits to include a lower dosage of pralidoxime is a simple process. Nevertheless, safety data from asymptomatic children accidentally administered adult atropine autoinjectors revealed anticholinergic symptoms without any serious side effects, and the doses required may be higher than expected in cases of severe poisoning from nerve agents or organophosphorus pesticides. In this case, the risk of toxicity is outweighed by the therapeutic benefit of giving a child a higher but instantly available dose. In 2004, the FDA approved N-acetylcysteine (NAC) in an IV formulation for the treatment of acetaminophen toxicity. The management of many acetaminophen-poisoned patients has been made simpler by the development of a specific IV formulation, which has eliminated the enteral formulation's problems with odor, unpalatability, and noncompliance. Nonetheless, a number of pediatric therapeutic errors have been documented, involving incorrect dosage and volume of diluent, underscoring the dangers associated with administering antidotes to children. Children who were accidentally given the adult diluent volume have experienced seizures and hyponatremia. In young children, an overdose of the IV formulation's NAC alone could be lethal. To guarantee proper administration, careful adherence to prescribing instructions and consultation with a toxicologist are recommended.

Alcohol dehydrogenase inhibition is the cornerstone of treatment for patients with toxic alcohol poisoning because it prevents the formation of toxic metabolites, which can cause metabolic acidosis and organ damage. The most popular method of achieving this treatment is the administration of fomepizole, which has demonstrated safety and efficacy in the pediatric population. In regions where fomepizole is not available, the same enzyme-inhibiting effects were previously achieved by IV or oral ethanol administration, which is still used today. Technically speaking, IV ethanol administration can be challenging. It involves central venous access, dose titration, mental status depression, and the possibility of fasting hypoglycemia. In the event of ethanol poisoning, young children are more susceptible to hypoglycemia and CNS depression; however, the side effects of therapeutic ethanol administration may be less severe. There was no symptomatic hypoglycemia or significant CNS depression in one study of 60 children who had been exposed to methanol and were treated with IV or oral ethanol; this finding probably reflects the benefit of close observation.

In the event of poisoning from fire smoke or other sources, having cyanide antidotes on hand is crucial for survival. In the past, amyl nitrite, sodium nitrite, and sodium thiosulfate have been the cyanide antidotes that were accessible in the US. On the other hand, there is a significant risk associated with the use of nitrites in pediatric medicine, as they produce methemoglobin, which can be excreted safely. When methemoglobin is administered with nitrite therapy, elevated levels of methemoglobin are caused by both a decreased activity of methemoglobin reductase and an increased proportion of fetal hemoglobin. A child's already diminished respiratory and metabolic reserve may be further depleted by the combined effects of methemoglobinemia, carboxyhemoglobinemia, and hypoxemia from breathing in fire smoke. Therefore, in cases of pediatric cyanide poisoning brought on by smoke inhalation, only sodium thiosulfate has historically been advised. The vitamin B12 precursor hydroxocobalamin, which has been used for a long time and has been approved by the FDA in IV formulation for this indication in 2006, appears to be as effective as sodium nitrite plus thiosulfate, if not more so. When it comes to treating cyanide toxicity, it is therefore the recommended agent. There are few but encouraging pediatric safety data for both sodium thiosulfate and hydroxocobalamin. 83 In cases of pediatric cyanide poisoning, where prompt antidote administration is essential, both agents should be deemed appropriate. Since its successful application in treating local anesthetic toxicity and later other poisonings leading to cardiovascular collapse, resuscitative IV lipid emulsion has been the subject of extensive research. Although the exact indications are still being determined, bupropion, calcium channel antagonists, and tricyclic antidepressants are among the lipophilic drugs that can cause severe poisoning. Pancreatitis, fat emboli, acute respiratory distress syndrome (ARDS), and digit amputation are among the side effects that have been reported. It appears to be a viable treatment for refractory cardiovascular collapse, despite the fact that the frequency of these events is unknown and pediatric data are even more sparse.

- **Enhanced elimination**. After multiple significant poisonings, the capacity to improve toxin elimination in particular circumstances may be a crucial adjuvant to therapy. The cornerstone of treatment for moderate to severe salicylate intoxication is urinary alkalinization. Through intestinal dialysis, it has been demonstrated that multiple-dose AC (MDAC) increases the clearance of a number of drugs, including barbiturates, salicylate, carbamazepine, and theophylline. However, using it was linked to side effects from repeated administration of AC, including aspiration, intestinal blockage, and vomiting. Moreover, it's unclear if the apparent pharmacokinetic benefit results in better clinical outcomes. We found that MDAC was most helpful when children had mild to moderate theophylline intoxications, and it sometimes prevented the need for hemodialysis (HD). However, as this is no longer the case, there aren't many clear-cut indications for MDAC in young children, though it might be taken into consideration for moderately severe intoxications caused by salicylate or carbamazepine. Extracorporeal toxin removal techniques help patients whose highly toxic substance has been absorbed and reaches a significant serum concentration avoid worsening of organ injury, metabolic compromise, or organ system collapse. High-flux HD is the main technique for quickly eliminating toxins from the blood by removing solutes and toxins through diffusion and convection across a semipermeable membrane. Other techniques like exchange transfusion, plasmapheresis, charcoal hemoperfusion, and peritoneal dialysis are not as useful and remove toxins at a much slower rate or with less volume. The only patients who should receive continuous renal replacement therapies—such as continuous venovenohemofiltration—are hemodynamically unstable and unable to handle acute HD. These therapies also have slower clearance rates.

Acute hemodialysis (HD) should be considered for removing toxins if there is a clinical benefit to faster removal than what the body can naturally do, if there is a clear relationship between toxin levels and toxicity, and if the toxin can be effectively removed. Toxins that are easily removed through HD are typically low in molecular weight, not bound to protein significantly, and have a low distribution volume. Common examples of these toxins include salicylates, toxic alcohols, lithium, and theophylline. HD can also be effective in removing valproic acid, barbiturates, and methotrexate, and can be life-saving for reversing metabolic and electrolyte imbalances, such as metformin-associated lactic acidosis.

In pediatrics, acute HD is commonly used for both chronic and acute kidney failure, and can be safely performed under the guidance of a nephrologist. Possible risks include complications from central venous access, electrolyte imbalances, and hemodynamic instability. Specific equipment and careful monitoring may be needed for very young infants to prevent hypotension. Despite technical challenges, most pediatric hospitals can perform HD, even for newborns. It should be used without delay in critically ill children requiring urgent toxin removal, even if transportation is required to a specialized center.

8.2.4. The Well-Appearing Child with Poison Exposure

Unlike a patient showing obvious signs of poisoning, an asymptomatic child who may have been exposed to a dangerous substance poses a different challenge. In cases of exploratory ingestions, children may have had access to a drug or chemical without supervision, and the ingestion may have gone unnoticed. Many substances involved in these cases are not harmful to young children under 6 years old, and a significant number of these cases do not require medical attention when reported to a poison control center. However, when the child is brought to the emergency department, the doctor must assess the seriousness of the exposure. A thorough history, including details about the timing, nature, and estimated amount of the exposure, is crucial. Typically, exploratory ingestions involve a small number of pills or a small amount of liquid. If the substance is more appealing, such as flavored liquids or chewable tablets, or if the child had more time unsupervised, they may have ingested larger amounts. The doctor will look for signs like missing pills, residue in the child's mouth or clothing, coughing or vomiting after ingestion, and what the child tells them happened, if the child can communicate effectively. They must also ask about all medications in the home, not just what the caregiver believes the child may have ingested. ¶If the child shows no symptoms of poisoning after a period of observation, they can usually be discharged safely. However, certain conditions must be met before discharge. The ingestion must have been of a harmless substance in a small amount, and the observation period should be sufficient to monitor the effects of the exposure (e.g., how long it takes for the substance to be absorbed and show clinical effects). The circumstances surrounding the ingestion should not raise any suspicions, as noted earlier. An appropriate follow-up plan should be in place, and consultation with a poison control center may be beneficial in determining the need for observation and discharge. They may also provide follow-up support over the phone as necessary.

8.2.5. Deadly in Small Doses: Persistent Perils and Emerging Exposures

While many substances consumed by small children may not be harmful, there are some exposures that need to be treated very carefully because they can have deadly effects even in small doses. In these situations, it is best to assume the worst-case scenario regarding the type and quantity of toxin consumed and admit kids for observation. This advice is particularly pertinent to sustained-release formulations of extremely hazardous medications. Emerging risks require the emergency physician to be aware of them. Ingestion of foreign bodies can lead to severe tissue damage, which is the first of these hazards. There has been a correlation between button batteries and a higher incidence of exsanguination deaths due to the formation of aortoesophageal fistulas. Button batteries are well known to require immediate endoscopic removal if lodged in the esophagus. The expanded availability of 20-mm lithium disk batteries appears to be the primary cause of this condition. Before the last ED visit, when the child presents with massive hematemesis, shock, or asystole, the child is frequently evaluated multiple times. There are multiple instances where battery ingestion is discovered after death and no prior history is known. Small magnet toys are another type of dangerous foreign body that can cause bowel obstruction and necrosis in the intestines by attracting one another. Expanding foam toys and flower fertilizer pellets present the same risk because they get bigger when submerged in water. Over the past few years, laundry detergent pods have become more and more popular in the US consumer market. They are a small, colorful, and highly concentrated package of detergent that is sealed in a thin membrane that dissolves when wet. Cases of pediatric exposures emerged shortly after the pods were made available; in these cases, aspiration, CNS depression, oral and aerodigestive tract burns, and respiratory distress were all brought on by merely getting a mouthful of the pod. Though they resemble dishwashing detergent packets in appearance, they appear to have more severe clinical effects, so treating these children with caution is advised as they may become toxic in the hours following exposure.

In order to improve the identification of patterns, prevention goals, and sentinel events in these most tragic cases, a specific review of pediatric poisoning fatalities was implemented in 2010 as a collaborative effort with the NPDS annual report. Even though there aren't many poison-related deaths each year that are related to pediatric poisoning, a closer examination of the exposure conditions reveals that many are clearly preventable. First, despite the increasing prevalence of opioid abuse, methadone and buprenorphine cases are disproportionately associated with opioid abuse, underscoring the ongoing danger to the youngest victims of the epidemic. Therapeutic errors are a recurring problem in healthcare settings, usually involving children with complex medical needs. Despite prompt and effective airway management, ventilator support, and intensive ICU care, ingestion of torch fuel and other hydrocarbons remains one of the leading causes of death. There have been multiple cases of toddlers ingesting their own antidysrhythmics, leading to rapid cardiac arrest, and several exploratory ingestions of refrigerated medications, including liquid methadone. Refrigerators are harder to keep safe than lone medicine cabinets because they are used throughout the day by several family members. This finding should raise concerns among prescribers, who might choose to use a different medication that doesn't need to be refrigerated. It should also prompt a closer examination of the actual need for refrigerated storage of these compounds and better anticipatory counseling for families who use these medications at home.

A Closer Look

Pediatric Pharmacogenomics

Genetic variations play a significant role in drug metabolism and response in pediatric populations, influencing individual susceptibility to adverse drug reactions (ADRs). The study of pharmacogenomics, which examines how genetic variations affect drug response, has shed light on the interplay between genetics and pharmacotherapy. Understanding the impact of genetic variations is crucial in pediatric medicine, as children may respond differently to medications compared to adults due to developmental changes in drug metabolism pathways and enzyme activity.

One key area of focus in pharmacogenomics is the role of polymorphisms in genes encoding drug-metabolizing enzymes, such as cytochrome P450 (CYP) enzymes, which are responsible for the metabolism of many drugs. Genetic variations in these enzymes can lead to altered enzyme activity, affecting the rate at which drugs are metabolized and cleared from the body. For example, genetic polymorphisms in the CYP2D6 gene can result in poor metabolizer phenotypes, where individuals metabolize drugs slowly, or ultrarapid metabolizer phenotypes, where individuals metabolize drugs rapidly. These variations can significantly impact drug efficacy and toxicity, particularly for medications with narrow therapeutic indices or those that require metabolic activation to exert their effects.

Pediatric populations are particularly vulnerable to the effects of genetic variations on drug metabolism and response due to their dynamic growth and development. Enzyme expression levels and metabolic capacity can vary widely throughout childhood and adolescence, influencing the pharmacokinetics and pharmacodynamics of medications. For example, infants and young children may have lower levels of drug-metabolizing enzymes compared to adults, leading to slower drug clearance and increased susceptibility to adverse effects. Conversely, enzyme activity may increase with age, resulting in differences in drug metabolism and response between pediatric age groups.

The impact of genetic variations on drug response extends beyond metabolism to include drug targets, transporters, and other pharmacodynamic factors. Polymorphisms in genes encoding drug receptors or signaling molecules can alter drug efficacy or sensitivity, leading to variations in therapeutic response or increased risk of adverse reactions. Additionally, genetic variations in drug transporters, such as P-glycoprotein (P-gp), can affect drug absorption, distribution, and elimination, influencing drug exposure and response.

Advances in pharmacogenomics have led to the identification of genetic markers associated with increased risk of ADRs in pediatric populations. For example, genetic variations in the HLA-B gene have been linked to severe cutaneous adverse reactions, such as Stevens-Johnson syndrome and toxic epidermal necrolysis, following treatment with certain medications like carbamazepine and abacavir. Pharmacogenetic testing can help identify patients at increased risk of these reactions, allowing for personalized medication selection and dosing to minimize adverse outcomes.

Summary

- Pediatric toxicology is a specialized branch of medicine dedicated to the study, diagnosis, and treatment of poisonings and toxic exposures in children. It encompasses a wide range of substances including medications, household products, chemicals, plants, and venomous creatures that can potentially harm children.
- Determining the severity of toxicity is crucial for guiding treatment decisions. Pediatric toxicologists evaluate various factors including the dose and duration of exposure, the child's age and weight, the toxic properties of the substance, and the presence of any underlying medical conditions.
- Poisoning in children usually happens at home, when they take in a poisonous substance, breathe it in, or their skin is exposed to it. The poisoning is usually accidental and involves children under the age of 5.
- Medicines are the most common cause of poisoning in children. Several medicines you or a family member are taking can be dangerous to children. Opioids and barbiturates are well-known dangers, but medicines for high blood pressure, mental health, and diabetes are also hazardous.
- Pesticides represent a broad classification of chemicals that are applied to kill or control insects, unwanted plants, molds, or unwanted animals (e.g., rodents).
- Children are uniquely vulnerable to uptake and adverse effects of pesticides because of developmental, dietary, and physiologic factors. Exposure occurs through ingestion, inhalation, or dermal contact.
- Proximity to pesticide-treated agricultural areas or household members that work with pesticides presents another opportunity for contamination of the residential environment for some children.
- Children may find alcoholic drinks and consume them. Sanitizers, perfumes, OTC cold medicines, and mouthwash also contain alcohol. At young ages, alcohol ingestion causes low blood glucose levels, seizures, and coma.
- Acute intoxications give rise to highly diverse clinical manifestations, often of a neurologic nature. Doses that are usually harmless to adults may lead to severe conditions in children, especially when different substances are consumed simultaneously.

References

1. Baltimore, C., & Meyer, R. J. (1969). A study of storage, child behavioral traits, and mother's knowledge of toxicology in 52 poisoned families and 52 comparison families. *Pediatrics, 44*(5), 816–820.
2. Beuhler, M. C., Gala, P. K., Wolfe, H. A., et al. (2013). Laundry detergent "pod" ingestions: A case series and discussion of recent literature. *Pediatric Emergency Care, 29*(7), 743–747.
3. Bond, G. R., Woodward, R. W., & Ho, M. (2012). The growing impact of pediatric pharmaceutical poisoning. *Journal of Pediatrics, 160*(2), 265–270.

4. Bronstein, A. C., Spyker, D. A., Cantilena, L. R., Jr, et al. (2010). 2009 annual report of the American Association of Poison Control Centers' National Poison Data System (NPDS): 27th annual report. *Clinical Toxicology, 48*(10), 979–1178.

5. Budnitz, D. S., & Lovegrove, M. C. (2012). The last mile: Taking the final steps in preventing pediatric pharmaceutical poisonings. *Journal of Pediatrics, 160*(2), 190–192.

6. Burghardt, L. C., Ayers, J. W., Brownstein, J. S., et al. (2013). Adult prescription uses and pediatric medication exposures and poisonings. *Pediatrics, 132*(1), 18–27.

7. Deeths, T. M., & Breeden, J. T. (1971). Poisoning in children–a statistical study of 1057 cases. *Journal of Pediatrics, 78*(2), 299–305.

8. Haddon, W., Jr. (1980). Advances in the epidemiology of injuries as a basis for public policy. *Public Health Reports, 95*(5), 411–421.

9. Henretig, F. M. (1994). Special considerations in the poisoned pediatric patient. *Emergency Medicine Clinics of North America, 12*(3), 549–567.

10. Henretig, F. M. (Ed.). (1997). Patient and family issues. In *Textbook of Pediatric Emergency Procedures* (pp. 3–7). Williams & Wilkins.

11. Hepner, J., & Vohra, R. (2013). Household "HazMat": A pair of sudsy siblings. *Pediatric Emergency Care, 29*(7), 773–777.

12. Litovitz, T., & Manoguerra, A. (1992). Comparison of pediatric poisoning hazards: An analysis of 3.8 million exposure incidents. *Pediatrics, 89*(6), 999–1006.

13. Litovitz, T., Whitaker, N., Clark, L., et al. (2010). Emerging battery-ingestion hazard: Clinical implications. *Pediatrics, 125*(6), 1168–1177.

14. Maragos, G. D., Greene, C. A., & Mitchell, J. R. (1971). Accidental poisoning of children in transit. *Journal of Pediatrics, 79*(1), 125–126.

15. Margolis, J. A. (1971). Psychosocial study of childhood poisoning: A 5-year follow-up. *Pediatrics, 47*(3), 439–444.

16. McFee, R. B., & Caraccio, T. R. (2006). "Hang up your pocketbook"–An easy intervention for the granny syndrome: Grandparents as a risk factor in unintentional pediatric exposures to pharmaceuticals. *Journal of the American Osteopathic Association, 106*(7), 405–411.

17. Osterhoudt, K. C. (2006). The lexiconography of toxicology. *Journal of Medical Toxicology, 2*(1), 1–2.

18. Russo, M., Pecker, L., Wood, J., et al. (2013). Grandparent involvement in exploratory pediatric poisonings: A hospital-based study [Abstract]. *Clinical Toxicology, 51*(6), 593.

19. Schille, S. F., Shehab, N., Thomas, K. E., et al. (2009). Medication overdoses leading to emergency department visits among children. *American Journal of Preventive Medicine, 37*(2), 181–187.

20. Schum, T. R., & Lachman, B. S. (1982). Effects of packaging and appearance on childhood poisoning: Vacor rat poison. *Clinical Pediatrics (Philadelphia), 21*(5), 282–285.

21. Sibert, J. R. (1975). Stress of families of children who have ingested poisons. *British Medical Journal, 3*(5971), 87–89.

22. Sibert, J. R., & Newcombe, R. G. (1977). Accidental ingestion of poisons and child personality. *Postgraduate Medical Journal, 53*(620), 254–256.

23. Sobel, R. (1969). Traditional safety measures and accidental poisoning in childhood. *Pediatrics, 44*(5), 811–816.

24. Spiller, H. A., Buehler, M. C., Ryan, M. L., et al. (2013). Evaluation of changes in poisoning in young children: 2000–2010. *Pediatric Emergency Care, 29*(6), 635–640.

25. Tenenbein, M. (2005). Unit dose packaging of iron supplements and reduction of iron poisoning in young children. *Archives of Pediatrics & Adolescent Medicine, 159*(6), 593–595.

26. Turbeville, D. T., & Fearnow, R. G. (1976). Is it possible to identify the child who is a "high risk" candidate for the accidental ingestion of a poison? *Clinical Pediatrics (Philadelphia), 15*(10), 918–919.

27. Walton, W. W. (1982). An evaluation of the Poison Prevention Packaging Act. *Pediatrics, 69*(3), 363–370.

28. Yin, S. (2010). Malicious use of pharmaceuticals in children. *Journal of Pediatrics, 157*(5), 832–836.

Chapter

ROLE OF ANALYTICAL TOXICOLOGY

9

Contents

Introduction

The detection, identification, and quantification of foreign substances, or "xenobiotics," in biological and other specimens is known as analytical toxicology. There are analytical techniques for a very broad variety of compounds, including chemicals, pesticides, medicines, illicit drugs, and naturally occurring poisons. Poisoning diagnosis, treatment, prognosis, and prevention can all be aided by analytical toxicology. Furthermore, analytical toxicology laboratories can be engaged in various other tasks like monitoring for drugs of abuse, forensic analyses, therapeutic drug monitoring (Hallworth, M. and Watson, I. (2007)), and exposure assessment after chemical incidents. They might also work on studies to find out the effectiveness of novel treatment plans or the pharmacokinetic and toxicokinetic characteristics of drugs. All areas of toxicology are seeing constant advancements in analytical methods, many of which, as previously indicated, are centered on environmental issues. These devices can be used to find new methods for collecting water samples or to find an automated instrument to measure the amounts of compounds containing sulfur in the air. Many times, advancements in environmental analysis can be applied to drug toxicity experiments or to forensic medicine to identify poisoning causes.

Orientation and Directional Terms

Term	Definition	Illustration
Xenobiotics	A chemical substance found within an organism that is not naturally produced or expected to be present within the organism. It can also cover substances that are present in much higher concentrations than are usual.	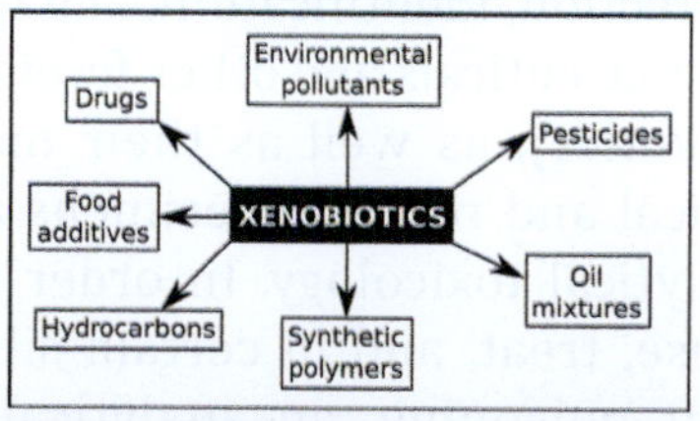
Forensic toxicology	A multidisciplinary field that combines the principles of toxicology with expertise in disciplines such as analytical chemistry, pharmacology and clinical chemistry to aid medical or legal investigation of death, poisoning, and drug use.	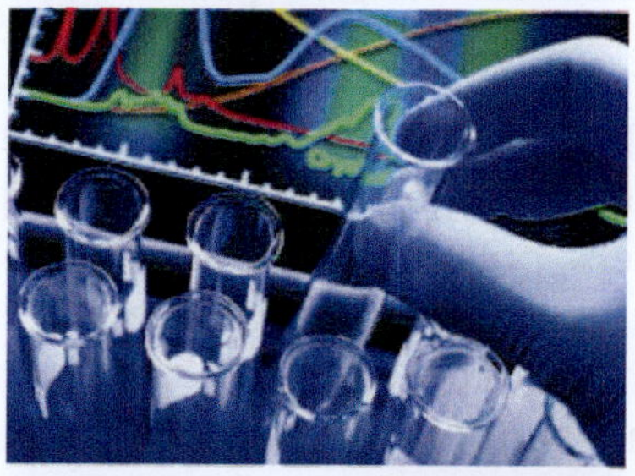
Clinical chemistry	A division in medical laboratory sciences focusing on qualitative tests of important compounds, referred to as analytes or markers, in bodily fluids and tissues using analytical techniques and specialized instruments.	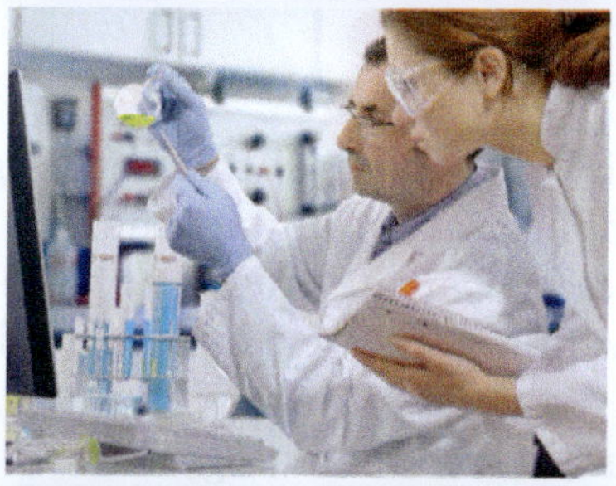
Pharmacokinetics	A branch of pharmacology dedicated to describing how the body affects a specific substance after administration. The substances of interest include any chemical xenobiotic such as pharmaceutical drugs, pesticides, food additives, cosmetics, etc.	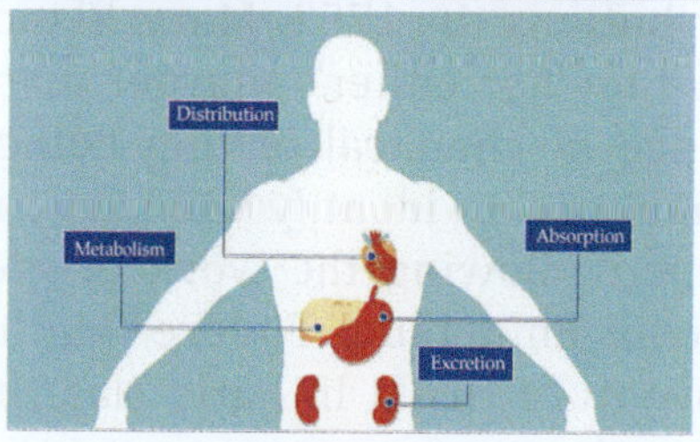
Alkaloids	A class of basic, naturally occurring organic compounds that contain at least one nitrogen atom. This group also includes some related compounds with neutral and even weakly acidic properties.	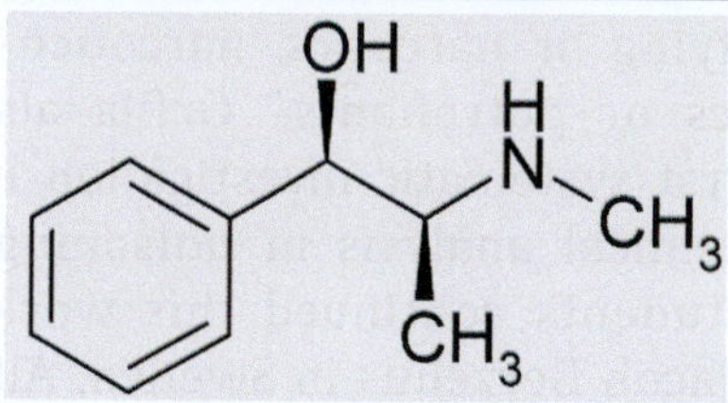

9.1 Basic Concept of Analytical toxicology

The detection, identification, and quantification of pharmaceuticals and other foreign substances (xenobiotics), as well as their metabolites, in biological and related specimens are the focus of analytical toxicology. In order to effectively diagnose, treat, and in certain situations even prevent poisoning, an analytical toxicologist must possess a foundational understanding of clinical and forensic toxicology (Jones, A.W. 1998). Additionally, the analyst needs to be able to communicate clearly with pathologists, coroners, police, and maybe other professionals. It's also preferable to have a solid grasp of pharmacology, clinical chemistry, and pharmacokinetics.

9.1.1 Historical Development

The field of forensic toxicology gave rise to the application of physicochemical techniques for the analysis of drugs and other poisons in bodily fluids, tissues, and related specimens. Later work on improving food safety and occupational toxicology made significant contributions. In 1752, Mary Blandy's trial at Oxford for her father's murder marks the first instance of chemical testing being used in a criminal trial to identify a poison—in this case, arsenic. Following the work of the physician François Emmanuel Fodere, Mathieu Joseph Bonaventure Orfila in Paris classified poisons into six classes: "corrosives, astringents, acrids, stupifying or narcotics, narcotico-acrids, and septics or putrefiants." Orfila also initiated the first systematic investigation into the use of chemical analysis in poisoning diagnosis. His students continued this work, including Jons Jacob Berzelius in Sweden, Alfred Swaine Taylor at Guy's Hospital in London, and Sir Robert Christison in Edinburgh. In the 1830s, sensitive and focused chemical techniques were developed for the detection of metallic poisons in biological specimens, including arsenic, antimony, bismuth, and mercury. Stas first described the use of solvent extraction to extract alkaloids, like nicotine, from biological specimens so that they could be more easily detected and identified through chemical or physiological tests. Otto then developed this method into a systematic way for extracting nonvolatile organic compounds from bodily fluids. Chemical and spectroscopic techniques for measuring blood ethanol concentration and carbon monoxide levels had also been developed by the late nineteenth century.

Additional noteworthy developments in chemical toxicology included the application of ammonium sulfate to "salt out" alkaloids and the development of a colorimetric method for quantifying barbiturates. The precipitation of protein with trichloroacetic acid, followed by kaolin adsorption and the elution of the drugs of interest, was described in 1937 as an alternative method for purifying basic drugs from biological specimens. Sodium tungstate protein precipitation was first introduced in 1946. In 1949, a synthetic magnesium silicate called Florisil was introduced as an alternative to kaolin for the adsorption of basic drugs like narcotics from biological specimens. Methods of microdiffusion (Conway, 1947) were created for volatile analytes. The development and use of refined physicochemical techniques like spectrophotometry and chromatography in the late 1940s led to significant advancements in analytical methodology. Particularly popular were visible spectrophotometry (colorimetry), infrared (IR) and ultraviolet (UV) spectrophotometry, as well as paper and ion-exchange column chromatography. Paper chromatography has been largely replaced in more recent times by thin-layer chromatography (TLC), which has the advantages of faster analysis and lower detection limits. These techniques are now widely applied to specific problems due to improved instrumentation for UV spectrophotometry (including facilities for derivative spectroscopy), spectrophotofluorimetry, atomic absorption spectrometry, anodic stripping voltammetry, electrochemistry, X-ray diffraction, mass spectrometry, nuclear magnetic resonance, and neutron activation analysis.

9.1.2 Analytical Toxicology in Present

Methods for locating, identifying, and quantifying drugs and other poisons in biological fluids have advanced significantly over the past 25 years, improving the accuracy and breadth of analytical results in the process. It is now clear how valuable some emergency assays are and how they fit into the therapeutic intervention process. While some of these assays are carried out for clinical purposes, they demand a high level of analytical reliability and have clear medicolegal ramifications. Examples include suspected cases of iatrogenic poisoning, screening for child abuse, and "brain death.". Furthermore, there is a growing need for laboratory analyses to track occupational exposure to specific chemicals, for drugs of abuse and laxative/diuretic screening, and for the measurement of plasma drug and occasionally metabolite concentrations to support treatment [therapeutic drug monitoring (TDM) (Hallworth and Watson, 2007)]. These days, the analytical toxicologist has access to a multitude of potent analytical techniques, most commonly chromatographic methods, ligand immunoassays, and other methods (Table 9.1). It is still not possible to search for every poison in every sample with the necessary level of sensitivity. Therefore, it is imperative that the purpose of any analysis be kept front and center.

While the fundamental concepts across the various subfields of analytical toxicology are consistent, there can be significant variations in the type and quantity of specimens available, the duration within which the result is needed, and the intended application of the result. Each of these elements could therefore have an impact on the method(s) selected for a given analysis. Particularly since the development of sensitive detectors like the flame-ionization detector (FID) and the electron-capture detector (ECD), gas-solid chromatography (GSC) and, more frequently, gas-liquid chromatography (GLC) have significantly improved the qualitative and quantitative analysis of pharmaceuticals and other organic poisons. These detectors work well together because the FID detects most organic compounds, whereas the ECD responds only to specific compounds or their derivatives, usually those containing a halogen or another electronegative or "electron-capturing" species like a nitro moiety.

Nitrogen-selective detectors (NSD), also referred to as alkali flame-ionization (AFID) and nitrogen-phosphorus (NPD) detectors, have expanded the application of GLC in more recent times. These detectors exhibit a more pronounced and focused response to compounds that contain phosphorus or C–N bonds. But the use of gas chromatography coupled with mass spectrometry (GC-MS) (Delves, H.T. and Campbell, M.J. 1988), sometimes called a "hyphenated technique," offers unmatched selectivity and high sensitivity, and it can identify numerous compounds with absolute certainty using only nanogram quantities of material. As a result, it has largely replaced the use of the NPD, at least in qualitative work.

Table 9.1. Some methods for the analysis of drugs and other organic poisons in biological samples

Principle	Technique
Chemical	Colour test
Electrochemical	Biosensors
	Differential pulse polarography (DPP)
Spectrometric	Mass spectrometry (MS), also known as mass fragmentography (MF)
	Nuclear magnetic resonance (NMR)
	Spectrophotofluorimetry (SPFM)
	Ultraviolet/visible absorption spectrophotometry (UV/Vis)
Chromatographic	Gas chromatography (GC), includes gas–solid chromatography (GSC) and gas–liquid chromatography (GLC)
	(High performance) liquid chromatography [(HP)LC]
	(High performance) thin-layer chromatography [(HP)TLC]
	Super(critical) fluid chromatography [S(C)FC]
Electrophoretic	Capillary (zone) electrophoresis [C(Z)E]
	Capillary electro-chromatography (CEC)
	Micellar electrokinetic capillary chromatography (MECC)
Immunoassay	Cloned enzyme donor immunoassay (CEDIA)
	Enzyme linked immunosorbent assay (ELISA)
	Enzyme multiplied immunoassay technique (EMIT)
	Fluorescence polarization immunoassay (FPIA)
	Latex agglutination tests (LAT)
	Microparticle enzyme immunoassay (MEIA)
	Radioimmunoassay (RIA)
Enzyme-based assay	Alcohol dehydrogenase – ethanol
	Aryl acylamide amidohydrolase – paracetamol

Source: https://uomustansiriyah.edu.iq/media/lectures/12/12_2021_12_02!11_08_44_PM.pdf

Since the early 1970s, high performance liquid chromatography (HPLC, formerly known as high pressure liquid chromatography) has found widespread use in analytical toxicology. While gases and extremely volatile solvents are acceptable, most analytes can be analyzed using HPLC or a variation of the standard protocol. This is not the case with GC, which can only be used to analyze both volatile and stable compounds at temperatures as high as about 350°C. Though there are now several reliable and sensitive detectors with different sensitivities and selectivities, including UV absorption, fluorimetric, electrochemical (ED), and MS, the use of HPLC in the qualitative analysis of drugs is somewhat limited due to the lack of a sensitive universal detector similar to the FID in GC. Furthermore, fractions of column effluent that match the relevant chromatographic peaks can be extracted and subjected to off-line analysis, such as immunoassay.

Whether using the more modern enzyme-multiplied immunoassay technique (EMIT) or the cloned enzyme donor immunoassay (CEDIA), or radioimmunoassay (RIA) (Baumgartner, et al., 1979), immunoassays have also found widespread use and are frequently very sensitive. There have also been reports of enzyme-based tests, like the one for acetaminophen (paracetamol). Nevertheless, the drawback of all these assays is that before an analysis can be conducted, antibodies, enzymes, or particular binding proteins must be prepared for each analyte or group of analytes. In contrast to chromatographic methods, which frequently call for some sort of purification procedure, such as solvent extraction, prior to the analysis, these and similar assays can frequently be used directly in small volumes of aqueous media (a process known as a "homogenous assay"). Despite the high sensitivity of immunoassays, some of them may have low selectivity, meaning that an antibody may detect multiple molecules with similar structures. At times, this cross-reactivity can be utilized for specific purposes, like identifying drug classes that are abused, like opiates.

9.1.3 Drugs and Pesticides

The assay of particular analytes and systematic toxicological analysis (STA) both frequently use capillary GC, which frequently has MS detection. However, packed column GC may still be useful in some circumstances. Specific compounds or groups of compounds are analyzed using HPLC, which is now frequently used in conjunction with MS. STA procedures based on diode-array detectors (DAD) and wavelength ratio techniques are also employed. In STA (poisons screening, drug screening, unknown screening), the challenge is to accurately identify the greatest number of compounds in the smallest amount of sample (plasma, serum, whole blood, urine, vitreous humor, stomach contents or vomit, tissues) at the highest sensitivity without producing any false positive results. In an ideal world, a small amount of sample would remain to allow for cross-checking the results with an alternative method and quantifying any poison(s) detected to help with the clinical interpretation of the findings. It is crucial to use a methodical approach when screening for unknown substances to rule out potential candidates and "home in" on the compound(s) that are present. There are three main phases to STA (Figure 9.1). The goal of the sample preparation step is to eliminate any potentially interfering sample matrix components while retaining all the substances that are toxicologically significant. Therefore, it is important to isolate a broad variety of analytes of interest, such as lipophilic and moderately polar, acidic, basic, and neutral species. The sample may be treated with -glucuronidase/arylsulfatase to hydrolyze conjugated metabolites, thereby increasing the yield of analyte(s).

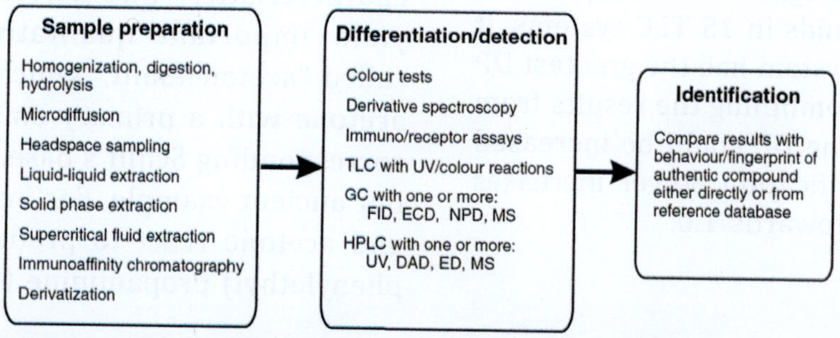

Figure 9.1 The three key steps in systematic toxicological analysis.

Source: https://uomustansiriyah.edu.iq/media/lectures/12/12_2021_12_02!11_08_44_PM.pdf

Finding the pertinent compounds in the shortest amount of time is the goal of the differentiation/detection stage. This necessitates combining highly specific techniques with comparatively nonspecific (or "universal") assays. Immunoassays can be used to identify drug classes, especially if the antibody has a broad cross-reactivity. The benefit of TLC is that all nonvolatile components of the extract stay on the plate, unlike GC and HPLC, where there's always a chance that some compounds haven't been eluted from the column. It goes without saying that no single analytical method can separate and identify every potential compound of interest; for instance, a single TLC plate can only resolve a limited number of compounds. Identification power is the capacity of a particular analytical technique to distinguish a compound from a given set of test compounds.

One approach in quantifying identification power is the use of discriminating power (DP):

$$DP = 1 - \frac{2M}{N(N-1)}$$

where M is the number of pairs of compounds which are not resolved and N is the number of compounds examined. The concept of discriminating power was introduced with the aim of quantifying the ability of paper chromatography, TLC and GLC to give unequivocal identification of unknowns. When this approach was applied to an investigation of the separation of 34 neutral compounds in 15 TLC systems, it was shown that one system had the greatest DP (0.75). However, by combining the results from two of the systems, the DP could be increased to 0.88. As the identification power increases so the DP increases towards 1.0.

The mean list length (MLL) is a second way to define the identification power. For a given analytical parameter (retention index in a GC system, for instance), the number of viable candidates is known as the list length. In that system, the MLL for that set of compounds is equal to the average of all list lengths. Calculating MLLs for a combination of systems is possible, just like in the previous example. MLLs are more than 1.0, but as identification power rises, they will get closer to 1.0. Analyzing a small number of test compounds will overestimate the identification power of the method in both the DP and MLL scenarios. The likelihood that an unknown substance(s) will be correctly identified increases with the analyst's toolkit's number and variety of techniques. Analyzing the ways in which different analytes react to distinct detectors—such as FID/ECD—can reveal important details about the makeup of an object. In addition to offering spectrum data, HPLC-DAD can verify peak purity by repeatedly scanning an eluting peak. When paired with computerized libraries of electron ionization (EI) fragmentation data that can be quickly searched to confirm compound identity, hybridized techniques like GC-MS can yield reliable analyte identification. Additionally, the Mr of a substance can be obtained using chemical ionization (CI) MS.

Analytes can be chemically changed to increase their "detectability" or chromatographic characteristics, but derivatization can also yield important qualitative data. The so-called "acetone-shift," which is the reaction of acetone with a primary amine to produce the corresponding Schiff's base, is one well-known but ancient example. For instance, amfetamine and acetone react to produce N-(1-methyl-2-phenylethyl) propanimine (Figure 9.2).

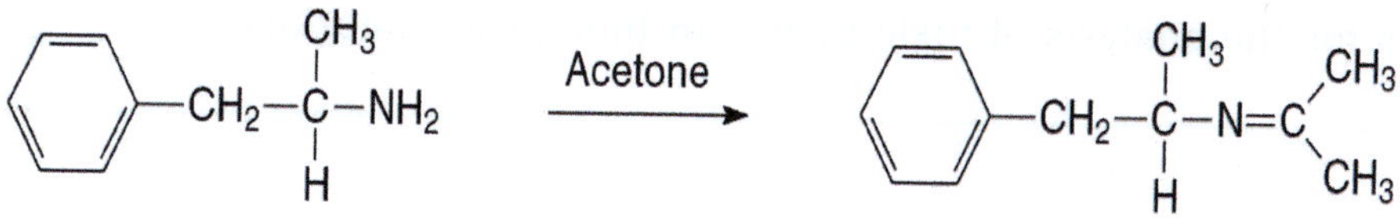

(±)-Amfetamine

N-(1-Methyl-2-phenylethyl)propanimine

Figure 9.2. Reaction of amfetamine with acetone.

Source: https://uomustansiriyah.edu.iq/media/lectures/12/12_2021_12_02!11_08_44_PM.pdf

Comparing the observed data with verified database information is the third step in the STA process. It is obvious that databases used for compound identification need to be updated frequently and should contain data on contaminants, common interferences, metabolites, and patent compounds. Reproducible analytical methods are crucial for creating these kinds of databases, both within and between labs.

9.1.4 Ethanol and Other Volatile Substances

Kits like the Abbott TDx/ADx are available that combine alcohol dehydrogenase with spectrophotometric measurement of a coenzyme to provide enzymatic methods for measuring blood ethanol. Additionally popular, especially in forensic work, is the GC analysis of ethanol, which can be performed by static headspace sampling or by directly injecting blood or urine that has been diluted with deionized water. The ability to separate and measure methanol, 2-propanol, and acetone simultaneously makes GC useful. One of the rare causes of acute poisoning "epidemics" is methanol poisoning from consuming synthetic alcoholic drinks; measuring blood methanol levels is crucial for both diagnosis and treatment monitoring. In acute poisoning cases resulting, for instance, from intentional inhalation of vapor to become intoxicated ['glue sniffing', solvent abuse, inhalant abuse, volatile substance abuse (VSA)], more than 20 additional volatile compounds may be encountered. Urine can be used to measure the metabolites of some volatile compounds, such as trichloroacetic acid (from trichloroethylene) and hippuric and methylhippuric (toluric) acids (from toluene and the xylenes, respectively). However, as most volatile chemicals are expelled unaltered as in the inhaled air, whole blood is the most suitable sample to find and identify these substances. (Machata, 1975).

9.1.5 Trace Elements and Toxic Metals

To aid in the diagnosis of persistent poisoning, elevations as low as a few g L−1 (parts per billion, ppb, i.e., parts per million) of serum or blood can be significant; however, repeatability and accuracy must be high. Contamination of the sample during collection (e.g., errors can come from sample tubes (or even from syringe needles in the case of manganese and chromium) and the actual laboratory. This is especially true for common elements like aluminum and lead. The complexity, cost, accuracy, and sensitivity of current techniques for determining toxic metal levels in biological materials vary greatly (Table 9.2). Some methods—such as neutron activation analysis and isotope dilution mass spectrometry—are reference methods. The use of flame or electrothermal atomization in a graphite furnace for atomic absorption spectrometry has been common, but inductively coupled plasma-mass spectrometry (ICP-MS) is replacing it. But when it comes to serum iron.

though this isn't always the case. When it comes to optically active (chiral) medications (Table 9.4), one isomer frequently possesses most of the desired clinical activity. In terms of the body, administering a racemate—a 50:50 mixture of enantiomers—is equivalent to giving different compounds because the other isomer might be pharmacologically inert or possess different qualities from its enantiomer. Sometimes the name used (dexamfetamine, dextropropoxyphene, levorphanol) indicates the availability of optically active compounds as pure enantiomers (optical isomers), but this is not always the case (hyoscine, morphine, and physostigmine).

Table 9.4. Summary of chiral nomenclature

Number of chiral centres	If n = number of optical centres there will be 2^n isomers. Molecules with 2 optical centres can exist as four molecules: two diastereoisomers (diasteromers), each consisting of two enantiomers, (i.e., there are *two pairs of enantiomers*). The exception to this is if two molecules have a *plane of symmetry* (a plane that divides a molecule into two parts, each a mirror image of the other) and therefore cancel out their net optical rotation. In such cases they are known as meso forms
Nomenclature	Enantiomers possess a unique property in that they rotate plane-polarized light in equal and opposite directions. This is the basis of the (+)/(−) or d/l notation, the former being preferred as it avoids confusion with D/L, however it does not unequivocally distinguish between enantiomers because some molecules may change rotation on forming salts. The notation tells nothing about the absolute configuration (i.e., the spatial arrangement) of the atoms
Rotation of plane polarized light	Rotates to the right: dextrorotatory (+ or d); rotates to the left: levorotatory (− or l).
Fischer	The absolute stereochemistry in the Fischer notation gives the absolute spatial arrangement by reference to D-glyceraldehyde. The letters D or L are used (not to be confused with lower case d or l). The Fischer convention is still used for carbohydrates and amino acids. The original choice of D-glyceraldehyde was arbitrary, but was proved correct by X-ray crystallography
Cahn–Ingold–Prelog (CIP)	The CIP system is the definitive method of assigning absolute configuration. The letters *R* and *S* indicate spatial arrangements as follows: 1. Assign values to the substituent groups by highest atomic number[a] 2. Point the lowest value away 3. If the remainder go from high to low clockwise then *R* (rectus) 4. If the remainder go from high to low anticlockwise then *S* (sinister) 5. In case of a tie go to the next atoms along The Fischer convention cannot be simply converted to the CIP system, that is *R* does not always equate to D. All naturally occurring α-amino acids in mammalian proteins are L. Using the CIP system, cysteine and cystine are *S* the others, without sulfur, are *R*

[a]The rules are in fact more detailed: Highest atomic number > highest atomic mass > *cis*- prior to *trans*- > like pairs (RR) or (SS) prior to unlike > lone pairs which are considered an atom of atomic number 0. [N.B. R* indicates a single enantiomer obtained, but with unknown stereochemistry].

Source: https://uomustansiriyah.edu.iq/media/lectures/12/12_2021_12_02!11_08_44_PM.pdf

Table 9.5. Some terms used in stereochemistry

Absolute stereochemistry	The absolute spatial configuration of the atoms of a molecule
Chiral	Hand-like, that is left- and right-handed mirror images
Enantiomer	One mirror image form of a pair of optically active compounds
Epimers	Optically active molecules with more than two chiral centres differing at only one chiral centre
Epimerization	Partial racemization of one chiral centre in a molecule with two or more chiral centres
Diastereoisomers	Structures with more than one chiral centre such that they are not mirror images (enantiomers)
Inversion	Conversion of one enantiomer to the other
Meso	Optically inactive isomer in which the optical activity of chiral centres are balanced
Racemate	Equimolar mixture of both enantiomers of an optically active compound
Racemization	Conversion of a single enantiomer to a racemate

Source: https://uomustansiriyah.edu.iq/media/lectures/12/12_2021_12_02!11_08_44_PM.pdf

Furthermore, it is estimated that up to 25% of pharmaceuticals currently in use are chiral and are supplied as racemates, typically with no warning. For example, the approved name of (±)-hyoscinamine is atropine. Although there are currently few compelling reasons to provide chiral methodology for routine analytical toxicology, it should be highlighted that chromatographic techniques, which offer ways to separate enantiomers in biological samples and on a preparative scale, have greatly aided in the development of pharmacology and therapeutics.

9.2.3 Chemical and Physical Methods

9.2.3.1. Sampling

The final data are only as representative as the samples used to derive the results, even with the most advanced analytical tools at hand. This is especially valid for samples taken in the environment. When sampling, it's important to ensure the outcome aligns with the study's goals. It is frequently necessary to pay extra attention to sampling procedures. Depending on the kind of subject being studied, sampling achieves a variety of goals. Regarding the environment (e.g., lakes, rivers, and wilderness areas) sampling can yield information on the degree of contamination as well as the concentration of pollutants. Sampling in urban areas can reveal the kinds of pollutants to which an individual is exposed through skin contact, inhalation, or ingestion over a specific time frame. It is possible to identify sources of pollution and identify hazardous conditions in industrial areas. Sampling is a tool used in the design of pollution controls and can be used to record changes in operating conditions over the course of control implementation. Documenting adherence to current US Environmental Protection Agency (US EPA) and Occupational Safety and Health Administration regulations is a significant additional use of sampling in industrial areas in the US. The numerous techniques for gathering environmental samples fall into four categories: soil, water, air, and tissue sampling. Forensic and experimental research are particularly interested in the fourth category.

- ***Air:*** Fuel combustion, industrial operations, and the disposal of solid waste are the main sources of pollutants that enter the atmosphere. The amount of atmospheric pollution is also influenced by other unidentified sources, including nuclear explosions, forest fires, dust storms, volcanoes, natural gas emissions, burning in agriculture, and pesticide drift. Particulate pollutants must fall into an aerosol, which is characterized as an airborne suspension of liquid droplets, or settle on solid particles small enough to have a low settling velocity to affect terrestrial animals and plants. Suspensions can be divided into two categories: solids, which include dusts, fumes, and smoke produced by crushing, metal vaporization, and combustion of organic materials, and liquids, which include mists (big particles) and fogs (small particles) produced by atomization, condensation, or entrapment of liquids by gases.

An adult human can breathe in between 5 and 20 m3 of air during an 8-h workday, depending on their level of physical activity. At rest, they can breathe in 6 to 8 L of air per minute (1 L = 0.001 m3). Aerosol particles must be between 0 and 5 μm in size in order to enter and stay in the lungs. Particulate matter (PM) in the size range of 2.5 to 10 μm has come under increased scrutiny as instrumentation used to collect atmospheric dust has become more accurate because many potential toxicants are adsorbed to their surfaces. When inhaled, these particles stay in the lungs, where they enable the compounds to enter the bloodstream.

To "trap" organic toxicants from the air or to gather particulate matter in the size range that is most harmful to humans, air samplers have been made smaller, and adsorbents have been created. An air sampler typically has an inlet to direct air through a filter to capture potentially interesting particles (e.g., dust); via the pump that draws air through the system, the flowmeter and valve that calibrate airflow, and the adsorbent that gathers organic vapors. Personnel samplers are battery-operated devices that can be worn on a person's clothing to enable continuous monitoring while they carry out their designated tasks in the workplace. This makes it possible to estimate each person's exposure.

Solid particulate matter, like asbestos, is collected by many air samplers using different kinds of filters. The asbestos is collected on glass fiber filters with pores of 20 μm diameter or less. Dust and silica are collected using membrane filters with pores ranging in diameter from 0.01 to 10 μm. Pesticides and mineral dusts are captured by impingers, which are collectors that hold liquid. Large impingers that can handle flows of 10 to 50 L of air per minute are used to collect mineral dusts, while smaller "midget" impingers that can handle flows of 2 to 4.5 L/ per min of air are used to collect insecticides. The entrapping liquid may be alcohol, distilled water, ethylene glycol, hexylene glycol (2-methyl, 2,4-pentane diol), or another solvent, depending on the pollutant being sought. Polyurethane foam (PUF) is quickly taking the place of midget impingers as a popular pesticide trapping medium due to its ease of handling and quick compound desorption. The US EPA has created a large-volume air sampler to detect polychlorinated biphenyls (PCBs) and pesticides. Insecticides and PCBs are trapped in the foam when air is drawn through a PUF pad at a rate of about 225.0 L/min. To capture organic vapors in the air, tiny glass tubes with an inner diameter of about 7.0×0.5 cm and filled with activated charcoal are utilized.

Many specialized businesses have developed and are still developing adsorbents to extract organic molecules from air samples. Industrial chemicals that are synthesized using commercially available adsorbents, or used in production processes, pesticides, and exhaust tower emissions are regularly monitored. Without the need for a pump, personnel monitoring can be carried out with a system made up of an adsorbent that collects compounds of interest and a porous membrane that allows air to diffuse through. Gaseous pollutants in trace amounts (e.g., CO_2, HNO_3), which have been in use for several years, are observed using infrared spectroscopy and direct reading instruments. These instruments remove substances like water vapor, which can mask the small quantities of these pollutants, by passively monitoring large areas and using extensive statistical evaluations. A direct reading device that can quantify any atmospheric gas or mixture of gases with a dipole moment in less than 10 seconds is being developed thanks to research in the millimeter/submillimeter area of spectroscopy and Russian technologies. This device works regardless of the amount or presence of water vapor in the atmosphere. It is anticipated that these gadgets will be accessible for purchase in the next five years.

- ***Soil***: The behavior of environmental pollutants that are deposited on land is complicated by multiple simultaneous interactions with existing liquid-gas phases, microscopic organisms, organic and inorganic components, and other soil constituents. Pollutants may be absorbed into plant tissue, move through the soil profile through random molecular motion, or stay in one place for variable lengths of time, depending on their physical and chemical makeup. Mass flow has an impact on movement as well because of outside factors like pollutants that dissolve in water, float there, or adhere to inorganic and organic soil constituents. To ensure representative samples, statistical methods must be used in the complex process of sampling for pollutants in soils. The chemical and physical properties of the site(s), potential interactions between the compound(s) of interest and soil constituents, and the degree of variability (i.e., variance in the soil profiles) at the location of the sample. The site(s) can then be divided into homogeneous areas and the necessary number of samples can be collected using these data. The functions of variance and accuracy level determine how many samples are needed. Sampling can start as soon as the proper protocol has been established.

Although there are many different kinds of soil samplers, coring devices are the best option because they make it possible to determine the vertical distribution of a pollutant. These devices can be either hand-operated 60- or 100-cm-long stainless steel tubes with a diameter of 2 to 7.6 cm. Additionally, 200 cm long, large, mechanically operated boring tubes are used. With these tools, samples can be taken to consistent depths, and the cores can be separated into different depths (e.g., 0–7–6 cm, 7–6–15–2 cm, and so forth) to ascertain motion. A different kind of coring device is a wheel with tubes attached, which enables the collection of numerous tiny subsamples and a more uniform sampling across a given area. A large diameter cylinder (about) can be used to gather soils from particular depths. 25 cm) that, once the sampler is inserted to the appropriate depth, has a blade to cut a core of soil.

- ***Water*:** Obtaining representative water samples requires careful consideration of numerous factors. The pollutant and the point of entry into the aquatic environment are the most crucial factors. Agricultural, industrial, municipal, and other sources—such as spills from accidents or train derailments—can all contribute to pollution. Other significant variables include temperature, thermal and salinity stratification, the direction and speed of the predominant wind, the velocity of stream or river flow, and the sediment content. Where to monitor or sample and how to get representative samples are two crucial questions. Samples of surface water are frequently taken using automated sampling equipment that is managed by a range of sensors. The "grab" technique is the most basic way to gather water; it involves lowering a container into the water, filling it, capping it, and then rinsing it out. Water at deeper depths is usually obtained using specialized samplers. Since the Clean Water Act of 1977 was put into effect in the US, ongoing monitoring has been necessary to gather information for management choices. In the US, there are numerous wells that are used for continuous monitoring. One way to collect samples from potable wells is by using an existing tap, which can be found inside the house or outside. Nevertheless, gathering samples from wells used for monitoring pollution necessitates a multi-step procedure. After determining the elevation of the water table, standing water needs to be removed. Conductivity and pH are the two factors that are used to decide how much water is removed before sampling if wells are utilized to monitor suspected pollutants. Bailers or pumps remove a predetermined number of well volumes until the conductivity and pH are both constant. The sample is then collected using a bottle that has been triple-rinsed. These kinds of devices can produce a lot of samples, so collectors with tiny-pore membranes (e.g., 45.0 μm) to trap contaminants that contain metals, ion-exchange resin cartridges, or long-chain hydrocarbons (e.g., organic pollutants (C18)) bound to silica for adsorption. By letting several liters of water pass through and trapping the pollutants in a tiny cylinder or container, these devices are frequently used to reduce the quantity and bulk of the samples. Moreover, disk technologies concentrate pollutants as water passes through the membrane using a filter with a Teflon matrix that has embedded C18 hydrocarbon chains. Polar evaporators, like e. g. They are removed from the disk using a solvent (such as methanol). Samples should be collected, frozen in solid CO2 (dry ice), and then brought back to the lab as soon as possible. They should be frozen at -20°C or less if they are not analyzed at that time. To keep the container from breaking, there needs to be enough headroom.

Tissues: Surveys of plants and animals are carried out when environmental areas are thought to be contaminated. Numerous surveys are carried out by federal and state laboratories during hunting and fishing seasons to ascertain the quantity of animals that are killed. Additionally, organs and other tissues are frequently removed for analysis of potential contaminants. Analyses can be used to ascertain the concentration, degree of contamination within a particular species, and areas of contamination. Sampling is done at random throughout an area. It is well known that a number of environmental contaminants concentrate in bone, particular organs, or particular tissues (e.g., fat). Animals that have recently died have these organs removed for examination. To ascertain the degree of potential contamination in the area sampled, the organs are frequently examined individually as single sub-samples rather than pooled with those of the same species. When collecting plant material for analysis, it is either separated into sections for the roots, stems, leaves, flowers, and/or fruit, or the entire plant is examined as a whole. A single sample for analysis can also be obtained by pooling samples from different sites. The selection is contingent upon the attributes of the putative pollutant.

9.2.3.2. Experimental Studies

Studies can be done in vivo or in vitro, with the latter being more common when they deal with the metabolism or mode of action of toxic compounds in animals (or, less frequently, plants). It is not as relevant to discuss random sampling techniques as it is with environmental samples because known compounds are used to treat organisms or enzyme preparations.

Recurring determinations on aliquots of the same preparation do not replicate the experiment; at most, they test the analytical method's reproducibility. Enough replication is required for statistical verification of significance. As opposed to metabolic studies, where the question of reactive (and hence unstable) products and intermediates is crucial, environmental studies focus on stable compounds or stable products. Hence, the sample needs to be treated with methods that minimize degradation after the reaction is stopped. The knowledge of the substrate and the various techniques available for determining the range of potential products make this easier.

Stopping the reaction, usually with a protein precipitant, is the first step in the sampling process. While conventional substances like trichloroacetic acid are efficient protein precipitants, they are typically unwanted. The application of a single organic solvent that is water soluble, like acetone or ethanol, is gentler than using a combination of solvents. The protein is denatured by the mixture of methanol and chloroform, which also causes a preliminary separation of the protein into organic-soluble and water-soluble components. A gentle way to stop reactions is by rapid freezing, but low temperature handling is required afterwards. It is essential to collect uncontaminated organ samples for toxicokinetic investigations that require consecutive animal sacrifice and tissue analysis. Aside from blood contamination, the organs can be carefully dissected and rinsed in ice-cold buffer, saline, or another suitable solution to obtain suitable samples. The process of obtaining blood samples involves puncturing the heart, and organ samples are protected from blood contamination by carefully bleeding the animal at the time of sacrifice or, if required, by perfusing the affected organ.

9.2.3.3. Forensic Studies

Since sudden or unexpected death is the main focus of forensic toxicology, there is a very wide range of potential toxicants. Typically, the analyst doesn't start looking through the samples until all preliminary investigations—such as autopsies and microscopic analyses of every tissue—are finished. As a result, the analyst can typically start with a working hypothesis regarding the range of potential toxicants involved. Adequate sampling and sample preservation are crucial because additional sampling typically requires exhumation, which makes it unlikely or impossible in the case of cremation. A sufficient sample size is crucial. Blood should be drawn in an amount of at least 100 milliliters so that substances such as ethanol, carbon monoxide, and other alcohols, barbiturates, and tranquilizers, can be examined.

The full contents of the bladder is retained, and urine is helpful for the analysis of both endogenous and exogenous chemicals. The liver and kidney are the two most important solid tissues for forensic analysis (Mitchell, C.A. (1938)); 100–200 g of the liver and the equivalent of one kidney are typically retained. The liver often contains high levels of toxicants and/or their metabolites. The application of polymerase chain reaction (PCR), which enables the analysis of ancient samples (e.g., bone marrow sampling and exhumation) to be examined and contrasted with surviving relatives; as a result, these data offer law enforcement and other stakeholders important information. Possession is a peculiar requirement that has significant legal implications. An uninterrupted line of distinguishable ownership (i.e., chain of custody) needs to be upheld. Every transfer needs to be signed by both parties and is noted on the samples with the time and date of collection, arrival at the lab, and other pertinent information. Legally speaking, the handling and security of samples while they are in possession must be verifiable.

9.2.3.4. Sample Preparation

Extraction: The majority of the time, physically removing a pollutant or other toxicant from the sample medium is necessary for analysis. The sample is chopped, ground, or blended to a consistent consistency before being subsampled to guarantee homogeneity. This subsample is extracted by intimately contacting it with an appropriate solvent, usually at a ratio of 5 to 25 volumes of solvent to 1 volume of sample. Depending on the sample matrix and the toxicant's physical and chemical properties, one or more of four methods may be applied. Less frequently, alternative extraction techniques like boiling, grinding, or distilling the sample with the right solvents are employed.

- *Blending:* Right now, the most popular technique for removing biologic materials from food is to use a blender that runs on electricity or air. After adding a solvent to a container containing the weighed sample, motor-driven blades homogenize the tissue. The majority of environmental toxicants can be extracted by blending for five to fifteen minutes, then blending again. Anhydrous sodium sulfate can be used as a filter to remove water from a homogenate in an organic solvent that could cause issues during the quantitation stage of the analysis. Sonication is a widely used technique for tissue sample extraction, especially when it comes to the binding of toxicants to subcellular fractions. Rapid cell rupture caused by sonicator probes enables the solvent to make close contact with every component of the cell. Fractions of interest can then be isolated using differential centrifugation. High-wattage compounds are extracted from environmental samples using sonifiers (450 watts), and sonification is recognized as a legitimate extraction technique by multiple US EPA methods.
- *Shaking:* Shaking with the right solvent or combination of solvents is usually how pollutants are removed from water samples and occasionally soil samples. Several water or soil samples are handled simultaneously by mechanical shakers. The analyst can perform lengthy extractions (e.g., 24,

if necessary). For total removal, two or more shakes are typically needed (i.e. more than 98%), of the poisonous substance from the matrix of samples.

- *Washing*: Washing with water-detergent combinations or with solvents can be used to remove surface contamination from environmental samples such as fruits or plants or from a worker's hands, if dermal exposure from industrial chemicals or pesticides is suspected.
- *Continuous Extraction:* Soxhlet extraction is the process that is carried out on solid samples (e.g., dirt) and calls for the use of one or more organic solvents in combination. Before being put inside the device, the sample is weighed into a cup (thimble) made of specialized porous material, like fiberglass or cellulose. This is made up of a water-jacketed condenser, an extractor that holds the thimble, and a boiling flask that contains the solvent. Boiling the solvent causes it to vaporize, condense, and fill the extractor, soaking the sample and removing the toxicant. The solvent is drained via a siphoning action, which restarts the cycle in the boiling flask. The duration of the extraction process can range from 2 h to four days, contingent upon the characteristics of the toxicant and sample matrix. There are now automated instruments available that complete the same task faster (e.g., 30 min) and employ significantly less solvent (e.g., 15-20 mL as opposed to 250 mL). They are more costly than the traditional approach, but still economical.
- *Supercritical Fluid Extraction:* Materials can be made to behave in ways that deviate from their natural state. Boiling points, for instance, are described as the temperature at which a liquid turns into a gas. The boiling point varies if the liquid is contained and pressure is applied. When a given liquid reaches what is known as the critical point—a particular combination of temperature and pressure—it is no longer a liquid and becomes a gas. There is a region above this one known as the supercritical region where the material will not be affected by increases in either pressure or temperature (i.e. it is not going to boil or condense). The characteristics of both a liquid and a gas will be present in this so-called supercritical fluid. The supercritical fluid has liquid-like solvent qualities and permeates materials like a gas.

Due to its chemical makeup, CO_2 has emerged as the material of choice among all those that can be used as a supercritical fluid. It has been possible to extract compounds from a range of sample matrices, such as soils, asphalt, and plant material, by using instruments that are designed to apply the principles mentioned. Pumped through the sample, the supercritical fluid passes via a filter or column to a trap where it vaporizes. Solvent is then added to transfer the analyses to a vial for analysis. More modern instruments gather data from complex samples by combining the supercritical fluid extraction system with multiple columns and detectors.

9.2.3.5. Separation and Identification

Numerous unwanted chemicals are also liberated from the sample matrix during extraction procedures; these need to be eliminated in order to get quantitative results from specific instruments. Plant and animal pigments, lipids, organic matter from the soil and water, and inorganic compounds are some of these constituents. If the impurities are left in place, they can mask peaks, create extraneous peaks on chromatograms, or reduce the sensitivity of the analytical instrument's detectors and columns. Some more modern devices are costly, even though they automatically eliminate these compounds and concentrate the samples into tiny volumes for quantitative analysis. Therefore, other techniques are used in the majority of laboratories. Solvent partitioning, thin-layer chromatography (TLC), and adsorption chromatography are a few of these. The preferred technique for removing co-extractives from the relevant compound is typically adsorption chromatography. (Figure 9.3).

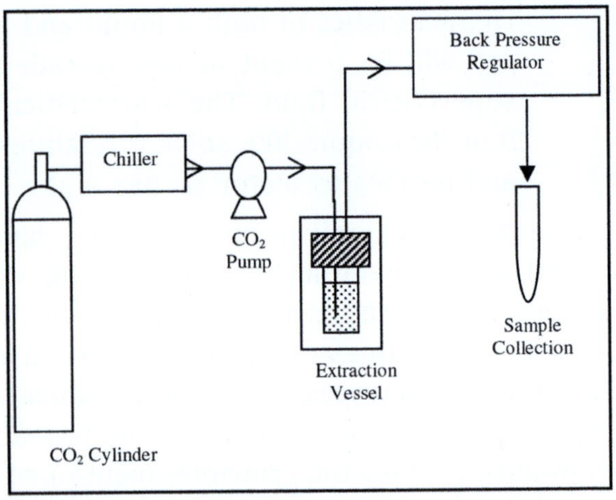

Figure 9.3. Supercritical fluid extraction.

Source: https://www.researchgate.net/profile/Cheng-Hock-Chuah/publication/26439786/figure/fig1/AS:671523945857039@1537115193721/Flow-diagram-of-supercritical-fluid-extraction-system.png

The solvent must be eliminated in order to obtain a working volume because most techniques require large volumes of solvent (e.g., 5–10 mL) that the analyst can easily handle. Distillation, evaporation under reduced pressure, or evaporation in an air stream or an inert gas like nitrogen are the methods used to achieve this. Extracts can undergo one or more procedures to further purify them once the working volume is reached. Apart from employing adsorbents, a lot of organic toxicants will split between two immiscible solvents (e.g., acetonitrile and hexane or chloroform and water). Some of the toxicant from the original extracting solvent will have moved into the other layer when the separatory funnel is shaken and allowed to equilibrate into the two original solvent layers. After several additions (e.g, 4 to 5 volumes), stirring, and elimination, the majority or all the target compounds will have been moved, leaving a large number of interfering compounds in the initial solvent. The amount of toxicant that is removed as described will result in a large volume of solvent, regardless of the method or combination of methods used for separation. Typically, final volumes utilized for compound identification and quantification fall between 250 µL and 100 mL.

Sensitive measurement of many toxicants at parts per billion and parts per trillion levels has been made possible by recent developments in circuit miniaturization, column technology, microprocessor development, and new concepts in instrument design. Since many hazardous materials present in trace amounts could not be detected until technological advancements reached the current state of the art, this increased sensitivity has drawn attention from the public to the extent of environmental pollution. Currently, chromatography, spectroscopy, and bioassays are used to identify and quantify the majority of pollutants. After the toxicant has been extracted and isolated from unnecessary components, the identification process can start. However, keep in mind that the purification steps are frequently utilized in identification as well (e.g., position of the peak in high-performance liquid chromatography (HPLC) and gas-liquid chromatography (GLC). Therefore, it is impossible to distinguish clearly between the two processes.

9.2.4 Method Implementation and Validation

Any approach chosen for a particular analysis needs to be validated, or it needs to be demonstrated to be "fit for purpose.". Knowing how to validate a method is crucial for both method development and routine method implementation. Table 9.6 provides several terms that are crucial to comprehending method validation. Obtaining certified pure reference material, or the closest possible approximation to such material, is a fundamental first step in any assay. When preparing primary standards, the Mr of salts and their level of hydration (water of crystallization) should be given special consideration. Instead of reporting a salt, analytical results are typically expressed in terms of free acid or base.

Table 9.6 Terms used when reporting method validation

Term	Notes
Accuracy	The difference between the measured value and the accepted ('true') value
Calibration range	The range of concentrations between the highest and lowest calibration standards. This should encompass the range of concentrations found in the test samples
Coefficient of variation (CV)	An obsolete term for RSD
Higher limit of quantification (HLoQ)	The highest concentration that can be quantified. Not always quoted, but important in assays with a clear upper 'cut-off', for example immunoassays and fluorescence assays
Internal standard	A second compound, not the analyte, added at an appropriate stage in the assay to correct for systematic errors in the analysis
Limit of detection (LoD)	The smallest amount of analyte that can be detected. Usually defined as some multiple (e.g. 5) of the baseline noise (signal to noise ratio = 5) or multiple of the SD of the blank signal
Linearity	A definable and reproducible relationship between a physicochemical measurement (e.g. UV absorption) and the concentration of the analyte. Not necessarily a straight line
Lower limit of quantification (LLoQ)	The lowest concentration that can be measured within defined limits. Usually a concentration for which the precision and accuracy have been set arbitrarily, for example RSD < 20 %
Precision	The scatter of measured values about a mean value
	Usually quoted as RSD – within-assay and between-assay precision is commonly given
Relative standard deviation (RSD)	The standard deviation of replicate measurements expressed as a percentage of the mean value:
	$RSD = SD/Mean \times 100\ \%$
	Useful when comparing precision at different concentrations
Selectivity	The ability to distinguish between the analyte and some other compound
Signal-to-noise (S/N) ratio	Strictly, the response to the analyte divided by the amplitude of random electronic noise of the detection system. In practice, the background signal due to interfering compounds is often greater than the electronic noise

Source: https://uomustansiriyah.edu.iq/media/lectures/12/12_2021_12_02!11_08_44_PM.pdf

It goes without saying that the approach needs to be sensitive enough for the job at hand. The lower limit of quantification (LLoQ) is a better term to use when referring to the limit of accurate measurement, which is sometimes referred to as the limit of sensitivity. A better term for the limit of sensitivity is the limit of detection (also known as the "cut-off value" or detection limit). Additionally, quantitative techniques need to be accurate and precise (reproducible), with the results having to accurately reflect the analyte's true concentration. When measuring a single species, selectivity (specificity, freedom from interference) is crucial; however, as was previously mentioned, broad specificity may be helpful when screening for the presence of a specific class of compounds. If sensitivity is a limiting factor, for example, the analyte recovery—that is, the amount of the target compound extracted from the sample matrix during the extraction—becomes significant; however, if the assay's limit of detection, accuracy, and precision are acceptable, this need not be a concern.

Regardless of the methodology used, standard solutions of each analyte (typically 6–8 concentrations across the calibration range) should be prepared in the same matrix and analyzed as a batch along with the test samples for quantitative assay calibration. The so-called "external standard" method of calculating the analyte concentration in the sample involves creating a graph of response against analyte concentration. Like all measurements, any quantitative analysis has both random and systematic errors associated with it. The "internal standard" approach is frequently used in chromatographic and other separation techniques to lessen the effects of systematic errors like changes in injection volume or extraction solvent evaporating during the analysis. Therefore, at the appropriate point in the analysis, a known quantity of a second compound (the internal standard) that behaves similarly to the analyte during the analysis but elutes at a different location on the chromatogram or is otherwise detected independently of the analyte is added. Then, when creating a calibration graph, the analyte's detector response in relation to the internal standard's response is plotted against the analyte concentration.

9.2.5 Quality Control and Quality Assurance

It's critical to demonstrate that an analytical method is still operating as intended after it has been validated and put into practice. Known positive and negative specimens should typically be examined alongside the test sample in qualitative research. In order to make sure that false positives (caused by, for example, e.g., glassware or tainted reagents) are not acquired. Incorporating a true positive also verifies that the reagents have been correctly prepared and have maintained their stability. The methodical examination of internal quality control (IQC) samples, which are separately made standard solutions with a known composition prepared in the same matrix as the samples but not used for assay calibration, is how assay performance is tracked in quantitative work. Plotting the IQC sample results on a chart makes it possible to keep an eye on the assay's daily performance and provides early warning of any issues. It is wise to make sure that the results of freshly prepared batches of calibration and IQC samples can be compared to those of previous batches or to results obtained with external QC material. It's also critical to take part in suitable proficiency testing (PT) and external quality assessment (EQA) programs (Wilson, 2002). Specimens of plasma, serum, whole blood, or urine—sometimes lyophilized—are sent to several participating laboratories in these schemes. The specimens are analyzed as real samples after reconstitution in deionized water, if appropriate, and the results are reported prior to the disclosure of the true or target concentrations.

A Closer Look

Environmental Toxicology

A multidisciplinary field that focuses on the study of the adverse effects of chemical, biological, and physical agents on living organisms and ecosystems in the environment. It encompasses the assessment, monitoring, and management of environmental pollutants to understand their sources, fate, transport, and potential impacts on human health and ecological integrity. Environmental toxicologists investigate a wide range of contaminants, including heavy metals, pesticides, industrial chemicals, air pollutants, and emerging contaminants such as pharmaceuticals and microplastics, to evaluate their toxicological effects on wildlife, plants, aquatic organisms, and humans.

One of the primary goals of environmental toxicology is to identify and assess the risks associated with exposure to environmental pollutants. This involves conducting toxicity testing and risk assessments to determine the concentrations at which contaminants pose adverse effects to organisms and ecosystems. Toxicity tests may involve laboratory experiments, field studies, and computer modeling to evaluate the effects of contaminants on various biological endpoints, such as growth, reproduction, behavior, and survival. Risk assessments integrate toxicity data with exposure estimates to quantify the potential risks to human and ecological receptors and inform decision-making and regulatory actions to protect public health and the environment. Environmental toxicology also plays a crucial role in environmental monitoring and surveillance to track the presence and trends of pollutants in air, water, soil, sediments, and biota. Monitoring programs involve the collection and analysis of environmental samples from different media to assess pollutant levels and trends over time. This information helps identify pollution hotspots, sources of contamination, and areas of concern, guiding pollution prevention and control strategies, environmental remediation efforts, and regulatory compliance. Additionally, biomonitoring studies measure the concentrations of contaminants and biomarkers of exposure and effect in biological samples from human populations and wildlife to assess potential health risks and inform public health interventions.

The field of environmental toxicology also addresses the fate and transport of pollutants in the environment, including processes such as bioaccumulation, bioconcentration, biomagnification, and ecological modeling. These processes influence the distribution, persistence, and bioavailability of contaminants in environmental compartments and food webs, impacting the transfer of pollutants from lower to higher trophic levels and potentially leading to human exposure through the consumption of contaminated food and water. Understanding the fate and transport of pollutants is essential for predicting their environmental behavior, identifying vulnerable populations and ecosystems, and developing effective risk management strategies to mitigate environmental contamination.

Summary

- Analytical toxicology is the detection, identification, and measurement of foreign compounds (xenobiotics) in biological and other specimens. Analytical methods are available for a very wide range of compounds: these may be chemicals, pesticides, pharmaceuticals, drugs of abuse and natural toxins.
- Analytical toxicology is concerned with the detection, identification and measurement of drugs and other foreign compounds (xenobiotics) and their metabolites in biological and related specimens.
- The use of physicochemical techniques in the analysis of drugs and other poisons in body fluids or tissues and related specimens has its origins in the development of forensic toxicology. Important contributions came later from work to improve food safety and from occupational toxicology.
- Gas–solid chromatography and, more commonly, gas–liquid chromatography have made a notable contribution to both the qualitative and quantitative analysis of drugs and other organic poisons, especially since the introduction of sensitive detectors such as the flame-ionization detector (FID) and the electron-capture detector.
- Immunoassays have also found wide application, whether radioimmunoassay or more recent variants, for example, enzyme-multiplied immunoassay technique and cloned enzyme donor immunoassay, and are often highly sensitive.
- Capillary GC, often with MS detection, is widely used both in systematic toxicological analysis and in the assay of specific analytes, although packed column GC may still find a place for certain applications.
- In analytical toxicology, clinical chemistry and related fields, the words 'sample' and 'specimen' are used to denote a portion of a body fluid, tissue, incubation medium, and so on obtained under defined conditions.
- Most pollutants entering the atmosphere come from fuel combustion, industrial processes, and solid waste disposal. Additional miscellaneous sources, such as nuclear explosions, forest fires, dusts, volcanoes, natural gaseous emissions, agricultural burning, and pesticide drift, contribute to the level of atmospheric pollution.
- An air sampler generally consists of an inlet to direct air through a filter to entrap particles that might be of interest (e.g., dust); through the adsorbent, which collects organic vapors, a flowmeter and valve to calibrate airflow, and a pump to pull air through the system.
- In toxicokinetic studies involving sequential animal sacrifice and tissue examination, it is critical to obtain uncontaminated organ samples. Apart from contamination by blood, suitable samples can be obtained by careful dissection and rinsing of the organs in ice-cold buffer, saline, or other appropriate solution.

References

1. ACGIH (American Conference of Governmental Industrial Hygienists). (2005). *TLVs and BEIs Based on The Documentation of The Threshold Limit Values for Chemical and Physical Agents and Biological Exposure Indices 2005*. ACGIH.
2. Baumgartner, A. M., Jones, P. F., Baumgartner, W. A., & Black, C. T. (1979). Radioimmunoassay of hair for determining opiate-abuse histories. *Journal of Nuclear Medicine, 20*(9), 748–752.
3. Boone, C. M., Franke, J. P., de Zeeuw, R. A., & Ensing, K. (1999). Evaluation of capillary electrophoretic techniques towards systematic toxicological analysis. *Journal of Chromatography A, 838*(1), 259–272.
4. Braithwaite, R. A., & Brown, S. S. (1988). Clinical and sub-clinical lead poisoning: A laboratory perspective. *Human Toxicology, 7*(6), 503–513.
5. Coley, N. G. (1998). Forensic chemistry in 19th century Britain. *Endeavour, 22*(4), 143–147.
6. Conway, E. J. (1947). *Microdiffusion Analysis and Volumetric Error* (2nd ed.). Crosby, Lockwood.
7. Curry, A. S., Walker, G. W., & Simpson, G. S. (1966). Determination of ethanol in blood by gas chromatography. *Analyst, 91*(1), 742–743.
8. Delves, H. T., & Campbell, M. J. (1988). Measurement of total lead concentrations and lead isotope ratios in whole blood by use of inductively coupled plasma source mass spectrometry. *Journal of Analytical Atomic Spectrometry, 3*(5), 343–348.
9. DFG (Deutsche Forschungsgemeinschaft). (2005). *List of MAK and BAT values 2005*. Commission for the investigation of health hazards of chemical compounds in the work area. Report 41. Wiley VCH.
10. Flanagan, R. J., Ruprah, M., Meredith, T. J., & Ramsey, J. D. (1990). An introduction to the clinical toxicology of volatile substances. *Drug Safety, 5*(5), 359–383.
11. Hallworth, M., & Watson, I. (2007). *Therapeutic Drug Monitoring and Laboratory Medicine*. ACB Venture Publications.
12. Jones, A. W. (1998). Historical developments and present status of forensic toxicology in Sweden. *Nordic Rettsmedisin, 4*(1), 35–44.
13. Kintz, P. (2004). Hair analysis. In A. C. Moffat, D. Osselton, & B. Widdop (Eds.), *Clarke's Analysis of Drugs and Poisons* (3rd ed., pp. 124–133). Pharmaceutical Press.
14. Machata, G. (1975). The advantages of automated blood alcohol determination by head space analysis. *Zeitschrift für Rechtsmedizin, 75*(3), 229–234.
15. Marsh, J. (1836). Account of a method of separating small quantities of arsenic from substances with which it may be mixed. *Edinburgh New Philosophical Journal, 21*, 229–236.
16. Mitchell, C. A. (1938). *Forensic Chemistry in the Criminal Courts*. Institute of Chemistry of Great Britain and Ireland.
17. Moffat, A. C., Smalldon, K. W., & Brown, C. (1974). Optimum use of paper, thin-layer and gas-liquid chromatography for the identification of basic drugs. I. Determination of effectiveness for a series of chromatographic systems. *Journal of Chromatography, 90*(1), 1–7.
18. Niyogi, S. S. (1981). Historical overview of forensic toxicology. In R. H. Cravey & R. C. Baselt (Eds.), *Introduction to Forensic Toxicology* (pp. 7–24). Biomedical Publications.

19. Orfila, M. P. (1821). *A General System of Toxicology, Or, A Treatise on Poisons, Drawn from The Mineral, Vegetable, and Animal Kingdoms, Considered as To Their Relations with Physiology, Pathology, and Medical Jurisprudence* (Vols. 1 & 2, 2nd ed.). Translated by Waller, J. A., & Cox, E. London.
20. Owen, P., Pendlebury, A., & Moffat, A. C. (1978). Choice of thin-layer chromatographic systems for the routine screening for neutral drugs during toxicological analyses. *Journal of Chromatography, 161*(2), 187–193.
21. Peng, G. W., & Chiou, W. L. (1990). Analysis of drugs and other toxic substances in biological samples for pharmacokinetic studies. *Journal of Chromatography, 531*, 3–50.
22. Plenck, J. J. (1781). *Elementa Medicinae et Chirurgiae Forensis*. Graeffer.
23. Reinsch, H. (1841). On the action of metallic copper on solutions of certain metals, particularly with reference to the detection of arsenic. *Philosophical Magazine, 19*, 480–483. (First published in *Journal of Practical Chemistry*, 1841, 19).
24. Stinson, J. C., O'Gharabhain, F., Adebayo, G., Chambers, P. L., & Feely, J. (1993). Pesticide-contaminated cucumber. *The Lancet, 341*(8845), 64.
25. Watson, K. (2004). *Poisoned Lives: English Poisoners and Their Victims*. Hambledon and London.
26. Wiley, J. F. (1991). Difficult diagnoses in toxicology: Poisons not detected by the comprehensive drug screen. *Pediatric Clinics of North America, 38*(4), 725–737.
27. Wilson, J. (2002). External quality assessment schemes for toxicology. *Forensic Science International, 128*(2), 98–103.

Chapter

TOXICOLOGY OF DRUG AND METABOLISM

10

Contents

Introduction

The breakdown of drugs by living things, usually through specialized enzymatic systems, is known as drug metabolism. All drugs and poisons that are not part of an organism's natural biochemistry are considered xenobiotics, and xenobiotic metabolism is, in general, the collection of metabolic pathways that change their chemical structure. Said to have originated in ancient times, these pathways represent a type of biotransformation found in all major groups of organisms (although occasionally the intermediates in xenobiotic metabolism can themselves cause toxic effects). These reactions frequently work to detoxify harmful substances. Call it pharmacokinetics: the study of drug metabolism. In pharmacology and medicine, the metabolism of pharmaceutical drugs is a crucial topic. The length and potency of a drug's pharmacologic action, for instance, are dictated by its rate of metabolism. Chemotherapy for cancer and infectious diseases is also impacted by drug metabolism, and dangerous drug interactions are frequently caused by certain medications acting as substrates or inhibitors of enzymes involved in xenobiotic metabolism. The xenobiotic metabolism of microorganisms, which determines whether a pollutant will be broken down during bioremediation or persist in the environment, makes these pathways significant for environmental science as well. Because they may result in pesticide and herbicide resistance, the xenobiotic metabolism enzymes, in particular the glutathione S-transferases, are also crucial to agriculture.

There are three stages to drug metabolism. Phase I involves the introduction of reactive or polar groups into xenobiotics by enzymes like cytochrome P450 oxidases. Phase II reactions then involve the conjugation of these modified compounds to polar compounds. Transferase enzymes, such as glutathione S-transferases (Commandeur JN, et al., 1995), catalyze these reactions. The conjugated xenobiotics may undergo additional processing in phase III before being recognized by efflux transporters and pumped out of the cells. Lipophilic substances are frequently changed by drug metabolism into hydrophilic products that are easier to excrete.

Orientation and Directional Terms

Term	Definition	Illustration
Biotransformation	A metabolic process that takes place mainly in the liver and helps to facilitate the excretion of both exogenous and endogenous substances.	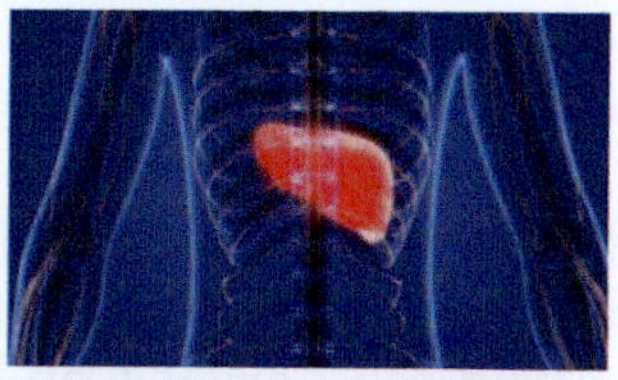
Penicllins	Penicillin is one of the most commonly used broad-spectrum antibiotics globally and has numerous clinical indications.	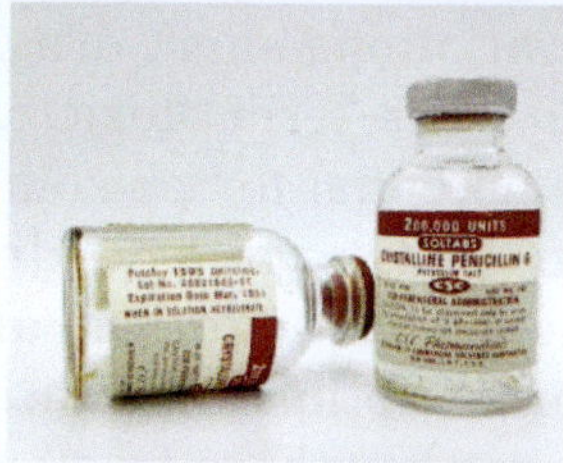
Antibodies	Antibodies are proteins that protect you when an unwanted substance enters your body. Produced by your immune system, antibodies bind to these unwanted substances in order to eliminate them from your system.	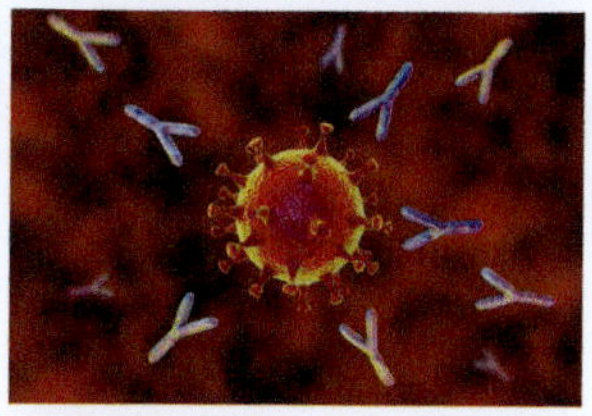
Polymorphism	Polymorphism is the occurrence of two or more clearly different morphs or forms, also referred to as alternative phenotypes, in the population of a species. To be classified as such, morphs must occupy the same habitat at the same time and belong to a panmictic population.	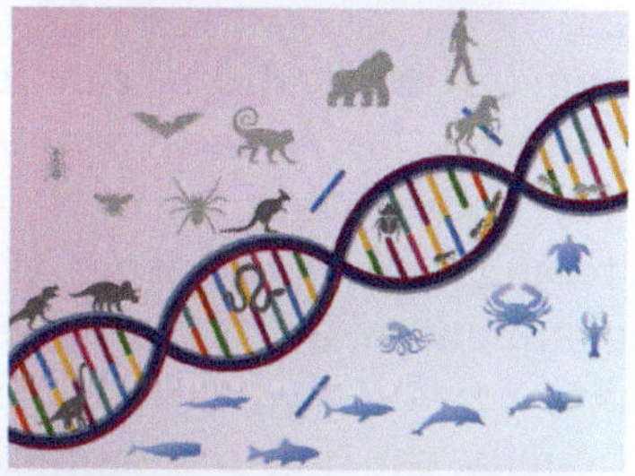
Detoxication	The physiological or medicinal removal of toxic substances from a living organism, including the human body, which is mainly carried out by the liver.	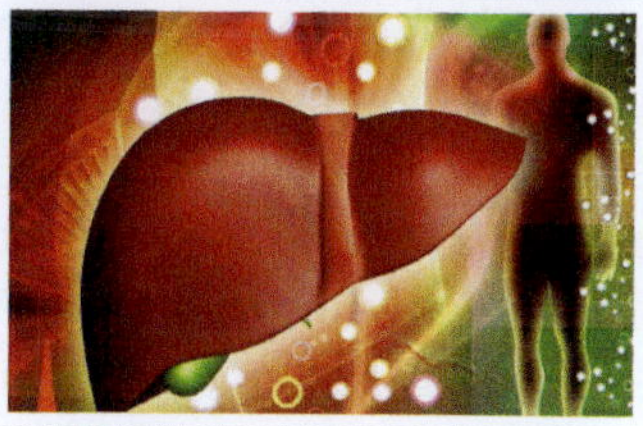

10.1. Drug Toxicology

Toxicology is the study of how drugs and chemicals in the environment cause unintended effects, while pharmacology is the scientific field that investigates how drugs change biological systems to promote health and treat disease. When taken as a whole, these fields cover the molecular underpinnings of drug action, how drugs affect cells, organs, and organisms, how genetic variations affect drug action, and drug discovery. The term "toxicity" describes a substance's potential for poisoning or harm. According to pharmacology, drug toxicity happens when a patient has an excessive amount of prescription medication in their system, which can have harmful effects. Formally speaking, drug toxicity is defined as a wide range of negative consequences that can result from using drugs at either therapeutic or non-therapeutic dosages.

10.1.1. Causes of Drug Toxicity

Overdosing on medications can lead to drug toxicity, where the excessive amount of the drug in the body causes harm. This can occur through taking more than the prescribed dose or if the recommended dosage is too high. Adverse reactions to certain medications can also result in drug toxicity, causing unintended side effects even at normal therapeutic doses. The line between an effective and toxic dose can be slim, with some individuals being more sensitive to medications than others. Accumulation of drugs with long half-lives in the bloodstream can also contribute to drug toxicity over time. Factors like age, kidney function, and hydration levels can affect how quickly the body processes and eliminates medications, making monitoring of drug levels necessary for certain medications like lithium.

10.1.2. Mechanisms of Drug Toxicity and Relevance to Pharmaceutical Development

The average cost of creating a successful drug has been estimated to be more than US $1.7 billion, which has been rising for many years in the pharmaceutical industry. On the other hand, a graph showing the annual number of newly approved medications is rather flat. Increasing regulatory barriers and the challenges of target validation in the face of increasingly complex disease areas are some of the causes of the issue. An average of 10,000–25,000 distinct chemicals are thought to be taken into consideration when developing a new medication. What are the main causes of lead compound attrition? Twenty-five years ago, poor human pharmacokinetics was a major problem. Advances in our understanding of transporters, human cytochrome P450 (P450) (Guengerich, 2001), and other enzymes have helped to address this aspect. Predictive in vitro assays have also been developed. On the other hand, toxicity issues have grown as metabolic issues have decreased (Figure 10.1). Roughly one-third of attrition cases are caused by the combined effects of pre-clinical toxicity (animal toxicity) and adverse events (human toxicity). If one excludes the "non-scientific" issues (e.g., if any) then the percentage is even higher (commercial, financial).

The true problem lies in investing time and financial resources in compounds with toxicity problems and must eventually be withdrawn from development. Numerous stages in the drug discovery and development process involve the assessment of toxicity and safety (Figure 10.2). Compounds with toxicity problems could cost hundreds of millions of dollars and years of research if they are not abandoned until it is too late. As a result, early choices are crucial to the development of new drugs, and these choices need to be made correctly. Most of the toxicity issues related to drugs will be covered in this review.

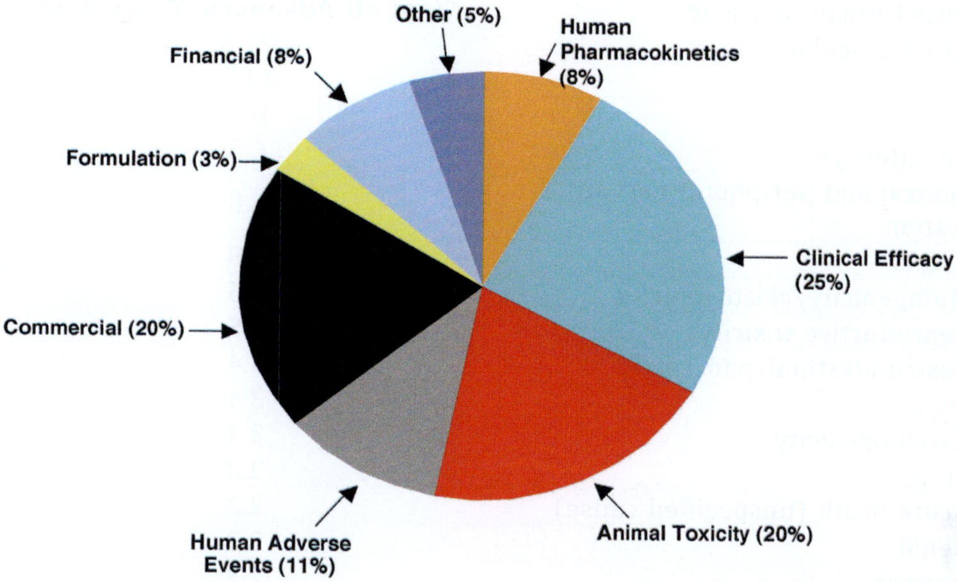

Figure 10.1. *Estimates of fractions of reasons for attrition of drug candidates in pre-clinical and clinical development (ca. 2000).*

Source: https://www.ncbi.nlm.nih.gov/pmc/articles/PMC4707670/bin/nihms749476f1.jpg.

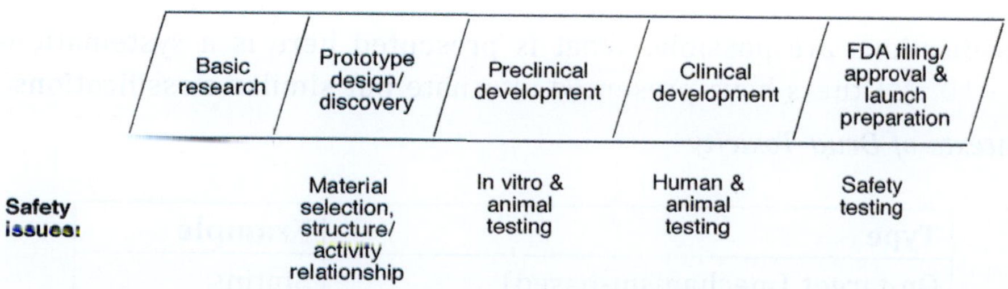

Figure 10.2. *Safety issues at different stages of drug discovery and development.*

Source: https://www.ncbi.nlm.nih.gov/pmc/articles/PMC4707670/bin/nihms749476f2.jpg.

10.1.2.1. Contexts of Drug Toxicity

Using the Paracelsus axiom, all compounds are safe at very low doses and toxic at high doses. Here, toxicity and adverse events at doses that are pertinent to patients taking a medication are what we are thinking about, not unintentional drug overdoses. How one approaches the problem of avoiding toxicity or creating substitute compounds that will not have this liability will depend on the context of toxicity. Hepatic and cardiovascular toxicity are the most often reported issues (Table 10.1).

Table 10.1. *Sites for Toxicology Attrition*

Target organ or tissue	% of all Advanced Molecules[a]
Cardiovascular	27.3
Liver	14.8
Teratogenicity	8.0
Hematologic	6.8
Central and peripheral nervous system	6.8
Retina	6.8
Mutagenicity/clastogenicity	4.5
Reproductive toxicity	4.5
Gastrointestinal/pancreatic	3.4
Muscle	3.4
Carcinogenicity	3.4
Lung	2.3
Acute death (unspecified cause)	2.3
Renal	2.3
Irritant	2.3
Skeletal (arthritis/bone development)	1.1

[a]*Total = 100%.*

Source: https://www.ncbi.nlm.nih.gov/pmc/articles/PMC4707670/.

Several classifications are possible. What is presented here is a systematic one previously described (Table 10.2). Others have presented alternate but similar classifications.

Table 10.2. *Contexts of Drug Toxicity*

Type	Example
On-target (mechanism-based)	Statins
Hypersensitivity and immunological	Penicillins
Off-target	Terfenadine
Biological activation	Acetaminophen
Idiosyncratic	Halothane

Source: https://www.ncbi.nlm.nih.gov/pmc/articles/PMC4707670/.

On-target, or mechanism-based, toxicity is the first type of toxicity. In other words, the drug's interaction with the same target that results in the intended pharmacological response causes the toxicity. Instead of focusing on competitive inhibition, the idea is that the drug's biological response to binding to its target is what causes both the toxic and effective effects. This kind of toxicity is challenging to manage in theory because it manifests in all classes of compounds created to treat the illness. It might be required to alter the disease's target. But statins provide an example of an alternative tactic. Because they block the liver's 3-hydroxy-3-methylglutaryl CoA (HMG CoA) reductase, all statins result in hypercholesterolemia. e. the objective. Muscle and potentially other tissues' inhibition of HMGCoA reductase is another reason why statins have negative effects. e. Protein geranylgeranylation is suppressed. Thankfully, different transport proteins can regulate the distribution of statins across tissues, and while on-target toxicity is a concern, it can be managed through inter-tissue distribution. The second context pertaining to drug toxicity involves immune responses and hypersensitivity. For example, penicillin allergy reactions have long been known to exist. The idea is that drugs (or their metabolites) interact with proteins in the body (as haptens) to produce antibodies and immune responses. This concept was largely developed based on the groundbreaking work of Landsteiner. Penicillin's are an example of a chemical that is not entirely stable and has the ability to bind covalently to proteins and start the production of antibodies.

Off-target toxicity is the third setting in which drugs can be toxic. The medication's lack of specificity in its interactions is the problem here. Toxic effects result from binding to a different target. Given what we currently know about the intricacy of multiple gene families and biological regulatory pathways (e.g., kinases), so it's understandable that a medication might not be entirely targeted. Terfenadine is used as an example in Table 10.2, as it binds to both the hERG channel and the H1 receptor, resulting in arrhythmias and the desired antihistaminic response. Since a lower dose may be able to avoid the specificity problem, this liability could theoretically be addressed by conducting additional screening and developing drug candidates with lower IC50 and Kd values. Bioactivation is the fourth context in which drugs can be toxic. Many medications are transformed into reactive products, which are frequently referred to as "metabolites." These substances alter the proteins they interact with and in some way produce toxicity, though the exact mechanisms are unknown (see infra). According to one theory, significant regulatory or other proteins undergo modification and lose functionality. An additional possibility that connects to the second context of toxicity is that the altered proteins trigger immunological responses. According to a review of medications at Bristol-Myers Squibb, "metabolism" was a factor in 28% of the cases where drug candidates were shelved from development (Table 10.3).

Table 10.3. *Mechanistic Causes of Toxicology Attrition.*

	% of all Advanced Molecules[a]
Biotransformation-related	27
Target-based	28
Single or multiple ion channel inhibition	18
Immune-mediated	7
All other mechanisms	36

[a]*n = 88. Because categories are partially overlapping, the total is > 100%.*

Source: https://www.ncbi.nlm.nih.gov/pmc/articles/PMC4707670/.

The fifth context of toxicity is idiosyncratic reactions. Idiosyncratic means "individual," and these are rare events ($1/10^3$ to $1/10^4$ individuals), which are not well understood. Such responses are highly problematic in that few (if any) animal models are very predictive. The low incidence makes such adverse events difficult to find, even in large clinical trials. However, with widely-used drugs for which millions of prescriptions may be written, even an incidence of $1/10^4$ can yield hundreds of problems.

The context of toxicity has bearing on how difficult it is to predict safety problems (Figure 10.3).

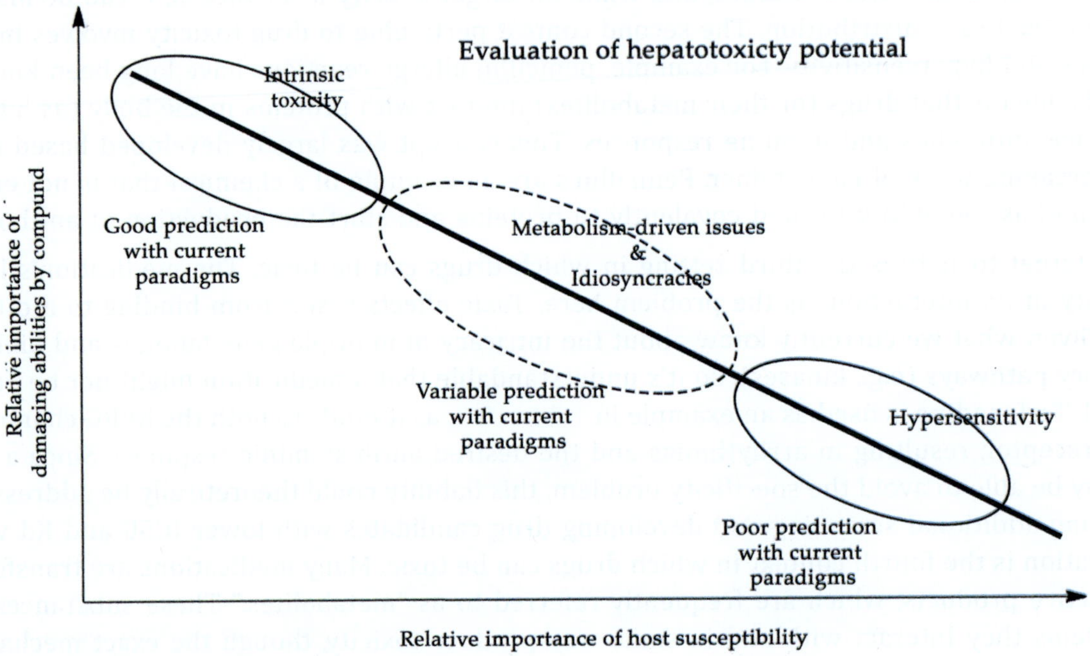

Figure 10.3. *Hypothetical relationship between the inherent toxicity of drugs and the variability of the response among hosts (e.g., test animals, humans). The dose is not a consideration in this treatment, adapted from Zimmerman. At toxic doses, the most readily understood compounds are those with high toxicity in all animal species. Variation among species introduces more uncertainty in extrapolation to humans. Predictions can be made if the issue is metabolism but idiosyncratic problems are very difficult to understand with animal models.*

Source: https://www.ncbi.nlm.nih.gov/pmc/articles/PMC4707670/bin/nihms749476f3.jpg.

10.1.2.2. Theories Regarding Mechanisms of Idiosyncratic Reactions

Others have reviewed this subject (Table 10.4). In order to account for all drugs for which idiosyncrasies have been reported, at least five theories have been put forth, and they might not be mutually exclusive (Table 10.5). Polymorphisms or uncommon alleles of metabolism-related enzymes are the first theory. (The term "rare alleles" refers to instances of less than 1–2%, so the term "polymorphism" might not be appropriate in this case. The idea is that sensitivity results from a drug's lack of metabolism, which includes a lack of detoxication. For example, a person may be the ~1% of the (Caucasian) population that has a high likelihood of activating a drug (e.g., the extremely quick metabolizers in the P450 2D6 group) and may also lack an enzyme necessary to detoxicate the product, such as glutathione transferase. Consequently, multiplying two polymorphisms at the 1% level would result in an incidence of 1/104. Although there are no reliable examples to support any observed idiosyncratic reactions, this scenario is plausible.

Table 10.4. *Intrinsic vs. Idiosyncratic Hepatotoxicity*

Intrinsic	**Idiosyncratic**
Predictable (?)	Unpredictable
Relatively common occurrence	Rare occurrence (< $1/10^4$)
Detected pre-clinically	Not detected until post-launch
Dose dependence	Occurs at any dose (?)
Acute or sub-acute onset	Delayed onset
No immune component	Immune/metabolic component (usually see fever, rash, eosinophilia)
Animal models useful	Few (any?) animal models available
Example: acetaminophen	Examples: isoniazid, halothane

Source: https://www.ncbi.nlm.nih.gov/pmc/articles/PMC4707670/.

Table 10.5. *Idiosyncratic Toxicity: Proposed Mechanisms*

- Metabolic
  - [Rare allele] × [rare allele] = unusual metabolism
- Hapten hypothesis
  - Reactive metabolites act as haptens —> immunological response
- Inflammagen model
  - Inflammation or other predisposing episodes render some individuals more sensitive
- Danger hypothesis
  - Injured tissue —> danger signals —> toxicological response
- Pharmacological intervention
  - Drugs —> immunological response by *reversible* binding (not electrophiles)

Source: https://www.ncbi.nlm.nih.gov/pmc/articles/PMC4707670/.

The second, which has already been discussed, is the happened theory. The idea is that while some people will activate a medication more than others to produce a hapten, only a small percentage of people will exhibit this response due to differences in immune systems. There is some evidence in the cases of tienilic acid and hydralazine, which cause hepatitis and produce anti-P450 antibodies in humans when activated by human P450s and bound covalently to P450s. The shortcoming is that it hasn't been able to establish whether these incidents are merely coincidental but unconnected or whether they are the cause of the hepatotoxicity. The inflammation model is another name for the third theory. The idea is that while many people experience bioactivation and other events, only some people become more sensitive to inflammation or other predisposing episodes. This phenomenon may be shown in rats given lipopolysaccharide treatments to induce oxidative stress. It's debatable, though, exactly how representative this is as a model for human peculiarities.

The danger hypothesis is the fourth (theory). Here, the damaged tissue sends out warning signals. It is not the medication or its metabolites but rather lipid oxidation products and cytokines that cause a toxic reaction. There is no concrete proof that this is a mechanism underlying clinical medication idiosyncracies, but as Uetrecht has noted, if an immunological response is involved, this hypothesis is not incompatible with the hapten theory. The model of pharmacological intervention is the fifth theory. According to this model, medications trigger immune reactions through reversible protein binding, i.e., without a covalent connection. Sulfamethoxazole, an arylamine that is prone to producing reactive metabolites, served as one of the foundations for this proposal. There is some evidence that the peptide-like compound ximelegatran may function in this way.

10.2. Drug Metabolism

Humans need medicines to treat illnesses, but they are also foreign substances to the body. Therefore, the body tries to eliminate them as soon as possible. It is ideal for medications to leave the body as soon as possible after they start to act as a drug. The longer a medication is in the body, the more adverse effects it causes. The human body naturally gets rid of these foreign substances, or medications. The drug metabolism process primarily facilitates this. The biochemical conversion of one chemical form to another, usually carried out by specialized enzymatic systems, is known as drug metabolism (Meyer, et al., 1997).

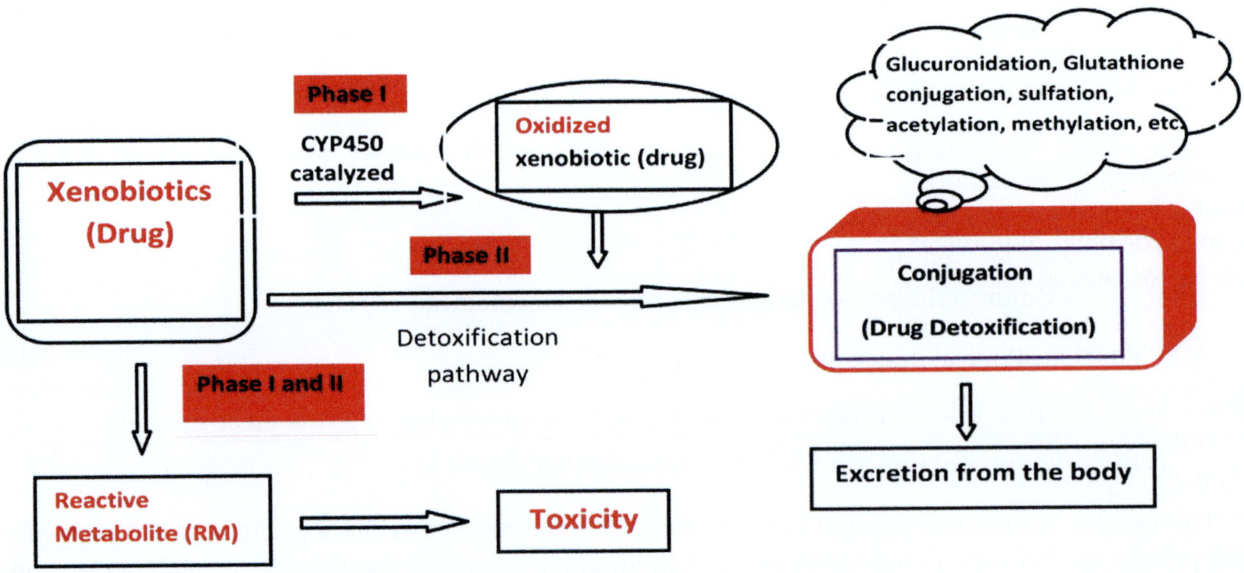

Figure 10.4. *General pathway of drug metabolism.*

Source: https://www.ias.ac.in/article/fulltext/reso/019/03/0259-0282#:~:text=Drug%20metabolism%20reactions%20comprise%20of,carbon%2C%20sulfur%20or%20nitrogen%20centre.

It frequently entails the transformation of lipophilic chemical substances—drugs—into highly polar derivatives that the body can eliminate with ease (refer to Figure 10.4).

Lipid soluble substances build up in the body and cause toxic reactions because they are passively reabsorption into the bloodstream from the renal tubules. The body has an arsenal in the form of a metabolic system to prevent the same. This system converts drugs that are lipophilic, water-insoluble, and nonpolar into metabolites that are more polar, water-soluble, and readily excretable from the body. Drug metabolism is therefore appropriately and fittingly referred to as a detoxification process. For a drug to take effect, some of the metabolites are necessary. Prodrugs are being designed with this phenomenon in mind. Reactive metabolites (RM), which are harmful to the human body, can also be produced by the same metabolic process. This process, known as drug bioactivation, is dependent on certain structural characteristics of the compounds in question. There are efforts underway to prevent the production of these reactive metabolites.

10.2.1. Metabolic Organs

Drug metabolism is a fascinating and intricate process that requires a deep understanding of chemistry. The smooth endoplasmic reticulum of the liver cell serves as the main location for drug metabolism. This is a result of the abundance of various types of enzymes in large quantities. The drug metabolism that takes place in the liver is called hepatic metabolism. Every biological tissue in the body has the capacity to metabolize drugs, except for the liver. Extrahepatic metabolism is the term for the drug metabolism process that takes place in organs other than the liver. The placenta, kidney, lungs, skin, adrenal glands, and gastrointestinal tract epithelial cells are among the other sites. These sites do, however, only have a small part in this process. The majority of drugs (roughly 70%) go through metabolism, which is facilitated by the enzymes found in the locations listed above (Lakshmanan, 2019).

10.2.2. Chemistry of Drug Metabolism

Enzymes are essential to the chemical process of drug metabolism because they facilitate the change of one chemical species into another. The cytochrome P450 family is the main enzyme family involved in these metabolic processes. The bioinorganic aspects of drug metabolism are made up of these enzymes' structural characteristics and functional activity.

10.2.2.1. Bioinorganic Chemistry of Drug Metabolism

Another name for the cytochrome P450 (CYP) enzymes is microsomal mixed function oxidases. The liver and other tissues' smooth endoplasmic reticulum contains membrane-bound proteins known as CYP enzymes. These are the most significant enzymes for the first stage of drug biotransformation. The iron-porphyrin unit is the heme group, which is present in these enzymes as a prosthetic group. The heme center, the oxidizing site in these enzymes, is in charge of converting hydrophobic substances into more polar or hydrophilic metabolites that can be excreted later. These are known as CYP450s because the reduced iron has a strong affinity for carbon monoxide and exhibits a significant UV absorbance at 450 nm when bound to the gas. As indicated by the equation below, CYPs catalyze the transfer of one oxygen atom to a substrate, resulting in an oxidized substrate and a water molecule.

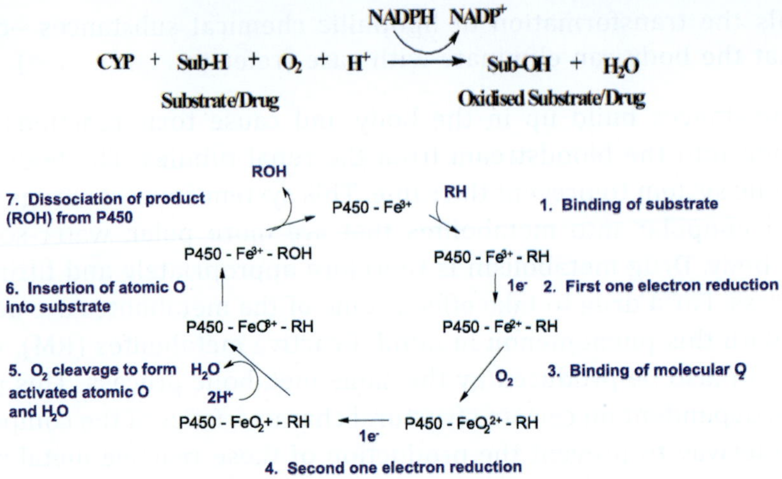

Figure 10.5. *The catalytic cycle of CYP450, leading to the oxidation of substrate.*

Source: https://www.ias.ac.in/article/fulltext/reso/019/03/0259-0282#:~:text=Drug%20 metabolism%20reactions%20comprise%20of,carbon%2C%20sulfur%20or%20nitrogen%20centre.

The comprehensive process of CYP metabolism has been explicated in the catalytic cycle depicted in Figure 10.5. Based on the amino-acid sequence, the more than 300 distinct CYP enzymes have been divided into a number of families and subfamilies. Of these, eighteen CYP families—mostly those of CYP1, CYP2, and CYP3—have been found in mammals. Figure 10.6 shows the percentage contribution of each CYP isoform to drug metabolism. Table 10.6 displays a chosen list of medications that are metabolized by different CYP enzyme families.

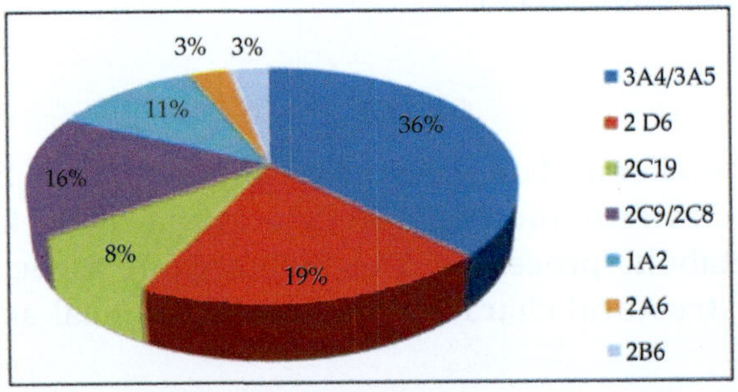

Figure 10.6. *The percentage contribution of various CYP isoforms in drug metabolism.*

Source: https://www.ias.ac.in/article/fulltext/reso/019/03/0259-0282#:~:text=Drug%20 metabolism%20reactions%20comprise%20of,carbon%2C%20sulfur%20or%20nitrogen%20centre.

Table 10.6. *A Selected List of Drugs Metabolized by various Families of CYP Enzymes*

With regard to the heme prosthetic group of CYP450, the iron atom can exist in Fe^{2+} (reduced) or Fe^{3+} (oxidized) states. These enzymes use one Fe-S (cysteine) covalent bond and ionic interactions to bind the heme prosthetic group to a polypeptide chain made up of several amino acids. The oxidation reactions carried out by CYP450 enzymes are caused by the active species of these enzymes, Cpd I. Figure 10.7 illustrates the heteroatom oxidation process that Cpd I catalyzes schematically.

In the initial step, the substrate binds to the enzyme's active site. As a result, a reactant complex is formed, and oxygen is then transferred from Cpd I to the substrate's heteroatom. This results in the product complex, where the oxygen atom is still attached to the heme-iron but the transfer of oxygen to the heteroatom is nearly complete. The next step involves the product containing the oxidized heteroatom exiting the enzyme's active site.

CYP	Drugs Metabolised
1A2	Amitriptyline, clozapine
2A6	Acetaminophen, amodiaquine, artesunate
2C8	Paclitaxel, torsemide
2C9	Diclofenac, ibuprofen, phenytoin
2C19	Diazepam, omeprazole, phenytoin
2D6	Amitriptyline, metoprolol, nortriptyline
2E1	Enflurane, halothane
3A4	Carbamazepine, erythromycin, zolpidem

Source: https://www.ias.ac.in/article/fulltext/reso/019/03/0259-0282#:~:text=Drug%20 metabolism%20reactions%20comprise%20of,carbon%2C%20sulfur%20or%20nitrogen%20centre.

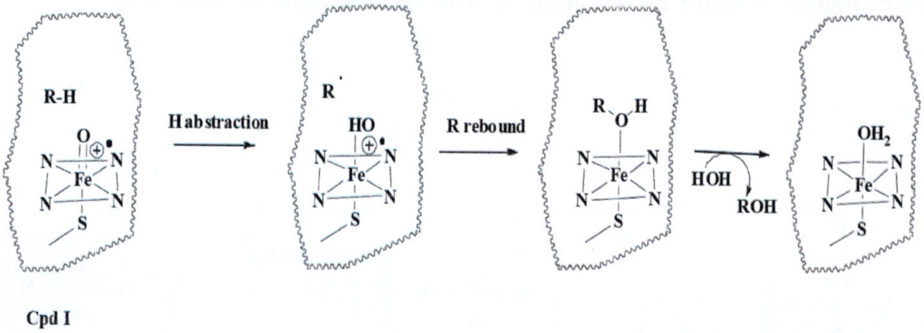

Figure 10.7. *The most important portion of the catalytic cycle of CYP450, leading to heteroatom oxidation of substrate.*

Source: https://www.ias.ac.in/article/fulltext/reso/019/03/0259-0282#:~:text=Drug%20 metabolism%20reactions%20comprise%20of,carbon%2C%20sulfur%20or%20nitrogen%20centre.

Studies have been done on additional drug metabolism reaction mechanisms that resemble heteroatom oxidation. Mechanistic information about the bioinorganic chemistry occurring inside the cytochrome active site cavity is provided by computational chemistry techniques. Quantum mechanical (QM) and QM/molecular mechanical (QM/MM) techniques are among these techniques. To clarify the mechanism, the computational studies make use of the active species Cpd I and theoretical techniques. Shaik and colleagues, for instance, have covered the processes of CH hydroxylation, N-oxidation, S-oxidation, olefin epoxidation, and N-dealkylation in a variety of substrates. Figure 10.8 illustrates the CH hydroxylation reaction mechanism. To create the ferric-alcohol complex, this first requires Cpd I to abstract hydrogen from the alkane (RH). Radical rebound then occurs on the iron-hydroxo intermediate. After that, this releases the alcohol and returns the body to its resting state (i.e., the water complex), as illustrated in Figure. 10.8.

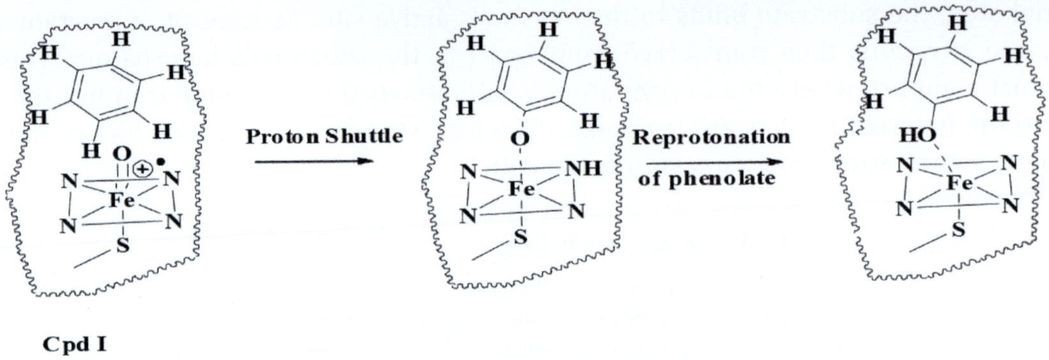

Figure 10.8. *The H-abstraction and rebound mechanism for CH hydroxylation.*

Source: https://www.ias.ac.in/article/fulltext/reso/019/03/0259-0282#:~:text=Drug%20metabolism%20reactions%20comprise%20of,carbon%2C%20sulfur%20or%20nitrogen%20centre.

Thiel and co-workers have further strengthened the mechanistic details through the use of QM/MM method, and established the basis behind several metabolic reactions, catalyzed by different CYP isoforms in the body. Visser and Shaik elucidated a novel mechanism of proton shuttle for CH hydroxylation of benzene. A brief description of the mechanism is shown in Figure 10.9.

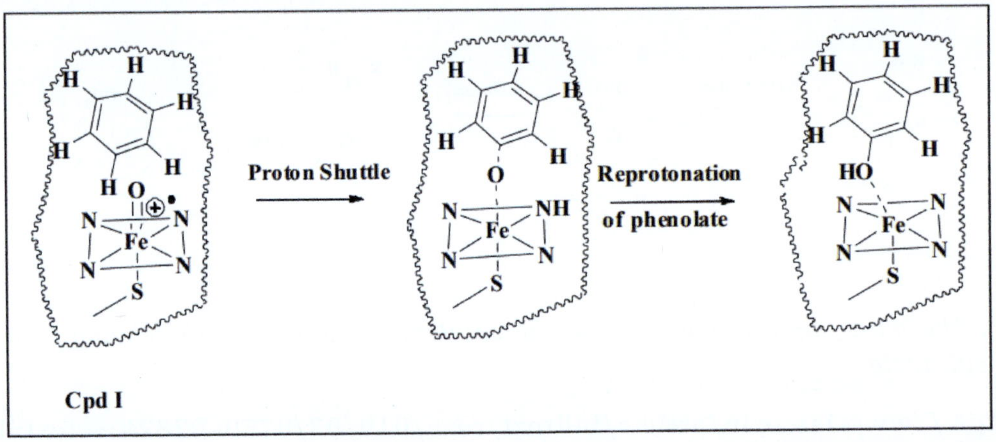

Figure 10.9. *The proton shuttle mechanism for CH hydroxylation in benzene.*

Source: https://www.ias.ac.in/article/fulltext/reso/019/03/0259-0282#:~:text=Drug%20metabolism%20reactions%20comprise%20of,carbon%2C%20sulfur%20or%20nitrogen%20centre.

In a similar vein, Figure 10.10 illustrates the mechanistic details that our group discovered during the S-oxidation of thiazolidinediones. As a result, while the mechanism differs depending on the reaction that CYPs are catalyzing, the active species (Cpd I) is always involved. These metabolic reactions have different mechanisms because they contain different functional groups, like S, N, alkyl, phenyl, alkene, alkyne, etc. Understanding the organic chemistry of metabolic reactions, the impact of steric hindrance, and the structure–toxicity relationship in brief, becomes crucial as a result.

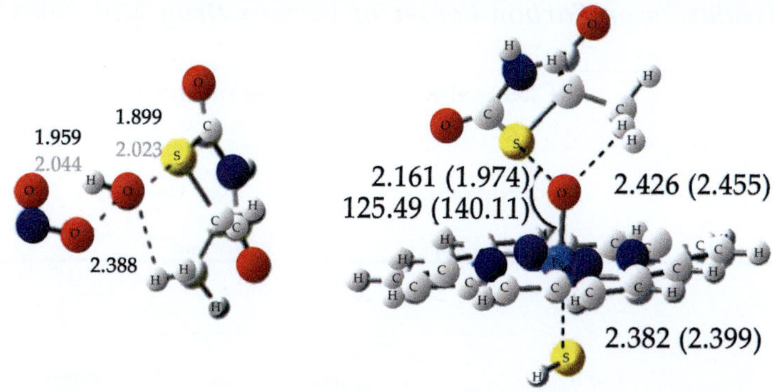

Figure 10.10. *The 3D structures of the transition state for S-oxidation of thiazolidinediones by HOONO and CPD I.*

Source: https://www.ias.ac.in/article/fulltext/reso/019/03/0259-0282#:~:text=Drug%20 metabolism%20reactions%20comprise%20of,carbon%2C%20sulfur%20or%20nitrogen%20centre.

10.2.2.2. Bioorganic Chemistry of Drug Metabolism

Understanding the different kinds of drug metabolism reactions is crucial to comprehending the idea of drug metabolism. As was previously mentioned, drug metabolism can result in a variety of outcomes, including detoxification or bioactivation. Phase I (functionalization) and Phase II (conjugation) reactions are the two main categories into which the detoxification reactions can be separated. The reactions could happen (i) in a sequential fashion, (ii) on their own, or (iii) all at once.

Detoxification Reactions: Phase I Reactions

The oxidation, reduction, hydrolysis, cyclization, and decyclization reactions are among the processes referred to as nonsynthetic reactions. These reactions, which typically involve CYP450, are primarily carried out by mixed function oxidases in the liver. A polar group is either introduced or, if it already exists, is unmasked in these reactions. Phase II reactions occur next to these reactions. Instead of being immediately eliminated, the majority of Phase I products go through Phase II reactions. The following list of Phase I reactions includes multiple examples:

- **Oxidation:** This reaction is the most frequent one and increases the hydrophilic content of substrates by adding a polar functional group, like –OH. Since this reaction can happen in drugs at multiple locations, oxidation reactions have been categorized appropriately. A compound's aromatic ring, olefinic center, and aliphatic groups can all be oxidized at the carbon center. Acetanilide, an analgesic, phenylbutazone, an antiepileptic, valproic acid, an antiepileptic, carbamazepine, and minoxidil, an antihypertensive, are among the significant medications metabolized by this reaction (see Table 10.7).

Table 10.7. *Metabolic Oxidation on Carbon Center of Various Drug Molecules*

Reaction Centre	Chemical Reaction on Drug substrate
Aromatic ring	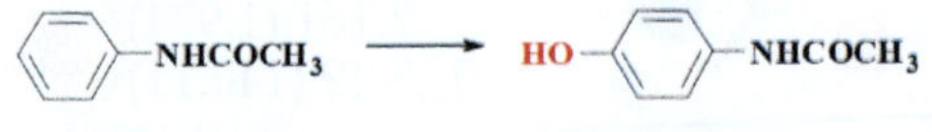 Acetanilide → Paracetamol
Olefinic centre	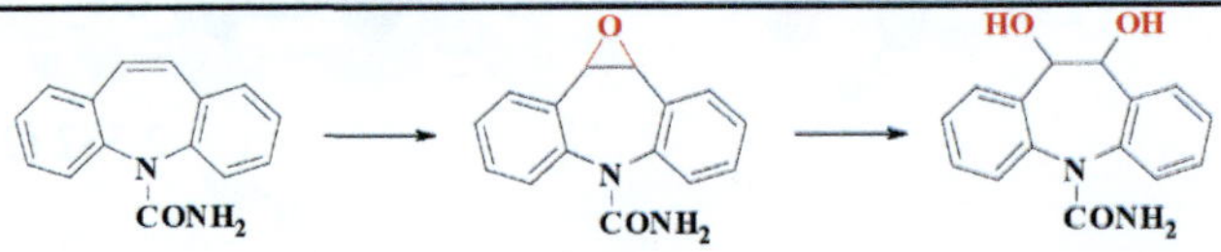 Carbamazepine → Carbamazepine-10, 11-epoxide → Trans-10,11-dihydroxy carbamazepine
Aliphatic groups	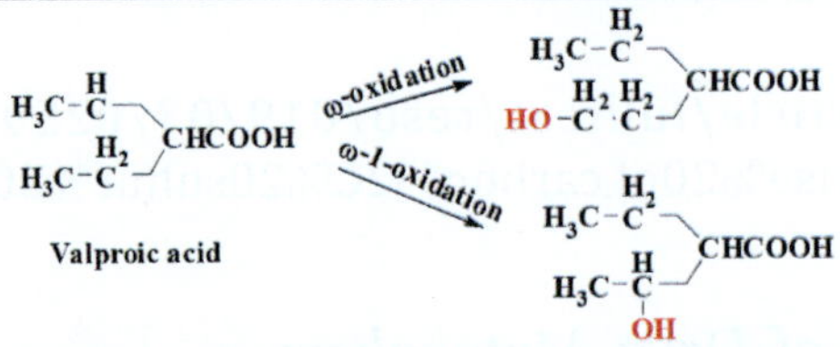 Valproic acid → (ω-oxidation) 5-Hydroxy valproic acid (minor product); (ω-1-oxidation) 4-Hydroxy valproic acid (major product)

Source: https://www.ias.ac.in/article/fulltext/reso/019/03/0259-0282#:~:text=Drug%20metabolism%20reactions%20comprise%20of,carbon%2C%20sulfur%20or%20nitrogen%20centre.

Table 10.8. *Metabolic Oxidation on Carbon-Heteroatom Systems of Various Drug Molecules*

Reaction	Chemical Reaction on Drug Substrate
Deamination	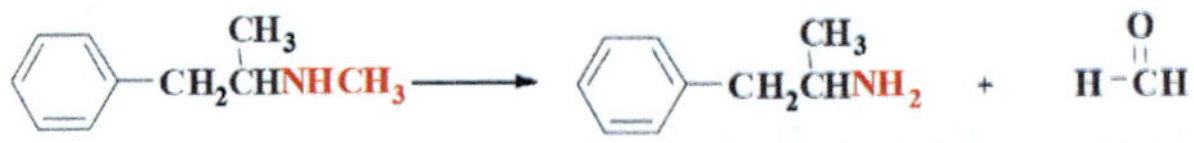 Methamphetamine → Amphetamine + Formaldehyde
	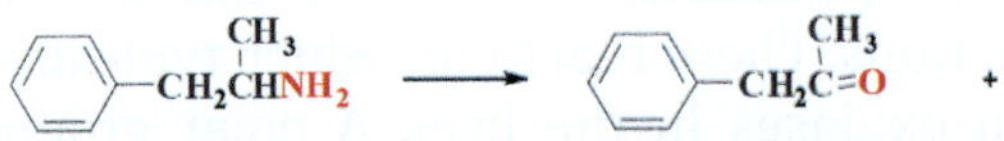 Amphetamine → Phenylacetone + Ammonia
Cyclization	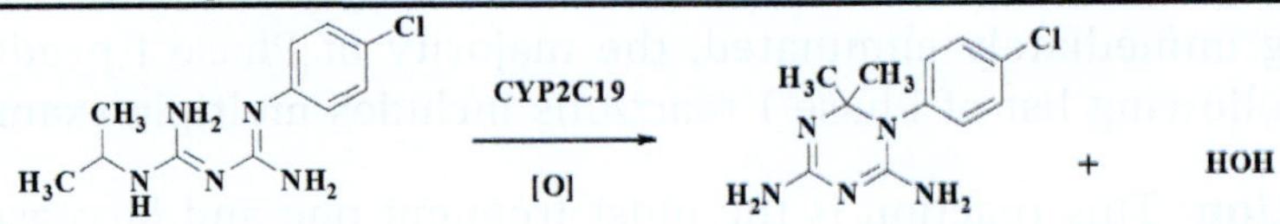 Proguanil (Prodrug) → (CYP2C19, [O]) Cycloguanil (Active Antimalarial metabolite) + Water
S-dealkylation	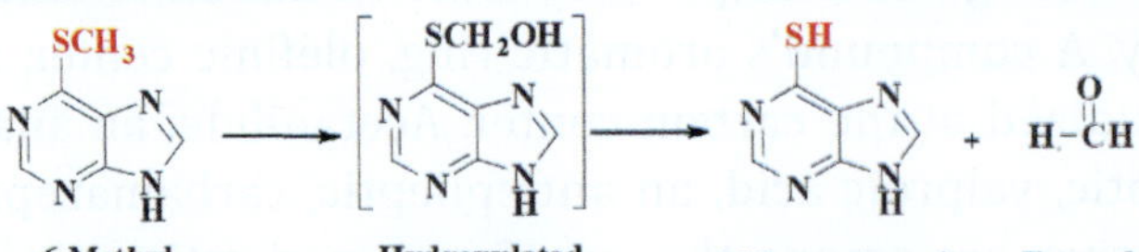 6-Methyl mercaptopurine → Hydroxylated intermediate → 6-Mercaptopurine + Formaldehyde

Source: https://www.ias.ac.in/article/fulltext/reso/019/03/0259-0282#:~:text=Drug%20metabolism%20reactions%20comprise%20of,carbon%2C%20sulfur%20or%20nitrogen%20centre.

Reactions on C–N, C–S, and C–O systems are involved in oxidation at carbon–heteroatom systems. N-dealkylation, oxidative deamination, N-oxide formation, and N-hydroxylation are the oxidation reactions that occur on C–N systems. Ndealkylation takes place in substrates where the nitrogen atom is directly connected to an alkyl group. Methamphetamine, an antidepressant, is one example of a substance that is converted to amphetamine through Ndealkylation. Oxidative deamination is the process by which amphetamine is further broken down into phenylacetone and ammonia (see Table 10.8).

Desulfuration, S-oxidation, and S-dealkylation are possible reactions in C–S systems. S-dealkylation proceeds through α-carbon hydroxylation, e.g., such as 6-methylmercaptopurine. Thiopental, a barbiturate medication, is changed into pentobarbital by the process of desulfuration, which results in the cleavage of the C=S bond and the formation of the C=O product. Sufide unit (-S-)-containing substrates exhibit the S-oxidation reaction. The antithyroid medication methimazole, the antihistaminic medications cimetidine and ranitidine, the antipsychotic medication chlorpromazine, etc. are a few examples of medications undergoing S-oxidation. Soxidation reaction is also a part of the thiazolidinedione class of antidiabetic medications, which includes pioglitazone and rosiglitazone. The use of theoretical chemistry has helped to clarify the mechanistic details of S-oxidation. Other significant oxidation reactions at the carbon center include oxidative dehalogenation, oxidative aromatization, and o-dealkylation. O-dealkylation is the process by which medications like the analgesic phenacetin and the antitussive codeine are metabolized. Oxidative dehalogenation is the metabolic process that halothane (a general anesthetic) goes through.

- **Reduction:** This reactions produce polar functional groups like amino and hydroxyl, which can then go through additional metabolic processes. These reactions can happen to a variety of functional groups, including hydroxyl and carbonyl. as displayed in Table 10.9.

Table 10.9. *Metabolic Reduction Reaction of Various Drug Molecules*

Reaction Centre	Chemical Reaction on Drug Substrate
Carbonyl	$Cl_3C-CHO.H_2O \longrightarrow Cl_3C-CH_2OH$ Chloral Hydrate → Trichloroethanol
Nitrogen (N=N)	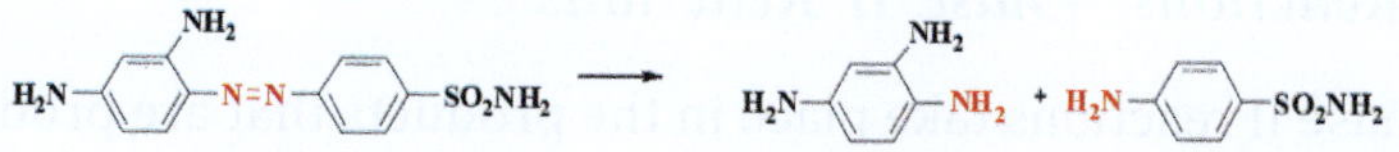 Prontosil → 1,2,4- Triaminobenzene + Sulfanilamide
Halogens	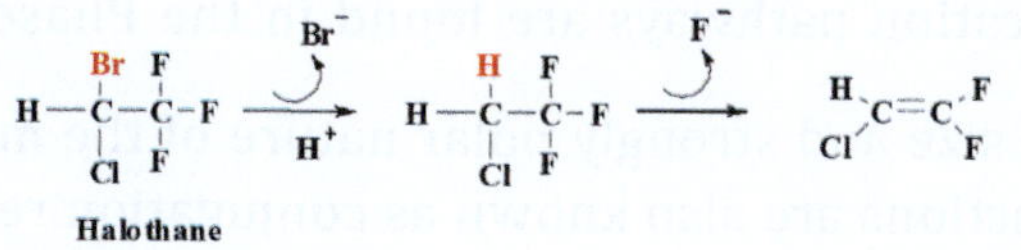 Halothane

Source: https://www.ias.ac.in/article/fulltext/reso/019/03/0259-0282#:~:text=Drug%20metabolism%20reactions%20comprise%20of,carbon%2C%20sulfur%20or%20nitrogen%20centre.

Ketones and aliphatic and aromatic aldehydes can undergo the reduction reaction. Drugs that go through this metabolic process include naltrexone (which treats alcohol dependence), methadone (an analgesic), and chloral hydrate (a sedative and hypnotic). This metabolic process is carried out by N-containing compounds containing nitro, azo, or N-oxide. Nitrazepam, a hypnotic and anxiolytic, and prontosil, an antibiotic that fights bacteria, are two examples of drugs that are reduced to their corresponding amines. Drugs containing halogen atoms can be reduced by substituting them with Hatom, e.g., halothane.

- **Hydrolysis:** The substrate undergoes a significant chemical change during these reactions. Table 10.10 lists the functional groups in which the hydrolysis reactions can take place. After being hydrolyzed, esters yield alcohols and carboxylic acids. Esters are typically administered as prodrugs, which are changed into active forms by hydrolysis e.g., aspirin (antipyretic, analgesic). Compared to esters, drug molecules with amide functionality hydrolyze more slowly. Amidases catalyze these reactions. It rarely happens in primary amides, but it does happen in secondary and tertiary amides, e.g., procainamide, an antiarrhythmic drug.

Table 10.10. *Metabolic Hydrolysis Reaction of Various Drug Molecules Having Different Functional Groups*

Reaction Centre	Chemical Reaction on Drug Substrate
Esters and ethers	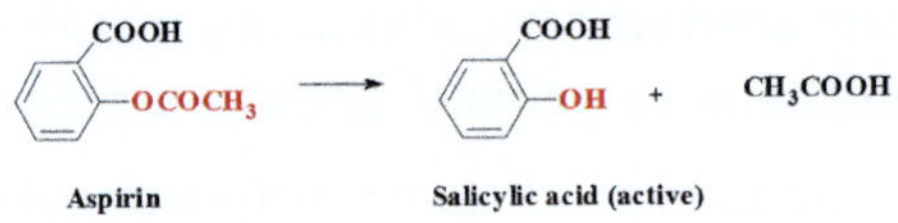
Amides	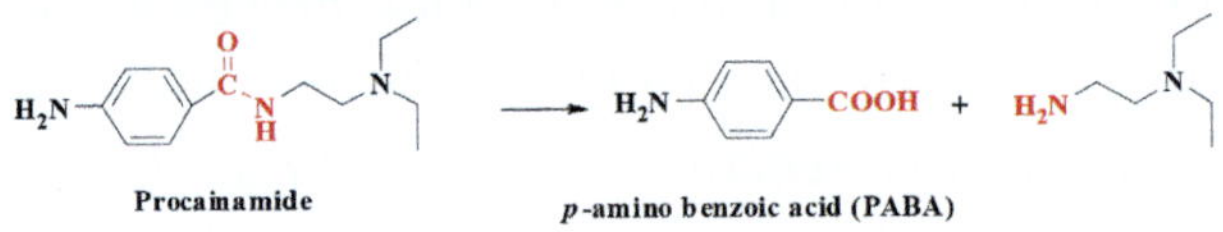

Source: https://www.ias.ac.in/article/fulltext/reso/019/03/0259-0282#:~:text=Drug%20 metabolism%20reactions%20comprise%20of,carbon%2C%20sulfur%20or%20nitrogen%20centre.

Detoxification Reactions: Phase II Reactions

The majority of Phase II reactions take place in the products that are produced from Phase I reactions and come after Phase I reactions. An appropriate moiety, like glucuronic acid, glutathione, sulfate, glycine, etc., is involved in these reactions. acquire conjugation to the Phase I reaction metabolites. The actual drug detoxification pathways are found in the Phase II reactions.

Because of the large size and strongly polar nature of the moieties with which the metabolites are conjugated, these reactions are also known as conjugation reactions. Many different transferase enzymes, including glutathione transferases, sulfotransferases, and uridine diphosphate (UDP)-glucoronsyltransferases, catalyze these reactions. These transferases are a subfamily of enzymes that is related to CYPs; however, they metabolize fewer drugs than CYPs. Table 10.11 enumerates several conjugation reactions, the enzymes involved, and instances of drugs that go through them. Figure 10.11 illustrates glutathione conjugation (Boyland E & Chasseaud LF. 1969).

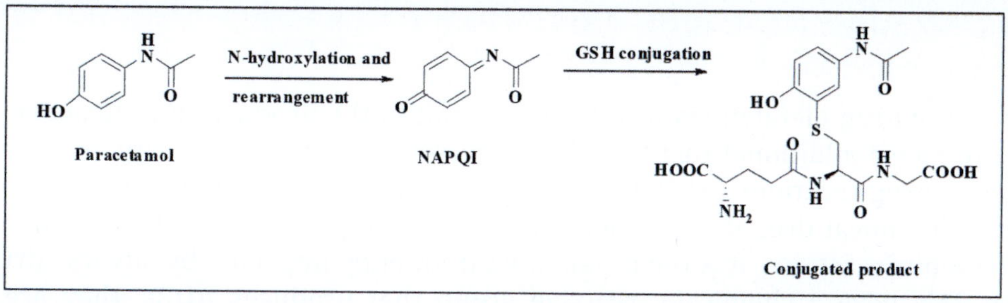

Figure 10.11. *A representative scheme showing glutathione conjugation as the Phase II metabolic reaction in the body.*

Source: https://www.ias.ac.in/article/fulltext/reso/019/03/0259-0282#:~:text=Drug%20metabolism%20reactions%20comprise%20of,carbon%2C%20sulfur%20or%20nitrogen%20centre.

Table 10.11. *The Conjugation Reactions Along with the Enzymes Involved and the Examples of Drugs Metabolized by the Same Pathway*

Conjugated Group	Endogenous Cofactor	Enzyme	Drugs
Glucuronidation	UDP glucoronic acid	UDP-glucuronosyltransferase	Chloramphenicol, morphine, paracetamol, salicylic acid, fenoprofen, desipramine, meprobamate, cyproheptadiene
Sulphation	Sulphate	Sulfotransferases	Paracetamol, salbutamol
Glycine/Glutamine conjugation	Glycine/glutamine	*N*-acyl transferases	Cholic acid, salicylic acid, nicotinic acid, phenylacetic acid
Glutathione conjugation	Glutathione	Glutathione *S* -transferases	Paracetamol, ethacrynic acid
Acetylation	Acetyl-CoA	*N*-acetyl transferases	Histamine, mescaline, procainamide, p-amino salicylic acid, isoniazid, phenelzine, hydralazine, dapsone
Methylation	*S*-adenosyl-L-methionine	Methyl transferase	Morphine, norephedrine nicotine, histamine, iso-prenaline, propylthiou-racil

Source: https://www.ias.ac.in/article/fulltext/reso/019/03/0259-0282#:~:text=Drug%20metabolism%20reactions%20comprise%20of,carbon%2C%20sulfur%20or%20nitrogen%20centre.

As a result, we have included a list of Phase I and II reactions along with the functional groups in the body that are involved in each reaction. We have discussed the drug metabolism's detoxification pathways, but we still need to comprehend how the bioactivation process causes harmful side effects from drug metabolism.

10.2.3. Bioactivation Reactions: Chemistry of Reactive Metabolites and Adverse Drug Effects

In certain cases, the drug metabolism process can result in the production of Reactive Metabolites (RM), which can cause additional toxicity. There are several types of toxicity, including immune-mediated adverse drug reactions (ADRs) and genotoxicity. Adverse drug reactions pose significant challenges to both clinical drug development and drug therapy. Since the liver is in charge of the majority of metabolic reactions, it is the organ most frequently impacted by adverse drug reactions. Because these RMs have a chemically reactive group that produces ADRs, they are specifically referred to as Chemically Reactive Metabolites (CRMs).

10.2.3.1. Structural Alerts

Several functional groups associated with the generation of CRMs constitute the structural alerts. Some well-known structural alerts are epoxides, furan, thiophene, anilines, anilides; arylacetic acids; hydrazines; thiophenes; terminal alkenes; nitroaromatics; quinones, quinone-methide, etc., as shown in Figure 10.12.

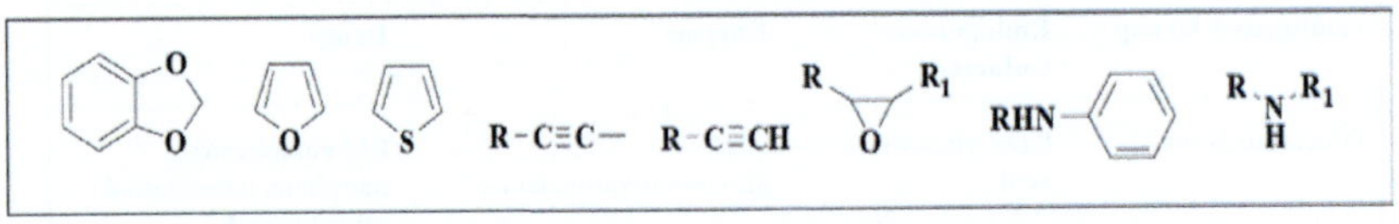

Figure 10.12. *Structural alerts associated with the generation of reactive metabolites in the body.*

Source: https://www.ias.ac.in/article/fulltext/reso/019/03/0259-0282#:~:text=Drug%20 metabolism%20reactions%20comprise%20of,carbon%2C%20sulfur%20or%20nitrogen%20centre.

But the kind and intensity of negative reactions might not always be indicated by the mere existence of these substructures that could form CRMs. Because they have a higher benefit-to-risk ratio than other drugs on the market, many of them have one structural alert or another. g. sulphonamides of aniline as anti-infective agents. Sometimes there is so much clearance that the toxic effects are not noticed. For instance, glucoronidation and sulphation of phenolic OH groups eliminate raloxifene (a medication used to treat osteoporosis), reducing the quantity of quinone and quinone-methide reactive metabolites that are produced. Early on in the drug discovery process, structural alerts have been effectively applied. One example of this is the ocular pain reliever bromofenac, which included aniline, arylacetic acid, and a bromophenyl ring as structural alerts. The carboxylic acid is a structural alert that has drawn everyone's attention. The majority of non-steroidal anti-inflammatory drugs (NSAIDs), including diclofenac and aspirin. , have a carboxylate function, and result in a variety of adverse drug reactions. Consequently, it's critical to comprehend the significance of a number of functional groups that could otherwise trigger harmful bodily reactions.

10.2.3.2. Structure–Toxicity Relationship

Certain functional groups can be qualified as the structural alerts using a variety of techniques. DEREK software is used in one methodology. Based on an examination of their chemical structures, the computer program DEREK, which stands for Deductive Estimation of Risk from Existing

Knowledge, is intended to help toxicologists and chemists anticipate probable regions of potential toxicological risk for novel compounds.

Table 10.12. *Differential Metabolism of Drugs, Where One is Toxic and the Other Non-Toxic, Representing Structure–Toxicity Relationship*

Predecessor Drug	Toxic Reaction Pathway	Successor Drug (devoid of toxicity)
Clozapine (hepatotoxicity, agranulocytosis)	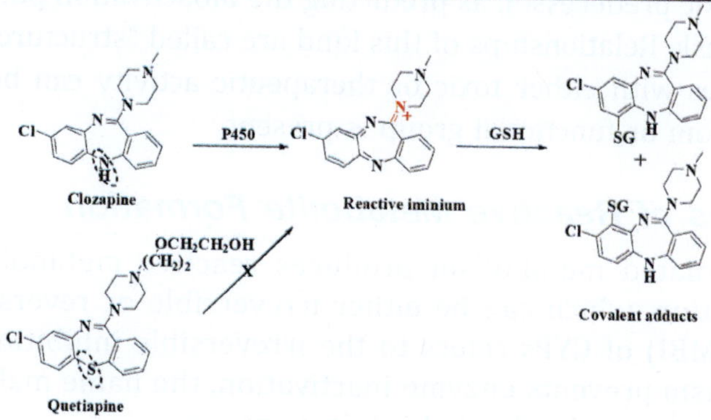	Quetiapine (rare agranulocytosis)
Halothane (hepatotoxin)	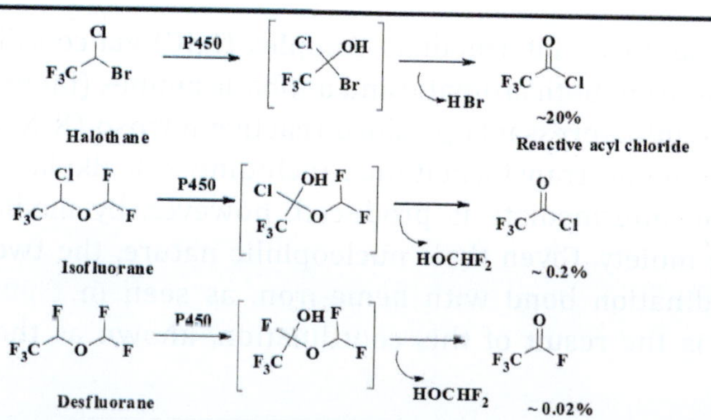	Isofluorane, desfluorane (no hepatotoxicity)
Tolcapone (idiosyncratic hepatotoxicity)	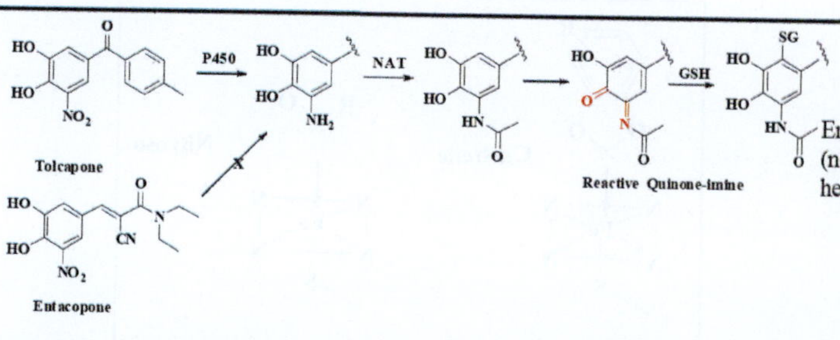	Entacopone (no hepatotoxicity)

Source: *https://www.ias.ac.in/article/fulltext/reso/019/03/0259-0282#:~:text=Drug%20 metabolism%20reactions%20comprise%20of,carbon%2C%20sulfur%20or%20nitrogen%20centre.*

The predictions of this knowledge-based expert system for identifying different structural alerts are partly derived from alerts that characterize structural characteristics or toxicophores linked to toxicity. But as of yet, no in silico tool exists that can be used to forecast when bioactivation and additional toxicity in a drug candidate will occur. There are computational tools available that can predict drug candidates' metabolic transformations, like MetaSite. The structure of the metabolites formed is provided by a computational process that uses a ranking derived from predictions of the site of metabolism. It helps chemists focus their compound design to reduce CYP-mediated metabolism by predicting "hot spots" in the molecule. In order to place the site of metabolism close to the catalytic center, it also draws attention to the molecular moieties that aid in directing the molecule within the cytochrome cavity. It cannot, however, foretell a drug candidate's bioactivation pathway. Understanding structural alerts would help with effective drug design, as it would ensure that a successful drug candidate lacks the structural alert found in a toxic predecessor, as predicting the bioactivation pathways of potential drug candidates is a challenging task. Relationships of this kind are called "structure–toxicity" relationships. A selection of drug molecules with either toxic or therapeutic activity can be found in Table 10.12, depending on whether an atom or functional group is present.

10.2.3.3. Consequences of Reactive Metabolite Formation

Most of the time, CYP-mediated metabolism produces reactive metabolites (RMs), which can cause an enzyme's inactivation, which can be either irreversible or reversible. Mechanism-based inhibition or inactivation (MBI) of CYPs refers to the irreversible inhibition or inactivation of an enzyme. Because a mechanism prevents enzyme inactivation, the name makes sense. Based on the mechanism, these inactivations can be divided into two groups:

- Formation of a metabolic-intermediate complex (MIC) via coordination between reactive species and heme-iron: Both aromatic and aliphatic amines (tamoxifen, an anticancer drug; nortriptyline, an antidepressant) produce reactive nitroso (R-N=O) intermediate through a variety of metabolic transformations, including Ndealkylation and N-hydroxylation. Reactive carbene intermediate is produced, however, by medications that contain the 1,3-benzdioxole moiety. Given their nucleophilic nature, the two intermediates combine to form a coordination bond with heme-iron, as seen in Figure 10.13. The inhibition of CYP activity is the result of this coordination, known as the metabolic-intermediate complex (MIC).

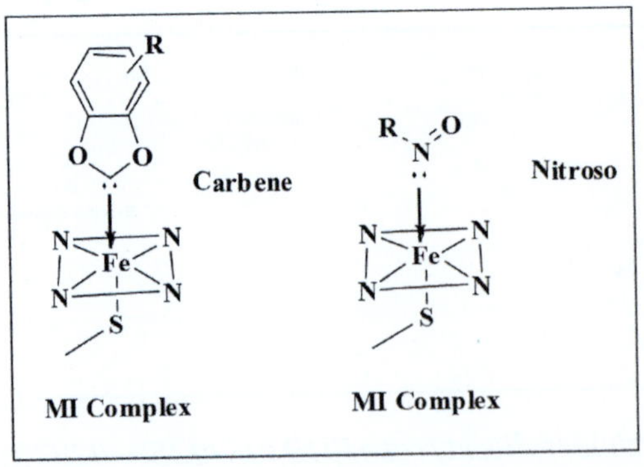

Figure 10.13. *A representation of coordination between reactive carbene/nitroso species and heme-iron, leading to formation of metabolic–intermediate complex (MIC).*

Source: https://www.ias.ac.in/article/fulltext/reso/019/03/0259-0282#:~:text=Drug%20metabolism%20reactions%20comprise%20of,carbon%2C%20sulfur%20or%20nitrogen%20centre.

Figures 10.14 and 10.15 shows the formation of reactive carbene intermediate from 1,3-benzdioxole moiety. Drugs such as stiripentol (antiepileptic), paroxetine (antidepressant), etc., possess this moiety, which acts as a perpetrator, and leads to mechanismbased inhibition of CYPs.

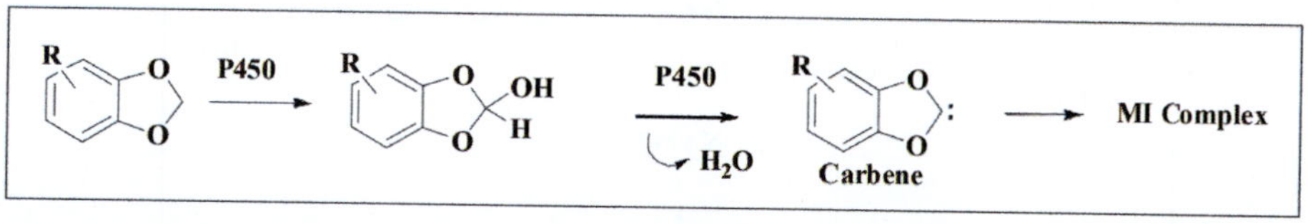

Figure 10.14. *Schematic pathway for the formation of reactive carbene species, starting from 1,3-benzdioxole moiety.*

Source: https://www.ias.ac.in/article/fulltext/reso/019/03/0259-0282#:~:text=Drug%20 metabolism%20reactions%20comprise%20of,carbon%2C%20sulfur%20or%20nitrogen%20centre.

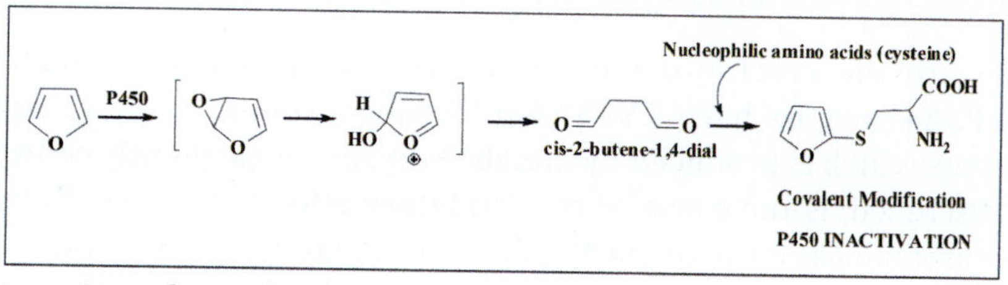

Figure 10.15. *Schematic pathway for the formation of reactive epoxide intermediate and nucleophilic adducts leading to MBI of CYPs, starting from furan moiety.*

Source: https://www.ias.ac.in/article/fulltext/reso/019/03/0259-0282#:~:text=Drug%20 metabolism%20reactions%20comprise%20of,carbon%2C%20sulfur%20or%20nitrogen%20centre.

- Covalent modification of reactive species with heme or amino acid residues: medications that produce reactive epoxide intermediate can cause mechanism-based inhibition of CYPs. These medications include thiophene, furan, olefin, and phenyl groups. Through the creation of a covalent bond as a result of nucleophilic active site residues opening the epoxide ring, CYP activity is inhibited. Additionally, quinone-imine and quinone-methide are reactive species that can form covalent bonds and cause MBI.. A few medications, including the HIV protease inhibitor L-754,394, form a reactive epoxide intermediate.

Another drug that lowers GSH levels by binding covalently to liver macromolecules is paracetamol, whose quinone-imine metabolite (N-acetyl p-benzoquinone-imine; NAPQI) is reactive (Figure 10.16). The body experiences hepatic necrosis as a result. Drug-drug interactions (DDIs) can result from this CYP inactivation and have potentially harmful effects on the body. For instance, hypertensive patients receiving simvastatin along with a calcium-channel blocker and a strong CYP3A4 inactivator, mibefradil, have been shown to exhibit a higher incidence of myopathy, or muscular weakness, and rhabdomyolysis, or the breakdown products of injured skeletal muscles released into the bloodstream. Here, the mechanism for DDI is the inactivation of the CYP-catalyzed simvastatin metabolism process by mibefradil, which further raises the plasma levels of statin and ultimately causes death. Because of these potentially fatal effects, mibefradil was eventually taken off the market.

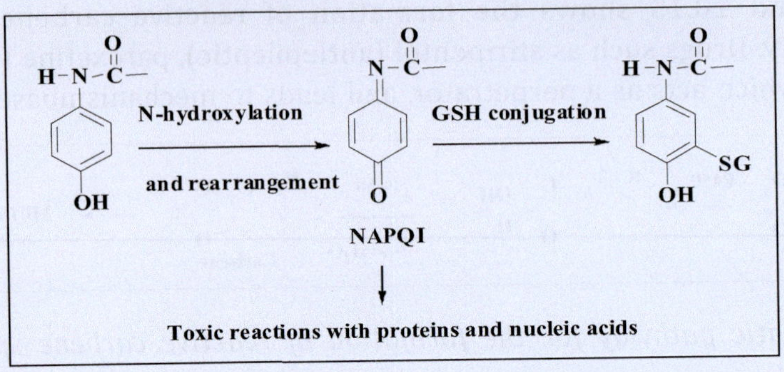

Figure 10.16. *Schematic pathway for the metabolism of paracetamol to the toxic NAPQI metabolite.*

Source: https://www.ias.ac.in/article/fulltext/reso/019/03/0259-0282#:~:text=Drug%20metabolism%20reactions%20comprise%20of,carbon%2C%20sulfur%20or%20nitrogen%20centre.

Other instances are the erectile dysfunction medication tadalafil, which is known to be metabolized by CYP3A4 and to have CYP3A4-inhibiting properties. It is suggested that the 1,3-benzodioxole group, which is produced by metabolism and subsequently coordinates with heme iron as previously discussed, is the cause of the inhibitory effects. As a result, long-term use of it may have negative consequences for patients. Parallel to this, paroxetine, an antidepressant, functions as a strong inhibitor of CYP2D6 by producing a reactive carbene intermediate that causes heme-iron to form a coordination bond with it. Since DDIs can result from the inactivation of enzymes, new compounds that target the major human CYP enzymes through mechanism-based inactivation are regularly evaluated within the context of drug discovery. Previously discussed topics included drug metabolism's fundamentals, detoxification, bioactivation pathways, and the bioinorganic and bioorganic chemistry of drug metabolism. The rate at which a drug is metabolized determines its pharmacological action, duration, toxicity, biological half-life, and intensity. Therefore, identifying the factors that impact this process is necessary.

10.3. Drug Metabolism: Approaches, Function and Education

The metabolism of both endogenous and exogenous substances is included in drug metabolism. Most medications lose their pharmacological effects and are eliminated from the body during metabolism. Dust, food, toxins, and air pollutants are just a few of the foreign particles to which the human body is exposed. We refer to these foreign particles as xenobiotics as a group. Xeno refers to something that is foreign to us and not typically found in our bodies. The body possesses a mechanism to alter foreign particles upon their entry and facilitate their expulsion from the body. Metabolism is the term for this process. Drugs are considered foreign particles, hence they are also considered xenobiotics. Biotransformation is another term for the drug metabolism process. Normally, metabolism reduces the pharmacological effect, but occasionally it generates active or toxic metabolites. Prodrugs are substances that go through a metabolic process in order to have a pharmacological effect. Certain medications are broken down into hazardous, mutagenic, or carcinogenic metabolites. The primary site of metabolism in the body is the liver. First-pass effects are caused by certain medications that are metabolized before entering the bloodstream. The kidney, skin, gastrointestinal tract (GIT), and other organs are also involved in drug metabolism. As chemical substances that the body does not naturally produce, most drugs are classified as xenobiotics. Through a variety of bodily processes, xenobiotics are detoxified, lowering their toxicity and making them more easily excreted. These procedures, also referred to as metabolic biotransformation or drug metabolism, enable the chemical conversion of pharmaceuticals into their metabolites.

These metabolites, which come in three different forms—toxic, inactive, and active—are the end products of drug metabolism. Inactive metabolites are biochemically inert substances that have neither toxic nor therapeutic effects, whereas active metabolites are biochemically active substances that have therapeutic effects. Similar to active metabolites, toxic metabolites are biochemically active substances that can cause a variety of negative consequences. A low concentration of active metabolites is found in the systemic circulation as a result of drug metabolism, which takes place at a particular site in the body. First-pass metabolism is the term given to this phenomenon, which restricts the bioavailability of drugs. Enzymes that catalyze metabolism are present all over the body, but first-pass metabolism mostly takes place in the liver. It is essential to comprehend these changes in chemical activity in order to choose the best pharmacological intervention for each patient. Any healthcare professional who regularly administers medication to patients should be interested in this topic.

10.3.1. Function

Drug excretion from the body is mainly carried out by the kidneys; however, lipophilic drugs are easily absorbed back into the bloodstream by passing through the renal tubules' cell membrane. Therefore, before the drug can be excreted, lipophilic drugs must first be metabolized in the liver. Phase I (modification), Phase II (conjugation), and occasionally Phase III (additional modification and excretion) are the different reactions that can occur during drug metabolism. Phase I modifications include oxidation, reduction, hydrolysis, cyclization/decyclization, and addition or subtraction of oxygen from more polar molecules in order to change the chemical structure of lipophilic drugs. This process can occasionally turn an inactive prodrug into a medication that is metabolically active. Most metabolites produced by oxidation still have some degree of pharmacological activity. Phase I modification, for instance, changes the popular anxiolytic medication diazepam into desmethyldiazepam and oxazepam. The physiological and psychological effects of diazepam and its metabolites are comparable. The majority of phase I reactions are catalyzed by the cytochrome P450 system, also referred to as microsomal mixed function oxidase. A drug molecule couples with another molecule in a conjugation reaction during phase II modifications. Conjugation typically makes the compound water soluble and pharmacologically inert, facilitating easy excretion. Methylation, acetylation, sulphation, glucuronidation, and glutathione or glycine conjugation are examples of conjugation mechanisms. These processes can take place in the kidney, liver, lungs, intestines, and other organ systems, among other places. Oxazepam is an example of phase II metabolism; it conjugates with glucuronide, a different molecule.

Without undergoing any additional chemical changes, the medication becomes physiologically inactive and is eliminated. Phase II metabolism, during which conjugates and metabolites are eliminated from the cells, may also be followed by phase III metabolism. Phase I and II process enzymatic catalysis is a crucial component of drug metabolism. For drugs to be efficiently metabolized, liver enzyme composition and concentration are essential. The two enzymes that are most frequently utilized in medicine are cytochrome P450 and monoamine oxidase. These two enzymes are in charge of breaking down numerous xenobiotic and biogenic substances. Monoamine oxidase, as its name implies, catalyzes the breakdown of monoamines, including dopamine and serotonin. Antidepressants called monoamine oxidase inhibitors (MAOI) raise dopamine and serotonin levels in the brain. The family of heme-containing isoenzymes known as the cytochrome P450 system is mainly found in the liver and gastrointestinal tract and is in charge of breaking down a wide range of medications and substances, including steroids and lipids. Amphetamines and opioids are among the many psychoactive substances that cytochrome P450 catalyzes the metabolism of.

10.3.2. Issues of Concern

Drug plasma concentrations can be impacted by drug metabolism, which needs to be taken into account. Drug interactions should worry prescribers because they can have a detrimental effect on the patient's health. For instance, imatinib's plasma concentrations may decrease if rifampin is taken concurrently with imatinib because rifampin can activate CYP3A4 and metabolize imatinib considerably more quickly. As a result, the anticancer effect of imatinib may be diminished. Similarly, imatinib's plasma concentrations rise when omeprazole is taken concurrently with imatinib to treat gastroesophageal reflux disease (GERD). This happens because imatinib is metabolized by CYP3A4, which is strongly inhibited by omeprazole. Imatinib builds up as a result of CYP3A4 inhibition, which can be toxic. Another element that influences drug metabolism is aging. Age-related slowing of drug metabolism increases the risk of side effects in elderly patients. The patient's age should be taken into consideration by prescribers when writing prescriptions. Patients may respond differently to different medications due to genetic polymorphism in the enzymes that break down drugs.

10.3.3. Clinical Significance

Any pharmacological intervention necessitates careful consideration of the drug's mode of elimination from the body by the prescribing physician. The majority of the time, first-order kinetics govern drug clearance; in other words, the drug's plasma concentration determines the clearance rate. In other words, the drug's concentration is directly correlated with the elimination rate. The chemical in question determines the rate of this type of clearance, which is frequently expressed as a half-life. This is how long it takes for the body to get rid of 50% of the medication. For instance, cocaine has a half-life of roughly 1 h, meaning that after 4 h, the body has only retained 6–25% of the initial dose. On the other hand, some medications are eliminated at a steady pace that is unaffected by plasma concentrations. As an illustration, ethanol is excreted from the body at a steady rate of roughly 15 milliliters/ h, independent of its bloodstream concentration. When low concentrations of an enzyme bind to its binding sites, a phenomenon known as zero-order kinetics takes place. Medicine is interested in kinetics because many medications require clinically significant drug concentration monitoring. Providers can modify patient-specific therapies by having a thorough understanding of pharmacokinetics (Bolton et al., 2004), specifically drug elimination. The goal of therapy is to reach a steady-state plasma concentration where drug elimination and metabolism happen at the same time.

A number of variables can affect metabolism, which is a highly variable process. Depot binding, which occurs when drug molecules attach to inactive sites in the body and become unavailable for metabolism, is a significant perturber of drug metabolism. Drugs that are susceptible to depot binding may have a shorter half-life as a result. One famous instance is the primary psychoactive ingredient in marijuana, tetrahydrocannabinol (THC) (Patilea-Vrana, et al., 2019). Users' adipose tissue is where THC binds because it is highly lipid-soluble. This interaction causes the drug's metabolism to be significantly slowed, which is why weeks after the patient's last use, THC metabolites can be found in their urine. Enzyme stimulation is another aspect of drug metabolism. The application of the same substance repeatedly induces enzymes. As a result of the drug's continuous presence, the body adjusts by producing more of the enzymes required for the drug's metabolism. Patients may require higher and higher dosages of some medications to achieve the same results, which is related to pharmacological tolerance. The main example is opioids. When prescribed opioid analgesics are used for an extended period, patients notice a decrease in the effectiveness of their medication. Notably, all drugs processed by the enzyme-induced method have a higher metabolic rate upon induction; chronic amphetamine use, for instance, results in elevated CYP2D6 concentrations. To achieve the intended result, a doctor prescribing oxycodone to a patient who uses amphetamines would need to prescribe a higher dose because this enzyme is also necessary for the metabolism of some opioids, including oxycodone.

On the other hand, certain medications can inhibit certain enzymes, increasing the patient's susceptibility to other medications that are metabolized by those enzymes. Monoamine oxidase inhibition caused by some antidepressants is a well-known example. These substances block the enzyme in the brain that breaks down "pleasure" chemicals, which has psychotherapeutic effects. But when people taking other medications while taking an MAOI, it can lead to abnormally high concentrations of these neurochemicals, which can cause issues. Cocaine, which increases serotonin, dopamine, and norepinephrine concentrations, will have a far more potent effect on a patient taking an MAOI. Numerous physiological issues, such as tachycardia, hypertension, and serotonin syndrome, can result from this interaction. Drugs with similar metabolic pathways may also "compete" for the same binding sites on enzymes, reducing the efficiency of the enzymes' metabolism. For example, the same cytochrome P450 family member metabolizes alcohol and some sedatives. There are very few enzymes that can degrade these substances. One reason that alcohol and other sedative or hypnotic drugs can work well together when given together is that pentobarbital would not be fully metabolized if it were given to a patient who is also metabolizing alcohol because alcohol molecules would occupy the majority of the necessary enzymes.

10.3.4. Enhancing Healthcare Team Outcomes

A critical clinical concern for the interdisciplinary healthcare team is drug metabolism. In order to avoid clinically significant drug interactions that could have an impact on patients' health, pharmacists and clinicians must collaborate. Nurses keep an eye out for any indications of a hazardous accumulation of metabolites or active medications in a hospital setting. This is particularly important in cases of hepatic or renal insufficiency. Pharmacists dose and oversee the administration of medications, including warfarin, aminoglycoside antibiotics, and fluoroquinolones, by keeping an eye on the drugs' serum levels and renal function. The best chance for achieving the best possible patient care is to use an interprofessional approach to drug dosing and administration in light of the effects of drug metabolism on patients, whether through impaired metabolism, drug-drug interactions, enzymatic induction, or other factors. With fewer unfavorable events, the interprofessional care approach produces better therapeutic outcomes. ..

10.3.5. Nursing, Allied Health, and Interprofessional Team Interventions

Positive results depend on interprofessional interventions and oversight. Researchers have found that interprofessional interventions work best when teams are willing and able to work together, communicate, share decision-making, coordinate care, and eventually integrate their competencies. An effective component of medication management through monitoring and interventions is the use of interprofessional teams. People react differently to medications, as was previously mentioned. Therefore, if the right steps are not taken, patients may be more vulnerable to unfavorable outcomes. When patients are not taking or administering medications safely, or if they are being taken improperly, teams need to keep an eye on things and take appropriate action. Patient safety should always come first. For interprofessional team monitoring to be effective, adverse events must be reported. Clinical teams should also receive training in order to perform monitoring and interventions correctly. Training can be given on a variety of subjects, including standardizing medication dispensing, recognizing medication errors to prevent adverse events, and effective team communication. Credits for Continuous Medication ought to focus on both monitoring and intervention. In order to provide healthcare, communication is essential. The methods used by interprofessional teams to follow patients through the continuum of care need to be improved.

Effective interprofessional education also fosters collaboration, interdisciplinary awareness, respect, and acceptance of the roles that various disciplines play in healthcare delivery. But one must also take the difficulties into account. Every discipline has a distinct methodology and culture. They differ in terms of professional language, qualifications, accountability, and routines as well as rules and regulations. This makes it challenging to standardize on any interventions or drug monitoring. But acknowledging these difficulties is the first step toward making a change. These issues can be resolved, and professionals in all fields—nurses, pharmacists, and doctors—will receive the necessary training to enable them to monitor medication for better health outcomes at any point during the course of treatment.

10.3.6. Drug Metabolism and Drug Design

In the design and development of new drugs, understanding drug metabolism is crucial. A few non-reactive groups that thwart drug metabolism are added if the new drug is rapidly metabolized by the body. For instance, the anti-diabetic medication tolbutamide (Figure 10.17) has a shorter half-life of 2.5 h. Its methyl group is changed into a carboxyl group during the metabolic process. Drug metabolism has a substantial impact on a drug's pharmacokinetic, pharmacodynamic, and safety. Chlorpropamide, when the methyl group is substituted with a chlorine atom, achieves a longer half-life (12–15 h) than tolbutamide. Prodrugs are pharmaceuticals that are given in inactive forms. A prodrug is a medication that has had its chemical makeup altered to address issues with excretion, metabolism, absorption, and administration. Liquid functional groups found in prodrugs are readily metabolized by the body. For instance, carbamate, phosphate, and ester. Oral bioavailability is enhanced by masking of polar functional. As an illustration, prodrugs of chloramphenicol and ampicillin are chloramphenicol palmitate and bacampicillin, respectively.

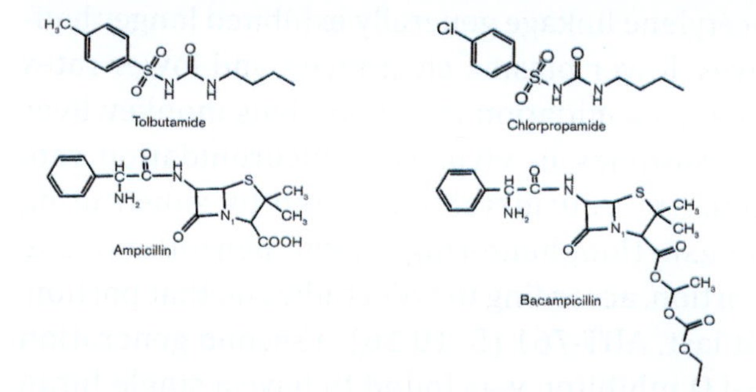

Figure 10.17. *Drug metabolism and drug design.*
Source: https://cdnintech.com/media/chapter/88053/1707895542/media/F18.png.

10.3.6.1. In silico Pharmacokinetic Studies

Poor pharmacokinetic properties account for about 40% of new drug failures in clinical trials. SwissADME, ADMETlab, and pkCSM web tools are now used to assess the pharmacokinetic properties of new compounds. Three-dimensional structures of compounds are created using online software, and calculations are made for their pharmacokinetic characteristics, or ADMET (absorption, distribution, metabolism, excretion, and toxicity). The oral activity of drug molecules depends on several properties, which can be predicted, including GI absorption, BBB permeation, P-gp substrate, cytochrome P450 enzyme inhibition/induction, and skin permeation. Understanding the behavior of drug molecules in the human body is aided by the prediction of pharmacokinetic properties. The expensive experimental approach is lessened with the aid of in silico predictions. The Lipinski Rule of Five also predicts the drug-likeness of novel molecules. This rule states that drug molecules with more than five hydrogen bond donors, more than ten hydrogen bond acceptors, more than five logP, and more than 500 daltons in molecular weight have a lower probability of being orally active. Drug molecules absorb poorly when they have a high lipophilicity. Compounds with large weights are also less likely to be absorbed by the GIT. Of the medications, 80% have a molecular weight of less than 450 daltons. Additionally molecules with polar surface areas less than 140°A and fewer rotatable bonds than 10 demonstrate good oral bioavailability. Pharmacological compounds that adhere to the RO5 have a higher chance of being approved for sale and a lower likelihood of failing clinical trials.

10.3.7. Improving PK and PD Properties

10.3.7.1. Metabolic Soft Spot

Drugs must enter the body and reach the site(s) of action to start having pharmacological effects. However, if drugs show inferior PK properties. Their PD effects are probably going to be less than ideal due to their high clearance, short half-life (t1/2), and low bioavailability after oral dosing. Studies of in vitro metabolism in animal and human tissue (e.g., drug metabolism pathways, or "soft spots," can be identified through the use of liver) preparations and/or in vivo metabolism studies in animals. The most preferred metabolic soft spots when these groups are not sterically hindered and are subject to P450 mediated metabolism are known to be the benzylic C–H bond, the allylic methyl, and the O–, N–, and S–methyl groups. Due to the nature of the hydroxylation reactions catalyzed by enzymes, the intrinsic reactivity of the substrate sites accessible to the ferryl oxidizing species in the P450-substrate complex plays a major role in determining the chemo- and regiospecificity of substrate oxidation as well as the rate of metabolism. The intrinsic reactivity of the functional groups and the substrate specificity of the specific molecule carrying this functional group (soft spot) in metabolizing enzyme systems will therefore determine the tendency to be metabolic soft spots. Replacing identified soft spots with bioisosteres is a common strategy to address the metabolic soft spot issue. Bioisosteres are substituents or groups with related molecular structures, comparable chemical or physical properties, and the potential to produce biological properties that are somewhat similar. For instance, in certain circumstances, a fluorine or chlorine atom, or a -CF3 group, could be utilized in place of a benzylic methyl group when it is determined to be a metabolic soft spot.

In research on the relationship between structure and metabolism, one method of reducing intrinsic clearance is to block a metabolic soft spot. This can result in a lower overall clearance and, if the volume of distribution remains unchanged, a longer half-life for affected molecules. Take Zelepton (1, Figure 10.18) as an example. Asthma maintenance therapy in humans involves the use of a 5-lipoxygenase (5-LO) inhibitor.". In vivo studies on cynomolgus monkeys, Zileuton demonstrated half-lives of 0 and 2 h. Glucuronidation at the N-hydroxyurea moiety to produce metabolite 2 is the main metabolism pathway for zileuton in cynomolgus monkeys and humans (Figure 10.18) and excreted in the urine afterwards. The N-hydroxyurea component is a pharmacophore necessary for activity, according to structure–activity relationship (SAR) studies. Only the linker and benzothiophene regions of zileuton could thus be the target of structural modification to reduce glucuronidation (3, Figure 10.18). A 6-fold increase in the intrinsic clearance (Clint) in cynomolgus monkey liver microsomes, a 2-fold decrease in the half-life, and a 4-fold increase in plasma clearance in cynomolgus monkey in vivo were observed in compound 4, which was the result of the methyl group being removed from the zileuton linkage group.

The glucuronidation at the N-hydroxyurea portion may have been lowered by the steric hindrance of the nearby methyl group from the zileuton linker. According to SAR studies on the linker portion, compounds containing an acetylene linkage generally exhibited longer half-lives, lower plasma clearances, and lower rates of glucuronidation in cynomolgus monkey liver microsomes in vivo. The glucuronidation rate could be considerably lowered by substituting a basic thiophene ring for the benzothiophene portion, according to SAR studies on that portion. At last, ABT-761 (5, 10.16), a second generation 5-LO inhibitor, was found to have a single furan ring and an acetylene linker. In cynomolgus monkey and human liver microsomes, the rate of glucuronidation was >12-fold and >29-fold lower, respectively, than zileuton. In cynomolgus monkeys and humans, ABT-761 demonstrated, respectively, >40- and >29-fold longer half lives than zileuton. Thus, compared to zileuton at the same dosage, ABT-761 demonstrated a markedly higher level of efficacy. ABT-761 only needs to be taken once daily in humans due to its enhanced potency and PK properties, while zileuton requires multiple daily doses. This work showed that it is possible to enhance the PK characteristics of a new chemical entity (NCE) without compromising or improving upon its pharmacological activity by blocking a metabolism soft spot.

Studies on 4-(3,4,5-trimethoxybenzoyl)-2-phenylthiazole SMART-H (6, Figure10.18) have examined 4-substituted methoxybenzoyl-aryl-thiozoles as novel anti-cancer agents was found to be a lead that exhibited strong inhibitory effects on tubulin polymerization and cancer cell proliferation. In contrast, SMART-H demonstrated significant metabolic instability in liver microsomes from humans, dogs, rats, and mice, with in vitro half-lives varying from less than five to thirty minutes. The reduction of the ketone functional group was the primary metabolism pathway, according to SMART-H metabolite profiling in human liver microsomes. O-demethylation of SMART-H methoxy groups was the second most common metabolic pathway. As a result, the ketone and methoxy groups of SMART-H were identified as metabolically sensitive areas. In the case of SMART-173A (7) and SMART-176A (8, Figure 10.18), the ketone group was substituted with an oxime group and a hydrazide group. In human liver microsomes, SMART-173A and SMART-176A showed a 3- and 2-fold, respectively, increase in metabolic stability.

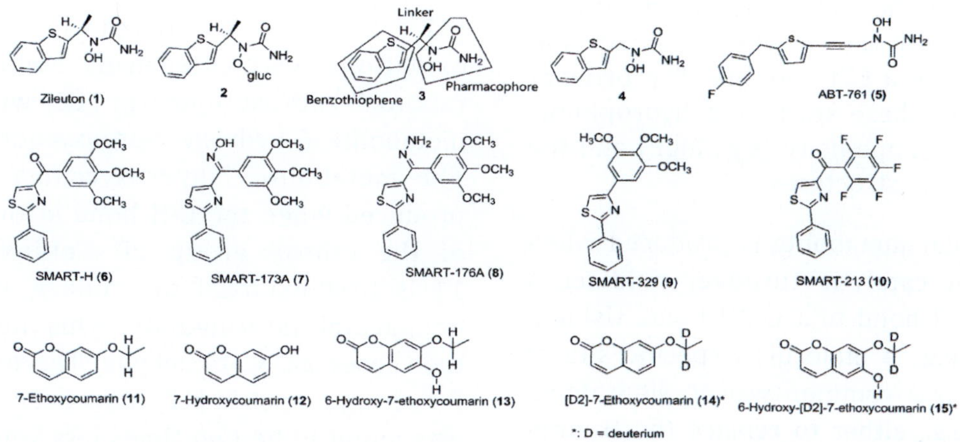

Figure 10.18. *Structures of zileuton (1), SMART-H (6), 7-ethoxycoumarin (11) and their analogs or metabolites.*

Source: https://www.ncbi.nlm.nih.gov/pmc/articles/PMC6146880/bin/gr1.jpg.

While SMART-176A significantly lost the anticancer activity with an average IC50 value of 1250 nmol/L, SMART-173A retained some of the anticancer activity against four prostate tumor cell lines, with an average IC50 value of 143 nmol/L (compared to 44 nmol/L for SMART-H). After removing SMART-H's most labile ketone functional group, SMART-329 (9, Figure 10.18) The metabolic stability was doubled by 2-fold. On the other hand, SMART-329 lost all anticancer activity, indicating that the ketone functional group is essential for anticancer action. Upon substituting fluorine atoms for the second soft spot (consisting of three methoxy groups) in SMART-H, SMART-213 (10, Figure 10.18). There was no anticancer activity and only a slight change in metabolic stability. This implies that the methoxy groups may be involved in the anticancer action as well. It is therefore plausible that structural alteration on or near a lead compound's metabolic soft spots could have a deleterious effect on biological activity.

10.3.7.2. Metabolic Switching And Deuterium Replacement

A large number of small molecule medications are processed by the body's cytochrome P450 (CYP) enzymes. CYPs are a class of enzymes that primarily reside in the endoplasmic reticulum of hepatocytes. They are responsible for a variety of oxidative and reductive biotransformations, such as halocarbon dehalogenation, carbon hydroxylation, bond oxidation, heteroatom oxidation, and hydrocarbon desaturation. When a drug is biotransformed into a metabolite by CYP-catalyzed biotransformation, it first binds to the enzyme's active site and then catalytically turns it into a metabolite via a process known as the P450 catalytic cycle. Although the relationship between the structure and metabolism of drugs involving CYPs is complicated and poorly understood, it is widely acknowledged that the main CYP enzymes that are involved in drug metabolism, such as CYP3A, which favors lipophilic substrates and has a large active site. Although substrates rarely interact with CYP through hydrogen bonding or ionic interactions, the binding and orientation of a substrate are frequently dictated by the hydrophobic and steric interactions of the substrate with the specific amino acids at the active site of a CYP enzyme. The primary determinant of these steric and hydrophobic interactions is lipophilicity (e.g., logP) and the substrates' steric structures.

A particular metabolite is produced when a subsequent catalytic turnover oxidizes a substrate's C-H bond to a C-OH bond. Using a substituent (e.g., a molecule's specific site of metabolism) is a common way to slow down or block it; e.g., either to replace the H-atom in the molecule's C-H bond or to move a bulky group into a nearby location to lessen or prevent the accessibility of the iron-bound oxidizing species of the P450 enzyme (a bioisostere, a bulky group, a halogen or a deuterium atom). Once the molecule is bound within the active site, the intrinsic reactivity of the sites on the molecule that are accessible to the iron-bound oxidizing species in the CYP active site then plays a major role in determining the specific site of metabolism in the substrate where the structural modification occurs. Because of the makeup of the CYP enzyme's active site(s) (e.g., Because CYP 3A4) has a large space binding pocket, blocking the soft spot (also known as the metabolically labile site) of a lead molecule with one of the substituents mentioned above may alter the binding and orientation of the newly synthesized molecule, changing the original metabolism site to a different C-H bond and causing the formation of other metabolite(s) to a greater extent than that of the lead compound. Because CYP enzymes can have multiple binding sites, it's also possible that a new molecule will bind to the metabolizing enzyme's alternative binding site if a lead molecule's soft spot is blocked by structural modification. This would result in metabolism of the new molecule on a different site.

The phenomenon of metabolic switching is not unusual. As an illustration, 7-ethoxycoumarin (11, Figure 10.18). Through CYP1A1-mediated oxidations, was extensively metabolized in rats to 7-hydroxycoumarin (12) with a minor metabolite 6-hydroxy-7-ethoxycoumarin (13). The metabolite 7-hydroxycoumarin (12) is produced when the C-H bond at the α-carbon of the ethoxy group of 7-ethoxycoumarin 11 is first oxidized to produce an unstable hemiacetal intermediate. This intermediate then loses an acetaldehyde. The formation of 7-hydroxycoumarin (12) in rat liver microsomes was found to be two times less when exposed to [D2]-7-Ethoxycoumarin (14), which is the product of substituting two hydrogen atoms with deuterium atoms at the α-carbon of the ethoxy group of 7-ethoxycoumarin 11. In contrast to 7-ethoxycoumarin (11) however, [D2]-7-ethoxycoumarin (14) demonstrated a 5-fold increase in the formation of 6-hydroxy-[D2]-7-ethoxycoumarinin (15) in rat liver microsomes, leading to nearly no change in overall metabolic stability. This finding implies that the oxidation of the C-H bond at the ethoxy group's α-carbon in 7-ethoxycoumarin 11 (Figure 10.19A) was changed to [D2]-7-ethoxycoumarin 14's C-H bond oxidation at position 6 (Figure 10.19B). Therefore, targeting a lead molecule's metabolically labile sites, also known as "soft spots," requires a methodical SAR process in which a number of variables, such as lipophilicity, stereochemistry, and intrinsic reactivity, should be taken into account during the drug design phase. The "isotope effect" is a technique used in the design of new bioactive molecules to block a metabolic soft spot or change the metabolism's path by substituting deuterium atoms for hydrogen atoms.

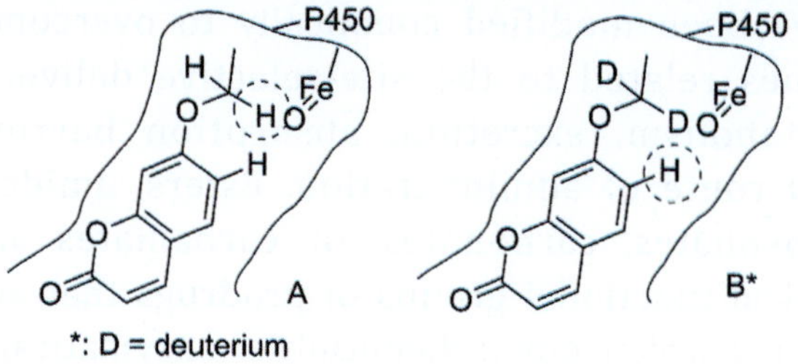

Figure 10.19. *Schematic presentation for oxidation of the C-H bond at the α-carbon of the ethoxy group of 7-ethoxycoumarin (A) and for oxidation of the C-H bond at the 6-position of [D2]-7-ethoxycoumarin (B) at the active site of a cytochrome P450 enzyme.*

Source: https://www.ncbi.nlm.nih.gov/pmc/articles/PMC6146880/bin/gr2.jpg.

The deuterated molecule may have decreased metabolism on the carbon atom where the deuterium atom is attached because the carbon-deuterium bond is more difficult to break than the carbon-hydrogen bond. This could potentially lower the in vitro and in vivo clearance or change the metabolism. The search for novel CNS-penetrant and mGlu3-selective negative allosteric modulators served as an example of this. Regarding SAR research, compound 16 (Figure 10.20) was found to be a lead possessing strong biological activity. Compound 16 was found to be metabolically unstable in liver microsomes of both humans and rats, with a calculated hepatic clearance of 18.9 mL/min/kg for humans and 54.01 mL/min/kg for rats. The primary O-demethylation pathway (soft spot) for 16 was CYP-mediated. The extremely shallow allosteric ligand SAR meant that traditional electronic or steric perturbations could not resolve this soft spot issue.

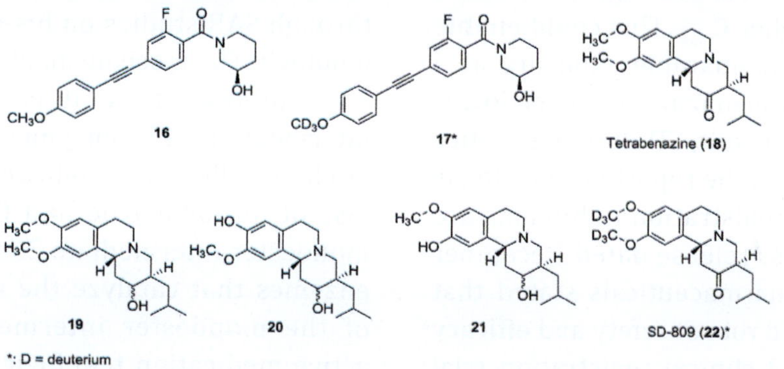

Figure 10.20. *Structures of compound 16, tetrabenazine (18) and their analogs or metabolites.*

Source: https://www.ncbi.nlm.nih.gov/pmc/articles/PMC6146880/bin/gr3.jpg.

Nevertheless, by substituting the deuterium atoms (17, Figure 10.20) for the hydrogen atoms in the -OCH3 group of 16, the computed hepatic clearance of rats fell from 54.1 mL/min/kg for compound 16 to 35.9 mL/min/kg for compound 17. Likewise, the plasma clearance of these rats dropped following IV dosing, going from 5.2 mL/min/kg for 16 to 2.9 mL/min/kg for 17. The potential metabolic switching for 17 may be the cause of the observed decreased deuterium effect. By replacing the deuterium, a novel compound was prepared, necessitating additional in vitro and in vivo biological testing.

Tetrabenazine (18, Figure 10.20) provides an additional example., where the new drug form with significantly better safety profiles is its deuterated version. One medication that is sold to treat chorea linked to Huntington's disease is tetrabenazine, which undergoes significant metabolism to produce an active metabolite 19 (Figure 10.20), which is subsequently converted to active metabolites 20 and 21 through additional metabolism by the polymorphic enzyme CYP2D6 (Figure 10.20). But the documented negative clinical outcomes, e.g., not only the drug's high $C_{ma}x$ but also the patients' varying levels of active metabolites because of CYP2D6 polymorphism may be linked to sedation, somnolence, fatigue, and insomnia. To find a dose that lessens chorea while still being well tolerated, it is necessary to individually monitor and gradually titrate the dosage over several weeks. The SD-809 (22, Figure 10.20), a deuterated tetrabenazine that aims to modify the O-demethylation reaction, is offered by Auspex Pharmaceuticals. In comparison to tetrabenazine in humans, SD-809 exhibited a longer half-life, higher exposure, and a marginally higher C_{max}. This could enable patients to receive comparable exposure at a lower Cmax than tetrabenazine at a much lower dose of SD-809. As a result, SD-809 might offer a better safety profile if the reported side effects of tetrabenazine administration in humans are C_{max}-driven. In a press release dated December 16, 2014, Auspex Pharmaceuticals stated that SD-809 demonstrated robust safety and efficacy outcomes in phase 3 clinical registration trial studies. SD-809 (Austedo) was approved by the FDA on April 3, 2017, to treat chorea linked to Huntington's disease. The FDA has indeed approved SD-809 (Austedo) as the first deuterated product for human use.

10.3.7.3. Prodrugs or Active Metabolites as New Drug Candidates

Prodrugs are a class of medications administered in an inactive pharmacological form and are converted to an active pharmacological form in vivo by chemical or enzymatic means. Traditionally, pharmacologically active molecules have been modified chemically to overcome issues related to the site-selective delivery, metabolism, excretion, absorption barrier, and route of administration. Esters, amides, phosphates, carbonates, or carbamates are typical functional groups of prodrugs that are readily broken down chemically or enzymatically in the body. Prodrugs are frequently used to improve oral bioavailability by masking the polar or ionizable functional groups of active molecules. One such nucleotide inhibitor of reverse transcriptase, an essential viral enzyme in human immunodeficiency virus 1 (HIV-1) infections, is tenofovir (26, Figure 10.21). Tenofovir had a very low oral bioavailability in humans (<5%) due to the high hydrophilicity of the phosphonic acid group, which restricted its use as a medication. Tenofovir disoproxil (23, Figure 10.21), a prodrug with an oral bioavailability of 39% in humans, was found through SAR studies on bis-carbonate esters of tenofovir. The mechanism of tenofovir disoproxil is as follows: first, it is hydrolyzed to the intermediate 24 by enzymes (carboxyesterases) or chemically; this is followed by a spontaneous loss of formaldehyde and CO_2 to produce the monoester intermediate 25 (Figure 10.21). The enzymes that catalyze the ultimate hydrolysis of the monoester intermediate 25 into the active medication tenofovir 26 are most likely phosphodiesterases (Figure 10.21).

Drugs will be eliminated from the body through metabolism and/or excretion in their intact form after being administered. The latter procedure, which is outside the purview of this work, occasionally involves active transport. The majority of the time, metabolism sites are erratic, and metabolites may exhibit no pharmacological activity at all, activity that is less than, equal to, or greater than the parent molecules' activity. Active metabolites are typically defined as those that possess comparable or superior pharmacological activity.

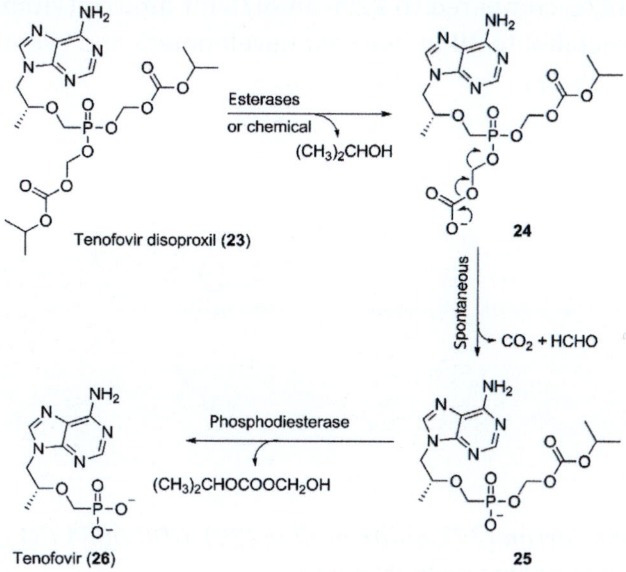

Figure 10.21. *Proposed mechanism for the formation of active drug tenofovir (26) from the prodrug tenoforvir disoproxil (23).*

Source: https://www.ncbi.nlm.nih.gov/pmc/articles/PMC6146880/bin/sc1.jpg.

The transformation of drugs into active metabolites differs from the transformation of prodrugs into active drugs in the following ways. Both pharmaceuticals and their active metabolites are pharmacologically active when it comes to this conversion process. Drugs are metabolized (biotransformed) by enzymes, and the sites of metabolism are unpredictable. Nonetheless, there are specific methods for converting pharmacologically inactive prodrugs into active medications, including enzymatic and chemical processes. The variability of metabolite formation during drug metabolism presents a potential avenue for the identification of active metabolites as novel compounds (NCEs) or novel structural templates for additional drug discovery optimization. A drug molecule's lack of PK–PD correlation or in vivo efficacy–in vitro potency correlation may be a sign of the presence of active metabolites. As an illustration, losartan (27, Figure 10.22) is used to treat hypertension in humans as an angiotensin II receptor antagonist. To produce the metabolite EXP3174, losartan's alcohol functional group is oxidized to a carboxylic acid group (28, Figure 10.22) in the body. One of the main metabolites that are circulating in humans is EXP3174. According to in vitro research, the IC50 of EXP3174 against the angiotensin II receptor is 0.2 nmol/L, while that of losartan is 4 nmol/L. The active metabolite EXP3174 may have contributed approximately 14 times the activity of in vitro–in vivo losartan itself by considering the in vitro potency, plasma exposure, and the free fraction in plasma. This suggests that more in vitro and in vivo studies on EXP3174 are necessary.

In some cases, active metabolites have been developed as new drugs. For example, amitriptyline (**29,** Figure 10.22) is a widely used drug for the treatment of mental disorders, including depression and anxiety. Amitriptyline is metabolized by CYP2D6, 3A4 and 2C19 to a demethylated metabolite **30** (Figure 10.22). This metabolite **30** is a more potent and selective norepinephrine reuptake inhibitor with K_i of 4.4 nmol/L, compared to 22.4 nmol/L for amitriptyline, against norepinephrine transporter. Consequently, metabolite **30** underwent development and eventually became a marketed drug, nortriptyline (Figure 10.22).

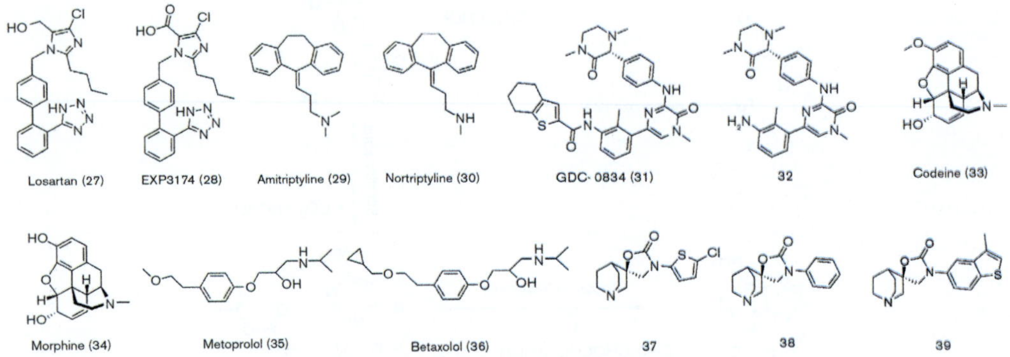

Figure 10.22. *Structures of losartan (27), amitriptyline (29), GDC-0834 (31), codeine (33), metoprolol (35), compound 37 and their analogs or metabolites.*

Source: https://www.ncbi.nlm.nih.gov/pmc/articles/PMC6146880/bin/gr4.jpg.

A Closer Look

Permeability Barriers and Detoxification

The exact compounds an organism is exposed to will be largely unpredictable, and may differ widely over time; these are major characteristics of xenobiotic toxic stress. The major challenge faced by xenobiotic detoxification systems is that they must be able to remove the almost-limitless number of xenobiotic compounds from the complex mixture of chemicals involved in normal metabolism. The solution that has evolved to address this problem is an elegant combination of physical barriers and low-specificity enzymatic systems.

All organisms use cell membranes as hydrophobic permeability barriers to control access to their internal environment. Polar compounds cannot diffuse across these cell membranes, and the uptake of useful molecules is mediated through transport proteins that specifically select substrates from the extracellular mixture. This selective uptake means that most hydrophilic molecules cannot enter cells, since they are not recognized by any specific transporters. In contrast, the diffusion of hydrophobic compounds across these barriers cannot be controlled, and organisms, therefore, cannot exclude lipid-soluble xenobiotics using membrane barriers.

However, the existence of a permeability barrier means that organisms were able to evolve detoxification systems that exploit the hydrophobicity common to membrane-permeable xenobiotics. These systems therefore solve the specificity problem by possessing such broad substrate specificities that they metabolise almost any non-polar compound. Useful metabolites are excluded since they are polar, and in general contain one or more charged groups.

The detoxification of the reactive by-products of normal metabolism cannot be achieved by the systems outlined above, because these species are derived from normal cellular constituents and usually share their polar characteristics. However, since these compounds are few in number, specific enzymes can recognize and remove them. Examples of these specific detoxification systems are the glyoxalase system, which removes the reactive aldehyde methylglyoxal, and the various antioxidant systems that eliminate reactive oxygen species.

Summary

- Drug metabolism is the metabolic breakdown of drugs by living organisms, usually through specialized enzymatic systems.
- The metabolism of pharmaceutical drugs is an important aspect of pharmacology and medicine. For example, the rate of metabolism determines the duration and intensity of the pharmacologic action of a drug.
- Medicines are required for humans to cure diseases but at the same time, they are foreign objects to the body. Hence, the human body tries to reject them at the earliest. It is highly desirable that the medicines get eliminated from the human body immediately after showing their drug action.
- The chemistry of drug metabolism needs an elaborate understanding – it is a fascinating and a complicated process. The primary site of drug metabolism is the smooth endoplasmic reticulum of the liver cell.
- The drug metabolism process can lead to the generation of Reactive Metabolites in some instances, which further lead to toxicity. The toxicity may vary from genotoxicity to immune-mediated Adverse Drug Reactions.
- Drug metabolism comprises the metabolism of endogenous and exogenous substances. During metabolism most drugs lose the pharmacological activity and are excreted from the body.
- Drugs that share elements of their metabolic pathways can also 'compete' for the same binding sites on enzymes, decreasing their metabolism's efficiency. For instance, alcohol and certain sedatives are metabolized by the same member of the cytochrome P450 family
- Drug metabolism is an essential clinical concern for the interprofessional healthcare team. Clinicians and pharmacists must work together to prevent clinically significant drug interactions that could affect patients' health.

References

1. Azzam, A. A. H., McDonald, J., & Lambert, D. G. (2019). Hot topics in opioid pharmacology: Mixed and biased opioids. *British Journal of Anaesthesia, 122*(6), e136–e145.
2. Bolton, A. E., Peng, B., Hubert, M., Krebs-Brown, A., Capdeville, R., Keller, U., & Seiberling, M. (2004). Effect of rifampicin on the pharmacokinetics of imatinib mesylate (Gleevec, STI571) in healthy subjects. *Cancer Chemotherapy and Pharmacology, 53*(2), 102–106.
3. Bortolussi, S., Catucci, G., Gilardi, G., & Sadeghi, S. J. (2021). N-and S-oxygenation activity of truncated human flavin-containing monooxygenase 3 and its common polymorphic variants. *Archives of Biochemistry and Biophysics, 697*, 108663.
4. Boyland, E., & Chasseaud, L. F. (1969). The role of glutathione and glutathione S-transferases in mercapturic acid biosynthesis. *Advances in Enzymology and Related Areas of Molecular Biology, 32*, 173–219.

5. Colizzi, M., Weltens, N., McGuire, P., Van Oudenhove, L., & Bhattacharyya, S. (2019). Descriptive psychopathology of the acute effects of intravenous delta-9-tetrahydrocannabinol administration in humans. *Brain Sciences, 9*(4).

6. Commandeur, J. N., Stijntjes, G. J., & Vermeulen, N. P. (1995). Enzymes and transport systems involved in the formation and disposition of glutathione S-conjugates: Role in bioactivation and detoxication mechanisms of xenobiotics. *Pharmacological Reviews, 47*(2), 271–330.

7. Eh-Haj, B. M. (2021). Metabolic N-dealkylation and N-oxidation as elucidators of the role of alkylamino moieties in drugs acting at various receptors. *Molecules, 26*(7), 1917.

8. Foye, W. O. (2008). *Foye's Principles of Medicinal Chemistry*. Philadelphia, USA: Lippincott Williams & Wilkins.

9. Guengerich, F. P. (2001). Common and uncommon cytochrome P450 reactions related to metabolism and chemical toxicity. *Chemical Research in Toxicology, 14*(6), 611–650.

10. Lakshmanan, M. (2019). Drug metabolism. In *Introduction to Basics of Pharmacology and Toxicology* (Vol. 12019, pp. 99–116). Singapore: Springer.

11. Marchitti, S. A., Brocker, C., Stagos, D., & Vasiliou, V. (2008). Non-P450 aldehyde oxidizing enzymes: The aldehyde dehydrogenase superfamily. *Expert Opinion on Drug Metabolism & Toxicology, 4*(6), 697–720.

12. Meyer, U. A., & Zanger, U. M. (1997). Molecular mechanisms of genetic polymorphisms of drug metabolism. *Annual Review of Pharmacology and Toxicology, 37*, 269–296.

13. Nebert, D. W., & Dalton, T. P. (2006). The role of cytochrome P450 enzymes in endogenous signalling pathways and environmental carcinogenesis. *Nature Reviews Cancer, 6*(12), 947–960.

14. Patilea-Vrana, G. I., Anoshchenko, O., & Unadkat, J. D. (2019). Hepatic enzymes relevant to the disposition of (-)-Δ9-tetrahydrocannabinol (THC) and its psychoactive metabolite, 11-OH-THC. *Drug Metabolism and Disposition, 47*(3), 249–256.

INDEX

C

D

E

F

L

M

N

O

P

Q

R

S

Printed and bound by CPI Group (UK) Ltd, Croydon, CR0 4YY
18/09/2026
14965061-0004